Instructional Design Exemplars in eHealth and mHealth Education Interventions

Suha R. Tamim
University of South Carolina, USA

IGI Global
PUBLISHER of TIMELY KNOWLEDGE

A volume in the Advances in Medical Education, Research, and Ethics (AMERE) Book Series

Published in the United States of America by
IGI Global
Medical Information Science Reference (an imprint of IGI Global)
701 E. Chocolate Avenue
Hershey PA, USA 17033
Tel: 717-533-8845
Fax: 717-533-8661
E-mail: cust@igi-global.com
Web site: http://www.igi-global.com

Library of Congress Cataloging-in-Publication Data

Names: Tamim, Suha R., 1964- editor.
Title: Instructional design exemplars in eHealth and mHealth education interventions / Suha R. Tamim, editor.
Description: Hershey, PA : Information Science Reference, [2022] | Includes bibliographical references and index. | Summary: "This book showcases design exemplars of ehealth and mheath interventions in health promotion and in education and support of health professionals with the goal to demonstrate the integration of theory and design principles that will benefit practitioners, educators, and researchers in the fields of health and education, and in particular, health professionals and instructional designers involved in the creation of ehealth and mhealth interventions"-- Provided by publisher.
Identifiers: LCCN 2021058143 (print) | LCCN 2021058144 (ebook) | ISBN 9781799894902 (hardcover) | ISBN 9781799894919 (paperback) | ISBN 9781799894926 (ebook)
Subjects: LCSH: Medical education. | Medical informatics.
Classification: LCC R735 .I56 2022 (print) | LCC R735 (ebook) | DDC 610.285--dc23/eng/20220106
LC record available at https://lccn.loc.gov/2021058143
LC ebook record available at https://lccn.loc.gov/2021058144

This book is published in the IGI Global book series Advances in Medical Education, Research, and Ethics (AMERE) (ISSN: 2475-6601; eISSN: 2475-661X)

British Cataloguing in Publication Data
A Cataloguing in Publication record for this book is available from the British Library.

Advances in Medical Education, Research, and Ethics (AMERE) Book Series

ISSN:2475-6601
EISSN:2475-661X

Mission

Humans are living longer now than ever as a result of advances in the medical field. Having the tools available to train knowledgeable and ethical future generations of doctors and medical researchers is essential to continuing to advance our understanding of the human body and develop new ways of treating and curing sickness and disease.

The **Advances in Medical Education, Research, and Ethics (AMERE)** book series highlights publications pertaining to advancements in pedagogical practice for developing future healthcare professionals, research methods, and advancements in the medical field, as well as moral behavior and practice of healthcare professionals, students, and researchers. Featuring research-based book publications that are highly relevant to the healthcare community, this series is ideally designed for library inclusion at medical universities and research institutions as well as personal use by medical professionals, researchers, and upper-level students entering the field.

Coverage

- Clinical Research
- Conflicts of Interest
- Ethics in Medicine
- Healthcare Pedagogy
- Medical Curricula
- Medical Simulation
- Patient Data
- Professional Development
- Research Methods
- Scientific Misconduct

IGI Global is currently accepting manuscripts for publication within this series. To submit a proposal for a volume in this series, please contact our Acquisition Editors at Acquisitions@igi-global.com or visit: http://www.igi-global.com/publish/.

The Advances in Medical Education, Research, and Ethics (AMERE) Book Series (ISSN 2475-6601) is published by IGI Global, 701 E. Chocolate Avenue, Hershey, PA 17033-1240, USA, www.igi-global.com. This series is composed of titles available for purchase individually; each title is edited to be contextually exclusive from any other title within the series. For pricing and ordering information please visit http://www.igi-global.com/book-series/advances-medical-education-research-ethics/132365. Postmaster: Send all address changes to above address.

Titles in this Series

For a list of additional titles in this series, please visit: www.igi-global.com/book-series/advances-medical-education-research-ethics/132365

Contemporary Issues in Global Medicine and Moving Toward International HealthcareEquity
Nick Comninellis (University of Missouri-Kansas City, USA) and Steven D. Waldman (University of Missouri-Kansas City School of Medicine, USA)
Medical Information Science Reference • © 2022 • 305pp • H/C (ISBN: 9781799884903) • US $295.00

Technological Adoption and Trends in Health Sciences Teaching, Learning, and Pactice
Samuel Marcos-Pablos (University of Salamanca, Spain) and Juan Antonio Juanes-Méndez (University of Salamanca, Spain)
Medical Information Science Reference • © 2022 • 387pp • H/C (ISBN: 9781799888710) • US $345.00

Global Production and Consumption of Fast Food and Instant Concentrates
Inna Vladimirovna Simakova (Saratov State Vavilov Agrarian University, Russia) Victoria Nikolaevna Strizhevskaya (Saratov State Vavilov Agrarian University, Russia) Roman Lvovich Perkel (Peter the Great St. Petersburg State Polytechnic University, Russia) and Galina Yuryevna Rakhmanova (Office of the Federal Service for Supervision of Consumer Rights Protection and Human Welfare in the Saratov Region, Russia)
Medical Information Science Reference • © 2022 • 253pp • H/C (ISBN: 9781799881971) • US $285.00

Advancing Health Education With Telemedicine
Mildred Lopez (Tecnologico de Monterrey, Mexico)
Medical Information Science Reference • © 2022 • 377pp • H/C (ISBN: 9781799887836) • US $295.00

Handbook of Research on Updating and Innovating Health Professions Education Post-Pandemic Perspectives
Channing R. Ford (Jacksonville State University, USA) and Kimberly B. Garza (Auburn University, USA)
Medical Information Science Reference • © 2022 • 462pp • H/C (ISBN: 9781799876236) • US $395.00

Handbook of Research on Assertiveness, Clarity, and Positivity in Health Literacy
Cristina Vaz de Almeida (Instituto Superior de Ciências Sociais e Políticas, CAPP, University of Lisbon, Portugal) and Susana Ramos (Centro Hospitalar Universitário Lisbon Central, Portugal)
Medical Information Science Reference • © 2022 • 423pp • H/C (ISBN: 9781799888246) • US $395.00

Pedagogies for Pharmacy Curricula
Isabel Vitória Figueiredo (University of Coimbra, Portugal) and Afonso Miguel Cavaco (University of Lisbon, Portugal)
Medical Information Science Reference • © 2021 • 248pp • H/C (ISBN: 9781799844860) • US $265.00

IGI Global
PUBLISHER of TIMELY KNOWLEDGE

701 East Chocolate Avenue, Hershey, PA 17033, USA
Tel: 717-533-8845 x100 • Fax: 717-533-8661
E-Mail: cust@igi-global.com • www.igi-global.com

Table of Contents

Detailed Table of Contents

This chapter provides an overview of the theoretical foundations of health education. Although health education theories and models are many, the chapter focuses on the most popular four: the health belief model, the theory of reasoned action and theory of planned behavior, the transtheoretical model of change, and the social cognitive theory. These models are explained through a scenario that highlights determinants of health behavior and how they can be used by health educators to plan behavioral change. The chapter continues with basic instructional design principles that guide the development of health education interventions, stressing the interplay between health education and instructional design. Lastly, the chapter ends with a brief synopsis of two widely used health education planning models, PRECEED-PROCEDE and intervention mapping, to provide a systems perspective to health education interventions.

The design of ehealth and mhealth interventions is grounded in interconnected fields, mainly education, health, behavioral psychology, communication, and technology. To provide an overview of these interconnections, this chapter begins with a presentation of key concepts and terms related to elearning, mlearning, ehealth, and mhealth, providing an overview of their definitions and understanding. This is followed by a discussion of ehealth and mhealth theories that shed the light on the factors that prompt health behavior. Next, elearning design principles are explained as they play an important role in the design of interventions. The last section of the chapter addresses ehealth and mhealth spread of use, prominent applications, their benefits, and their challenges.

The importance of telehealth applications reached a critical nature during the COVID-19 pandemic of 2020. Telehealth allowed for a continuum of care while maintaining patient satisfaction during times of complete lockdown, quarantine, or isolation. The likelihood of a full audio-video telehealth visit for Black patients or those on Medicaid, however, was reduced. In fact, the Black patient population experienced two-times the rate of incomplete visits or telephone only visits compared to non-Hispanic White patients. Rivera et al. identified several significant barriers. Platform and portal designers must consider these barriers when creating telehealth tools. Framing the design on critical race theory can work towards equity in access to telehealth services.

Needs assessment and analyses allow for organizations and individuals to identify any gaps or discrepancies between a current state of performance and a desired state. In regards to m-health technology, needs assessment can be used to help healthcare providers identify specific gaps or areas that could benefit from m-health technologies such as reducing the cancellation of appointments, improving health records, consolidating paperwork, and improving patient education efforts. The purpose of this chapter is to explore how needs assessment strategies can be leveraged to support healthcare providers' abilities to identify, select, and in implement m-health technologies into their patient plans. This chapter will review the types of needs healthcare providers must consider when implementing m-health technologies, as well as strategies that can support their decisions.

Obesity and insufficient physical activity represent ongoing pandemics. These cases describe the design process of two different electronic and mobile health interventions in the areas of behavioral weight loss and physical activity promotion. An interdisciplinary team of experts followed several guidelines of an established intervention framework to ensure the interventions were addressing significant research gaps and grounded in theory and empirical evidence. Intervention strategies were guided by the intervention mapping taxonomy of behavior change methods and integrated both custom-built and commercially available technologies. These cases detail how the chosen theories, methods, and intervention strategies were connected. Challenges and opportunities in relation to both the interventions and the fields of technology-based behavioral weight loss and physical activity more broadly are also discussed.

Digital health tools have been used in a wide variety of healthcare services including promoting healthy behaviors and improving health outcomes in people with chronic conditions including cardiovascular disease. However, there is no "one size fits all" approach for these digital health tools. The need for individualized designs in order to maximize usability, effectiveness, and sustainability of use among patients has been highlighted. Intelligent health solutions are used to guide the design of effective and personalized tools for patients with cardiovascular diseases. The integration of health behavior theories and well-defined care plans in the intervention/tool are key to ensure maximum effectiveness and benefits to the patients. To this end, this chapter aims to provide a background on digital health tools in cardiovascular health and a detailed overview of the various components of intelligent health solutions that guide the tool design process.

Data analytics reflects trends on the particular subject based on comparison with historical dataset and present dataset. With the advancement of technology, healthcare predictive analytics at periodic intervals affords insights into diseases collectively, identifying risk of the patients' health in the future. The novelty of this project is to analyze symptoms and healthcare datasets, to predict the risk of the mentioned diseases using machine learning algorithms to better time management and convenience for physicians and the general population. Hence, the proposed model provides the provision to save patients directly from risk to the particular disease based on the periodic trend analysis. On the contrary, the hospital will utilize the proposed model to control future disease outbreaks.

The COVID-19 pandemic precipitated several mental health effects on people such as stress, depression, irritability, anger, and confusion. Especially affected were school-aged children whose daily routines were disrupted by school closure and isolation. Hamilton et al. reported that the social-emotional health of 30-40% of students in the USA was impacted negatively, especially those learning remotely and historically marginalized. The virtual learning environment for students needed an intervention to help alleviate the impacts of isolation during remote and virtual learning. Social emotional learning curriculum was implemented in the virtual learning environment for students in a seventh grade English class. Theories of mindfulness and social emotional learning are addressed to show the academic and mental health benefits for implementing social emotional learning in the classroom for adolescents learning in the virtual environment.

Section 3
eHealth and mHealth Education Interventions: Exemplars in Higher Education

The intersection between higher education, technology, and mHealth is growing at a rapid pace, bringing with it an array of implications for data privacy. It is important for instructional designers to attend to these new and constantly shifting data privacy considerations when developing mHealth interventions. Therefore, with a connection to both extant instructional design literature and sociocultural theory, the authors of the current work provide strategies for developing more privacy-conscious mHealth interventions for the higher education community.

This chapter considers social constructivism as an educational theory for the development of multimedia content to assist primary-care providers, particularly those in HIV clinics and other clinicians, and support staff involved in the care of patients with substance use disorders in better understanding the intake processes at the Methadone clinics. Main aspects of social constructivism with its focus on the collaborative and generative learning and the importance of a cultural and social context are elaborated within the framework of the multimedia design. A series of four videos were developed that feature interviews with patients who describe their experience on Methadone. In addition, medical providers and medical staff describe the intake procedures for Methadone. Also discussed is the instructional design process and the Bergman and Moore instructional design model that informed the design.

Medical educators often receive minimal formal pedagogical and technological training. The COVID-19 pandemic made this gap even more apparent, necessitating the development of a multidisciplinary

Preface

This book is an outcome of my professional journey that began in public health with a focus on health behavior and health education and later transitioned to education with a focus on instructional design and technology and curriculum studies. I realized that although scholars in these fields strive to improve behavior, whether health or academic, they often delve into parallel theoretical spaces and work in silos. I recognized the commonalities despite the different discipline-related identities, cultures, and professional languages. Moreover, through my research on how health professionals create ehealth and mhealth interventions, I found variability in design and development that stems from the varied backgrounds, resulting in gaps that could be bridged through an understanding of the common threads between the different fields. These factors inspired the work on this book to disseminate best practices while providing an overview of the instructional design process, the theoretical foundations, and the design principles for virtual interventions.

CHALLENGES IN eHEALTH AND mHEALTH EDUCATION INTERVENTIONS

The use of ehealth and mhealth interventions for purposes of health promotion and education of and support for health professionals is on the rise. Their wide reach and the advantages they present in tailoring to specific needs, overcoming barriers of time and distance, and facilitating engagement, interactivity, and collaboration give them significant potential for learning and behavioral change. Health professionals and instructional designers create ehealth and mhealth interventions drawing from several disciplines such as education, behavioral psychology, instructional design, elearning, plus public health and medicine. Although well invested in the quality and effectiveness of their ehealth and mhealth interventions, they vary in their use of theory and instructional design principles based on the perspectives of the disciplines that influence their work. The literature varies in the description of the effectiveness of ehealth and mhealth interventions and few reports show ties to theoretical foundations, evidence supporting how theory relates to program components, or describe how the interventions work through the adopted theoretical constructs. With the absence of a clear theoretical picture, the rationale of the interventions is lost, and measures of success are difficult to track. Additionally, the absence of a clear instructional design process creates unanswered questions about the rigor, efficacy, effectiveness, and relevancy of the interventions. Therefore, a compilation of design exemplars grounded in theory and instructional design principles is a useful resource to practitioners, educators, and researchers in the fields of health and education.

AIM OF THE BOOK

This book aims to showcase design exemplars of ehealth and mheath education interventions in health education. These exemplars focus mainly on the goals of the intervention, the theory that frames the design, and the systematic instructional design process. Readers will notice varied levels of emphasis on the design elements, stemming from the academic backgrounds of the authors and the contexts of the interventions. Some exemplars revolve around a specific intervention in a specific context, others provide a wider lens for large scale interventions. Some are situated in communities, others in educational settings. Preceding the exemplars are four chapters that provide theoretical grounding and conceptual guidance to facilitate the understanding of the different approaches used in the chapters that follow.

TARGET AUDIENCE

The book targets health professionals, instructional designers, educators, professors, and researchers working in the field of instructional design and technology, public health, medicine, and other health-related fields. Moreover, it provides design insights to students specializing in the fields of instructional design, health promotion, and health professions education. The book can be used as a resource in academic and practice settings.

BOOK ORGANIZATION AND CHAPTER DESCRIPTION

The book is divided into three sections, each consisting of four chapters as described below. The reader will notice that chapters vary in structure. Some are intended to give a theoretical and conceptual overview of ehealth and mhealth education, other show different design processes in different settings that underscores the notion of having many perspectives based on many disciplines that drive the design of ehealth and mheatlh interventions.

The first section focuses on the theoretical underpinnings of ehealth and mhealth education. It serves as an encompassing introduction to the exemplars discussed in sections two and section three. It covers major theories that pertain to ehealth and mhealth education, it also clarifies corresponding terminologies and definitions, in addition to addressing equity in ehealthcare access and the importance of determining needs in designing these types of interventions.

- In Chapter 1, *The Interplay Between Health Promotion, Health Education, and Instructional Design*, Dr. Suha R. Tamim gives an overview of the theoretical foundations and models of health education. The selected models are explained through a scenario that highlights determinants of health behavior and how they can be used to plan behavioral change. The chapter also covers basic instructional design principles to stress the interplay between health education and instructional design. Lastly, the chapter ends with a brief synopsis of two widely used health education planning models, PRECEED-PROCEDE and Intervention Mapping to provide a systems perspective to health education interventions. This introductory chapter lays the foundation for the book presenting to the reader the different perspectives and scopes of health education interventions.

- In Chapter 2, *eHealth and mHealth-Definitions, Theories, Models, and Applications*, Dr. Suha R. Tamim and Dr. Hadi Danawi build on Chapter 1, focusing on ehealth and mhealth. The authors begin by describing the landscape of definitions and terms used in ehealth, mhealth, elearning, and mlearning to address the inconsistencies present in the literature in order to facilitate the understanding of the exemplars chapters that follow. Adding to the theories presented in Chapter 1, Dr. Tamim and Dr. Danawi give an overview of theories particular to ehealth and mhealth that focus on the technological aspects of the interventions. This is followed by a discussion on ehealth and mhealth uses, prominent applications, their benefits, and their challenges.
- In Chapter 3, *Framing eHealth Design on Critical Race Theory to Mitigate Barriers in Access to Healthcare*, Dr. Christina B. Gunther, Dr. Bronwyn Cross-Denny, Ms. Melanie M. Reyes, and Ms. Danielle Provenzano draw attention to the importance of equity in healthcare access, specifically telehealth access. They discuss existing barriers for various marginalized communities in the United States of America and worldwide, which were exacerbated by the COVID-19 pandemic. They propose framing the design of interventions in critical race theory that can work towards equity in access to telehealth services.
- In Chapter 4, *Determining Needs to Support m-Health Interventions,* Dr. Jill E. Stefaniak highlights the importance of needs assessment and analysis in identifying gaps or discrepancies between a current state of performance and a desired state. Focusing on mhealth technology, she explains how needs assessment strategies can be leveraged to support healthcare providers' abilities to identify, select, and implement mhealth technologies. Therefore, she discusses the purpose of needs assessment in mhealth, the theories that support it, the needs assessment process, and the different types of needs and data sources. Additionally, she examines patient, provider, and environmental affordances.

The second section presents exemplars in health behavior change. These exemplars aim at improving the health of specified populations. What is particular about this section is the variation of approaches, scopes, and stages of the interventions. While Chapters 5, 6, and 8 describe completed interventions, Chapter 7 proposes a web-based innovative prototype based in machine learning. Moreover, Chapters 6 and 7 illustrate wide-scale community-based interventions that are complex, multilayered, and leaning heavily on theory while Chapter 8 presents a context-specific school-based intervention, localized in one classroom. Though different in approaches, each chapter shows a systematic design process that fits best the nature of the intervention.

- In Chapter 5, *Promoting Behavioral Weight Loss and Physical Activity: The Case of Two Interventions*, Dr. Courtney M. Monroe presents two ehealth/mhealth interventions addressing behavioral weight loss and physical activity, guided by the Intervention Mapping taxonomy of behavior change. After a rich literature review, Dr. Monroe, details how the chosen theories, methods, and intervention strategies are connected in each case. She grounds the interventions in social cognitive theory, self-determination theory, and social network theory, aligning intervention strategies with corresponding theoretical constructs.
- In Chapter 6, *Exemplars in eHealth Education Interventions: The Case Study of Cardiovascular Health,* Dr. Patrick J. Dunn and Dr. Hadi Danawi present a background on digital health tools in cardiovascular health and a detailed overview of the various components of intelligent health solutions that guide the tool design process. They propose a creative layered approach that is highly

personalized by identifying and addressing the social, medical, lifestyle and behavior, learning and digital preferences, and even personality traits of the individual, aligned with artificial intelligence and machine learning. They describe a theoretically based intervention that gives users access to the American Heart Association's digital Care Plans. The intervention is a collection of evidence-based content, data collection, communication, and decision rules designed to assist a patient in their self-management care. They explain how the intervention has a modular approach, is adaptive, person-centered, and multi-lingual and culturally appropriate.

- In Chapter 7, *Predictive Healthcare Web Analytics Using Machine Learning,* Ms. Anjali Agarwal, Dr. Anjata Das, and Dr. Ravish Kumar Bansal illustrate an innovative application using machine learning algorithms to analyze symptoms and healthcare datasets to predict the risk of certain diseases. Their proposed model provides periodic trend analysis to forecast illnesses based on a patient's treatment history and health information, which can also help health providers control future disease outbreaks.
- In Chapter 8, *Implementing Social Emotional Learning in the Virtual Environment for K-12 Classrooms*, Dr. Erika L. Patterson describes the design of a social-emotional learning virtual intervention, based on mindfulness, as a strategy to address the mental health impacts of school closure and online learning imposed by the COVID-19 pandemic. Through a systematic instructional design process aligned with the social cognitive theory, Dr. Patterson discusses how she mitigated challenges to support her students during the pandemic.

The third section offers exemplars in higher education. These exemplars are contextualized in health professions education. As in section two, the exemplars differ in stages, theoretical frameworks, and purposes. While Chapter 10 describes the instructional design process for developing online videos to facilitate communication and collaboration between providers, Chapter 11 discusses a multidisciplinary approach to improve the quality of online teaching in a medical school, and Chapter 12 proposes a model for facilitating virtual clinical encounters for graduate level health professions students. Framing these chapters is Chapter 9 that provides an overview of mhealth in higher education with mhealth examples and challenges.

- In Chapter 9, *mHealth, Data, and Privacy: The Case of the Higher Education Community*, Dr. Stephanie J. Blackmon, and Ms. Tiera J. Lanford offer strategies for developing privacy-conscious mhealth interventions for the higher education community, making connections to extant instructional design literature and sociocultural theory. They begin with an overview of the growth of mhealth in higher education, in the United States of America, describing several mhealth interventions. Furthermore, they highlight the urgency of students' data privacy, stressing the need for awareness, transparency, inclusivity, and proactivity. Additionally, they provide examples of the interplay between technology and instructional design.
- In Chapter 10, *Methadone Referrals Demystified: A Client's Journey Into Methadone Treatment – Social Constructivism and the Use of Video-Based Content in Medical Provider Education*, Dr. Katarzyna M. Sims, Mr. Ralph Brooks, Ms. Lisa Nichols, Mr. Maximilian D. Wegener, and Dr. Merceditas S. Villanueva expound on the design process of a video-based intervention aimed at assisting primary care providers in better understanding the intake processes at Methadone clinics, filling provider-identified gaps in knowledge, and improving communication between HIV and Opioid Use Disorder providers to optimize patient treatment. The intervention consists of a series

of four online videos that feature interviews with patients who describe their experiences while on Methadone. Grounded in social constructivism, the videos combine personal experiences from patient interviews with medical expertise from substance abuse disorder staff interviews to promote collaboration and discussion. The authors present the systematic instructional design of the intervention following the Bergman and Moore Instructional Design Model.

- In Chapter 11, *Leveraging Instructional Technology to Design Diverse Learning Experiences Through Collaborative Stakeholder Engagement*, Ms. Jessica A. Giraldo, Dr. Samantha Marina Lemus-Martinez, and Mr. Gáramis E. Campusano describe the development of a multidisciplinary team approach to design and implement quality online learning interactions, offering pedagogical and technical support for medical faculty. Based on the Technological Pedagogical Content Knowledge, their intervention aims at assisting faculty in shifting from lecture-based instruction to active learning methods, providing medical educators a form of reverse faculty development, informing faculty about cognitive load and the science of learning, and cultivating positive experiences. The authors present the systematic instructional design of the intervention that followed the ADDIE model and resulted in self-paced modules, online, synchronous modules that facilitate collaborative learning, gamification activities, and instructor-led training.
- In Chapter 12, *Telehealth Use in Interdisciplinary Health Professions Student Groups to Support Improved Outcomes,* Dr. LuAnn Etcher and Dr. Donna Faye McHaney propose an interdisciplinary telehealth intervention for clinical encounters to address the challenges of securing clinical placements for graduate level health professions students, exacerbated by the COVID-19 pandemic. They outline a systematic instructional design process and ground the intervention in the Quality-Caring Model, the Community of Inquiry, and the Trauma Informed Approach to Education.

CONCLUSION

The design of ehealth and mhealth education interventions draws from many disciplines, which poses a challenge for instructional designers and health education professionals. On one hand, these interventions need to be grounded in health behavior and learning theories to clarify how they act on behavior and learning. On the other hand, they need to follow a systematic instructional design process to ensure the quality and achievement of outcomes. This book highlights the interplay between these two essential foundations to serve as a guide for professionals interested in the design of ehealth and mhealth education interventions, regardless of their professional backgrounds and experiences in the fields. The book also illustrates the array of theories, concepts, and terms that are inherent to ehealth and mhealth to serve as a resource in the design of interventions and to clarify ambiguities and confusion.

Suha R. Tamim
University of South Carolina, USA

Acknowledgment

I would like to thank the members of the advisory board for their support and encouragement that made this book possible. The expertise of Dr. Jill E. Stefaniak and Dr. Max C. Anderson in instructional design in medical and other health professions, the expertise of Dr. Samantha J. Blevins and Dr. M. Aaron Bond in instructional design, distance learning, and systems thinking, and the expertise of Dr. Christina B. Gunther in social determinants of health and social justice in the global arena were invaluable in the review process and in supplementing chapters to the book.

Many special thanks to all the authors for their rich contributions and their painstaking work on the chapters to ensure alignment with the aim of the book. Additionally, special thanks to them and to other invited colleagues for their help with the review process.

Suha R. Tamim
University of South Carolina, USA

Section 1

eHealth and mHealth Theoretical Underpinnings

Chapter 1
The Interplay Between Health Promotion, Health Education, and Instructional Design

Suha R. Tamim
https://orcid.org/0000-0002-1664-747X
University of South Carolina, USA

ABSTRACT

This chapter provides an overview of the theoretical foundations of health education. Although health education theories and models are many, the chapter focuses on the most popular four: the health belief model, the theory of reasoned action and theory of planned behavior, the transtheoretical model of change, and the social cognitive theory. These models are explained through a scenario that highlights determinants of health behavior and how they can be used by health educators to plan behavioral change. The chapter continues with basic instructional design principles that guide the development of health education interventions, stressing the interplay between health education and instructional design. Lastly, the chapter ends with a brief synopsis of two widely used health education planning models, PRECEED-PROCEDE and intervention mapping, to provide a systems perspective to health education interventions.

INTRODUCTION

The interest in studying the interplay between disease, human behavior, and the environment dates to the 19th century when the notion of public health began to emerge, instituting regulations and laws aimed at controlling the spread of disease and improving health conditions. However, the resistance to these laws and the persistence of unhealthy behavior gave rise to the need for health education (Palfrey, 2018) to “educate people of all ages about healthful living” (Willgoose, 1985/2010, p.18). Previously, the definition of health education comprised a wide range of activities such as advocacy and social mobilization, but it was later narrowed down to differentiate it from the broader scope of health promotion and to focus it on communicating information related to health risk factors and behaviors (World Health Organization, 1998).

DOI: 10.4018/978-1-7998-9490-2.ch001

As in many fields, a variety of terms are used in public health, sometimes meaning different things to different people. To facilitate communication between diverse health agencies, the World Health Organization (WHO) published a glossary of terms in 1986 that was later revised in 1998, entitled Health Promotion Glossary (Smith et al., 2006). For the interest of this chapter, the following definitions are highlighted:

- *Health* is "a state of complete physical, social and mental well-being, and not merely the absence of disease or infirmity" (WHO,1998, p. 1). This definition is still the one most widely used in the literature (Sharma & Romas, 2011; Simons-Morton et al., 1995; Smith, 2010) and has not been amended since its formulation in 1946 (Word Health Organization, 2011). This is due to its emphasis on the positive aspect of well-being and the health dimensions beyond the physical ones (Simons-Morton et al., 1995; Stroebe, 2000).
- *Health Promotion* is "the process of enabling people to increase control over, and to improve their health" (WHO, 1998, p.1).
- *Health Education* "comprises consciously constructed opportunities for learning involving some form of communication designed to improve health literacy, including improving knowledge, and developing life skills which are conducive to individual and community health" (p.4).
- *Health Behavior* is "any activity undertaken by an individual, regardless of actual or perceived health status, for the purpose of promoting, protecting or maintaining health, whether or not such behaviour is objectively effective towards that end" (WHO, 1998, p.8).
- *Public Health* is the science and art of promoting health, preventing disease, and prolonging life through the organized efforts of society (WHO,1998, p.3).

Lately, the 2020 Joint Committee on Health Education and Promotion Terminology undertook a similar effort and proposed similar definitions for health education, health behavior, and health promotion (Joint Committee on Health Education and Promotion Terminology, 2021). In this chapter, the terms health education will be used as defined above to underscore the educational component of interventions.

THEORETICAL FOUNDATIONS OF HEALTH EDUCATION

Multiple factors determine the health status of people. These are called determinants of health (Nutbeam, 1998). Some of these determinants are changeable while others are not. An example of a changeable determinant is a certain skill one needs to improve their health, such as planning a healthy meal, while an example of an unchangeable determinant is age. These determinants are also situated at different levels. Some are individual, some are societal and interpersonal, and others are structural and environmental (Cleland et al., 2010). The complexity of the interplay between these health determinants and health behavior led to the emergence of several theories and models that explain why people behave the way they do in health-related matters (Glanz et al., 2008).

Indeed, theory guides practice and builds scientific knowledge (Goodson, 2010). A theory is "[a] coherent and systematic ordering of ideas, concepts, and models with the purpose of constructing meaning to explain, interpret and shape practice" (Garrison, 2000, p. 3) while practice represents "field-based or research-tested actions intended to effect a positive change" (Spencer et al., 2013, para 7). Consequently, the absence of a clear theoretical grounding brings fragmented and isolated activities that blur the interconnectedness between research and practice (Timmreck et al., 1988/2010). Using behavioral change theories in the design of health education interventions allows the targeting of specific behaviors and the determinants that drive them. Additionally, it provides operationalized constructs that can be used to analyze the effect of the interventions (Michie & Prestwich, 2010; Simoni et al., 2018). In other words, behavioral change theories help set measurable program objectives, select health education methods and strategies, and facilitate communication between professionals (Sharma & Romas, 2012).

Health behavior theories explain the "underlying factors that lead to behavior helping us to understand and to predict them" (Simoni et al., 2018, p.430). Models on the other hand, are informed by theory and are used to guide the systematic design of interventions with respect to selection of strategies and messages as well as evaluation (Glanz, et al., 2015; Green et al.1994, Simoni et al. 2018). Although theories and models differ in definition, they are often used interchangeably in health education (Tabak et al., 2012). Moreover, the corresponding constructs are intricately connected but can be viewed in different ways, resulting in a myriad of theories and models (Weinstien, 2007). Additionally, models and theories can be categorized differently. Individual models focus on the individual factors that affect health behavior, interpersonal models focus on the social influences, ecological models focus on the dynamic relationships between the different levels (Dustin et al. 2009; Glanz et al., 2008; Glanz et al., 2015; Sharma & Romas, 2012), and planning models that "exist at a macroscopic level …serve as an organizing framework for an entire health promotion effort aimed at fostering reduction in a given disease" (Crosby & Noar, 2011, p. S7). Moreover, theories and models could also differ in the flexibility of their constructs, ranging from broad to operational; the activity level, whether they disseminate or implement evidence -based interventions; or the levels at which they address change, ranging from single to multilevel (Tabak et al., 2012).

Moreover, health education promotes a holistic view of health, drawing from a variety of disciplines such as behavioral sciences, medicine, and education, "resulting in a jungle of theories" (Timmreck et al., 1988/2010, p. 68) and challenging health professionals to determine "which and how much of the theory of related or supportive fields to accept and apply while avoiding becoming or duplicating that discipline" (Timmreck et al., p. 68). Moreover, the field is expanding rapidly, "reflect[ing] an amalgamation of approaches, methods, and strategies from the social and health sciences" (Glanz et al, 2015, p. 6).

Glanz et al. (2008) reminded researchers about the challenges posed by the multitude of health behavior theories and models. Similarly, Mitchie et al. (2013) noted that the complex nature of health behavior interventions makes them difficult to replicate and blurs their effective components and the mechanism of behavior change, recommending a taxonomy of components to allow for accurate replication, faithful implementation, access to a comprehensive list of components for intervention development, and links to theory to investigative mechanisms of action.

Although more than 60 health behavior change theories and models are reported in the literature (Glanz et al., 2015), few are most widely used and "have weathered the test of time" (Glanz et al., 2015, p.67). These are the health belief model (HBM), the theory of reasoned action and theory of planned behavior (TRA/TTM), the transtheoretical model of change (TTM), and the social cognitive theory (SCT) (Glanz et al, 2015; Sharma & Romas, 2012; Simoni et al., 2018). It is important to note that the health belief model, the theory of reasoned action and the theory of planned behavior, and the transtheoretical model of change explain health behavior at the individual level and that the social cognitive theory looks at the interpersonal aspect of health behavior in addition to the individual level. Despite their popularity, these theories and models do have limitations that are discussed later in the chapter.

Figure 1. Ryan's health determinants

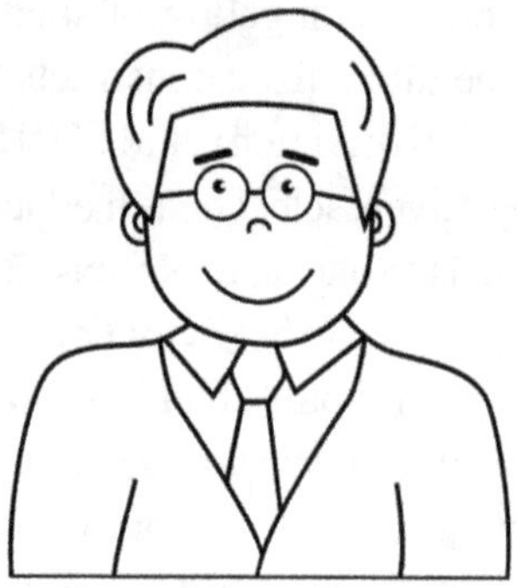

•Male.
•Middle age.
•Stressful work environment.
•Sedentary lifestyle.
•Family history of heart disease.
•Smoker.
•Does not eat enough fruits and vegetables.

To clarify the constructs of these theories and models and how they can be used to analyze and promote health behavior, the following scenario will be used.

The Scenario

Ryan, a middle-aged male, went for his yearly physical checkup. His doctor revealed to him results that show a high level of blood cholesterol, an elevated blood pressure, and excess body weight. He was told that he needed to make changes in his daily lifestyle to prevent potential health problems in the future such as heart disease. How would a health educator approach the development of an intervention addressing middle-aged men at risk of cardiovascular diseases, educating them on adopting healthy behaviors?

Let's take Ryan as an example of the target population and see what we know about him (Figure 1).

All these characteristics represent Ryan's health determinants. Obviously, characteristics such as age, gender, genetics, and work environment cannot be changed, and these are the non-behavioral determinants. On the other hand, activity level, smoking, and diet are directly linked to Ryan's behavior and therefore are changeable, and these are the behavioral determinants. Let's sort out Ryan's non-behavioral and behavioral determinants (Table 1).

Since non-behavioral determinants are not changeable, the role of the health educator, the instructional designer helping with the design of the intervention, or both is to focus on the behavioral determinants and to analyze them in order to address them successfully and reach the desired health behavior change.

Let's look at each of these three characteristics and see how they can be approached (Figure 2).

Looking closely at these factors, we can categorize them as shown in Table 2.

Therefore, to address health behavior change, we need to look at all these factors. Knowledge encompasses facts, concepts, principles, rules, and other cognitive skills (Dick et al., 2015; Morrison et al., 2013). Beliefs are "conviction[s] that a phenomenon or object is true or real. (Green & Kreuter, p.

Table 1. Categorization of Ryan's behavioral determinants

Non-behavioral	Behavioral
• Male • Middle age • Family history of heart disease • Stressful work environment	• Sedentary lifestyle • Smoker • Does not eat enough fruits and vegetables

Figure 2. Ryan's behavioral determinants analysis

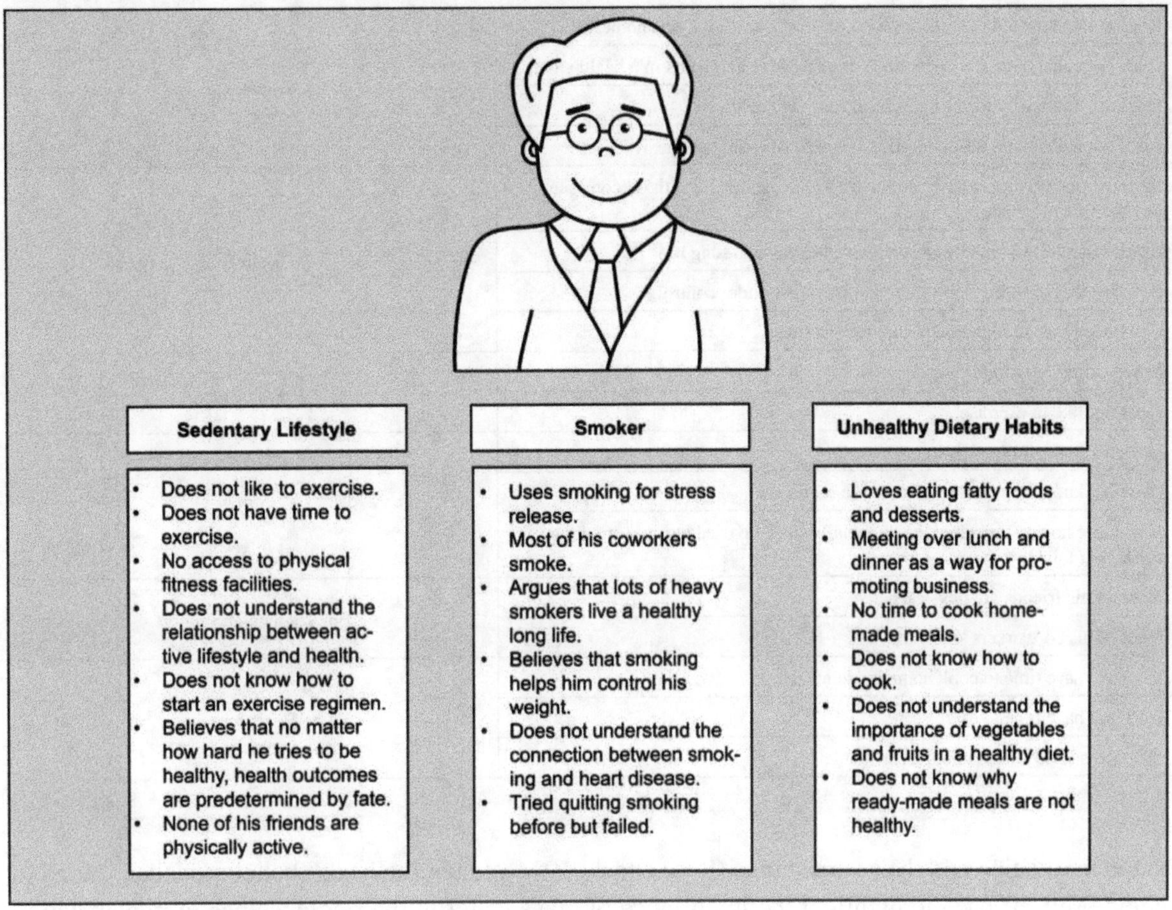

157). Attitudes carry an affective element and are defined by Green and Kreuter (2005) as "constant feeling[s] that [are] directed towards an object (be it a person, an action, a situation, or an idea)" (p. 159). On the other hand, skills refer to mental and physical activities needed to perform actions (Dick et al., 2015). As for the resources and support, these are socially and environmentally connected. Access and availability of facilities, equipment, time, and information are examples of resources while family members, friends, and coaches are examples of support.

This is a simplistic view of the roots of health behavior. Since the interplay between health determinants and health behavior is complex, these determinants must be explored from the lens of each of the four theories and models stated above: the health belief model, the theory of reasoned action and theory of planned behavior, the transtheoretical model of change, and the social cognitive theory. What follows is a brief overview of each and a corresponding analysis of Ryan's health behavior.

Health Belief Model

The health belief model (HBM) originated in the 1950s when scholars attempted to explain the health behavior of people to plan effective health behavior interventions (Champion & Skinner, 2008), focusing

Table 2. Categorization of Ryan's behavioral determinants

Determinant	Category
Does not understand the relationship between active lifestyle and health.	Knowledge
Does not understand the importance of vegetables and fruits in a healthy diet.	
Does not know why ready-made meals are not healthy.	
Does not understand the connection between smoking and heart disease.	
Believes that no matter how hard he tries to be healthy, health outcomes are predetermined by fate.	Beliefs
Argues that lots of heavy smokers live a healthy and long life.	
Believes that smoking helps him put his weight under control.	
Convinced that smoking helps him relieve stress.	
Loves eating fatty foods and desserts.	Attitudes
Does not like to exercise.	
Does not know how to cook.	Skills
Does not know how to start an exercise regimen.	
Is not sure how to quit smoking, especially since he tried quitting smoking before but failed.	
None of his friends are physical active.	Environmental Support
Most of his co-workers smoke.	
Does not have time to cook home-made meals.	Resources
Does not have time to exercise.	
No access to physical fitness facilities.	

on the motivation and their perceptions (Rosenstock, 1974). Later, the health belief model expanded to include self-efficacy to highlight the importance of one's belief in their competence in implementing health behavior change (Champion & Skinner, 2008; Rosenstock et al.,1988).

HBM focuses on six constructs (Champion & Skinner, 2008; Rosenstock, 1974; Sharma & Romas, 2012). These constructs are:

- Perceived susceptibility: belief in acquiring a disease.
- Perceived seriousness: belief in the severity of the consequences of a disease.
- Perceived benefits: belief in the positive returns of a health action, including reducing perceived threats.
- Perceived barriers: One's beliefs in the unfavorable aspects and costs resulting in taking a health action.
- Cues to action: External or internal triggers to action.
- Self-efficacy: One's belief in competence in achieving a change.

The Health Educator Diagnosis. A health educator choosing to design an intervention based on HBM would try to analyze where Ryan stands with respect to each construct. Table 3 below expands the scenario further.

Based on the analysis guided by HBM, the health educator would then start to design the appropriate intervention accordingly.

Table 3. Analysis of Ryan's health determinants through HBM

Construct	Ryan's Position	The Health Educator
Perceived susceptibility	What are my chances of acquiring a cardiovascular disease? Could I get it?	Does Ryan believe that he might get heart disease?
Perceived seriousness	If I develop it, how likely is it for me to have a heart attack? How damaging would it be to my health? Could I die?	Does Ryan believe that heart disease might have serious implications on his health?
Perceived benefits	If I change my dietary habits and if I exercise and stop smoking, could I avoid it, become physically fit and strong, and feel and look better?	Does Ryan believe that quitting smoking, increasing physical activity, and changing his diet will reduce his risks of heart disease?
Perceived barriers	But how can I eat healthy if I do not know how to cook? How can I exercise if I do not have time nor access to gym?	How difficult is it for Ryan to stop smoking, increase physical activity, and change his dietary habits? Could it be that he does not have coping mechanisms to deal with stress other than smoking, that he can't fit physical activity in his daily schedule, and that eating healthy means additional expenses that he can't afford?
Cues to action	One cue to action is the test results revealed by the doctor, which might trigger Ryan to act, or a close friend dying of heart disease, or a neighbor or friend starting to exercise inviting Ryan to a daily walk after dinner.	What will trigger Ryan to change his behavior? The doctor's warning, chest pain, a death of friend from heart disease, advertisements about heart disease?
Self-efficacy	Would I be able to resist not having sweet desserts after every meal? Would I be able to exercise at least 3 times a week without quitting?	What strategies can I use to increase Ryan's sense of self-efficacy?

Theory of Reasoned Action and Theory of Planned Behavior

The theory of reasoned action (TRA) that later evolved into the theory of planned behavior (TPB) stems from the work of Martin Fishbein that focused on the relationship between beliefs and attitudes (Sharma & Romas, 2012). Fishbein was later joined by Icek Ajzen to develop TPB, linking behavioral intentions to attitudes and beliefs (Glanz et al., 2008) and to perceived control (Fishbein & Ajzen, 2010).

Central to TRA/TPB is the construct of intention. Fishbein and Ajzen (2010) explained, "behavioral intentions are indicators of a person's readiness to perform a behavior" (p. 39). They increase the probability of the behavior but do not necessitate its occurrence. According to Fishbein and Ajzen (2010), intentions are governed by attitudes, perceived norms, and perceived behavioral control. Attitudes provide an evaluative component towards behaviors. Perceived norms are "the perceived social pressure to perform or not to perform" (p.130). Perceived behavioral control represents the perceived control over performance of a behavior and is the strongest predictor of behavior (Fishbein & Ajzen, 2010). Indeed, perceived behavioral control is strongly linked to Badura's (1977) concept of self-efficacy. However, the TRA/TPB constructs are also the result of beliefs: beliefs about the behavior outcomes, beliefs about social norms, and beliefs about behavioral control.

The Health Educator Diagnosis. Through the lens of TRA/TPB, the health educator might examine Ryan's intention for healthy dietary habits as shown in Figure 3.

Figure 3. Analysis of Ryan's health determinants through TRA

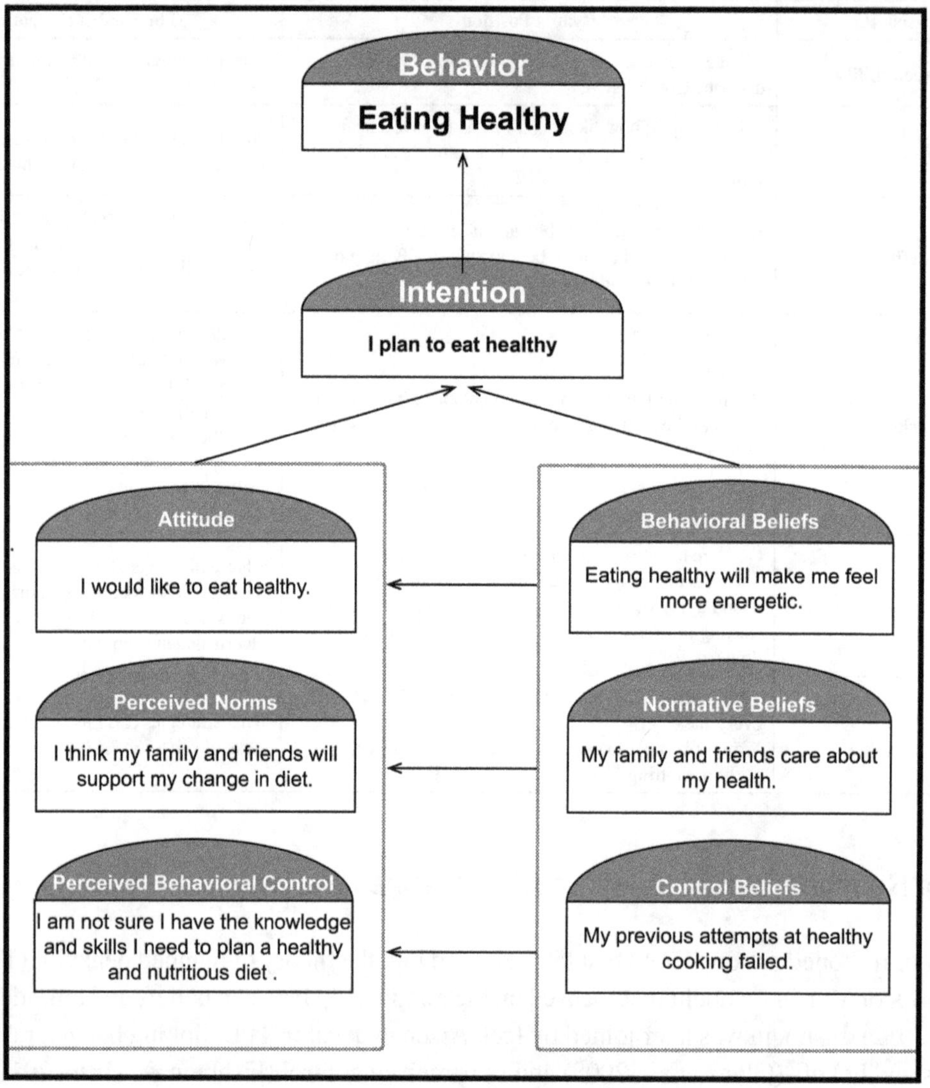

Fishbein (2008) stressed the importance of defining intended behaviors. He urged to differentiate between specific behaviors such as eating five servings of fruits and vegetables a day, and behavioral categories, such as eating healthy. Additionally, he pointed to four elements of behavior to be considered: action, target, context, and time. For example, the health educator will need to consider Ryan's action of eating fruits and vegetables, targeting five servings every day, at home and at work. Once Ryan decides to have five servings a day (intention), the health educator will examine his underlying beliefs about the behavior itself, the norms that surround it, and his perceived control over the behavior.

Based on the analysis guided by TRA/TPB, the health educator would then start to design the appropriate intervention accordingly.

Figure 4. Analysis of Ryan's health determinants through TTM' stages of change

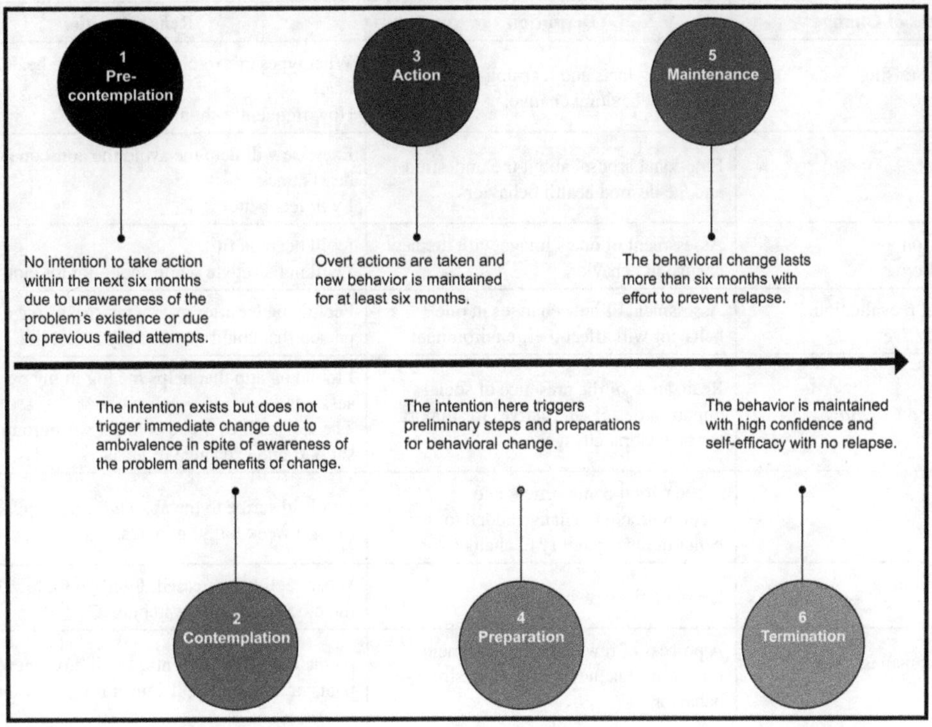

Transtheoretical Model of Change

Prochaska and DiClemente (1986) developed the transtheoretical model (TTM), describing "a three-dimensional model that integrates stages, processes, and levels of change" (p.4). The purpose of this comprehensive approach to change was to emphasize the change in people from the moment they become aware of their problem to the moment they take action and change their behavior (Grimley, et al., 1994). TTM consists of four main constructs: stages of change, processes of change, decisional balance, and self-efficacy.

Stages of change reflect a temporal dimension to how people's behavior changes over time, cyclically and spirally with relapses and progressions (Prochaska & DiClemente, 1986; Sutton, 2005). The temporal sequence of the stages of change consists of six stages (Prochaska & Norcross, 2001; Prochaska et al., 2008) shown in Figure 4.

Processes of change describe the covert and overt actions exhibited during change (Prochaska & DiClemente, 1986; Prochaska et al., 2008; Sutton, 2005). Understanding these processes informs intervention planning (Prochaska et al., 2008). Ten processes have been identified, varying between affective, cognitive, and behavioral (Prochaska et al., 2008; Sutton, 2005). These are clarified through the diagnosis below.

The Health Educator Diagnosis. Through the lens of TTM, the health educator might examine Ryan's intention for exercising as shown in Table 4.

However, the transtheoretical model of change has two additional constructs: decisional balance and self-efficacy.

Table 4. Analysis of Ryan's health determinants through TTM process of change

Process of Change	Definition	Ryan's Position
Consciousness raising *Cognitive*	Collecting facts and learning about the desired behavioral change.	What types of exercise improves the health of my heart? How frequently should I exercise?
Dramatic relief *Affective*	Emotional arousal about the undesired and the desired health behaviors.	Exercise will help me avoid the consequences of a heart attack I will feel better.
Self-reevaluation *Cognitive-Affective*	Assessment of one's image with the new change in behavior.	I will become fit I will not struggle while shopping for clothes.
Environmental reevaluation *Cognitive-Affective*	Assessment of how changes in one's behavior will affect their environment.	Feeling better after exercising makes me a happier person that could improve my social life.
Social liberation *Cognitive*	Realization of the presence of social opportunities or alternatives to support the behavioral change.	I found an app that helps me log in my exercise sessions. The app enables me to connect with groups for support and exchange of ideas.
Self-liberation *Behavioral*	A behavioral commitment and recommitment to change added to the belief in the capability to change.	I will subscribe to the app and start exercising three times a week for 30 minutes.
Counterconditioning *Behavioral*	Learning the new behavior.	When feeling depressed, I will go for a walk around the block instead of watching TV.
Reinforcement management *Behavioral*	A process of reward and punishment for actions taken towards the desired behavior.	At the end of each month, I will buy a new pair of pants or a new shirt, if I meet my exercise goals.
Stimulus control *Behavioral*	Changing the environment to support the behavioral change.	I bought new exercise shoes and renewed my gym membership.
Helping relationships *Behavioral*	Development of interpersonal relationships that help support the behavioral change.	I will seek support from my gym buddies.

Decisional balance is the process of weighing advantages versus disadvantages of behavioral change (Prochaska & DiClemente, 1986; Prochaska et al., 2008; Sutton, 2005), like perceived benefits in HBM and outcome expectations and barriers in SCT discussed next.

Self-efficacy that appears in HBM and SCT as well, represents one's confidence in changing behavior (Prochaska & DiClemente, 1986; Prochaska et al., 2008; Sutton, 2005).

Based on the analysis guided by TTM, the health educator would then start to design the appropriate intervention accordingly. The health educator will first determine where Ryan is with respect to stages of change and how close he is to making the change. Then, they will study his position across the processes of change to design an intervention that targets his cognitive, affective, and behavioral readiness to change. Simultaneously, the health educator will try to show Ryan how the advantages of exercising outweigh its disadvantages and will seek to boost his sense of self-efficacy.

Social Cognitive Theory

Alfred Bandura, the leading theorist behind social cognitive theory (SCT), explained behavioral change and learning through the environmental effects on cognition and self-regulation (Sharma & Romas, 2012; Simons-Morton et al., 1995). He believed self-efficacy to be a pivotal element in behavioral change

Figure 5. Interplay of behavior, personal characteristics, and environment in SCT

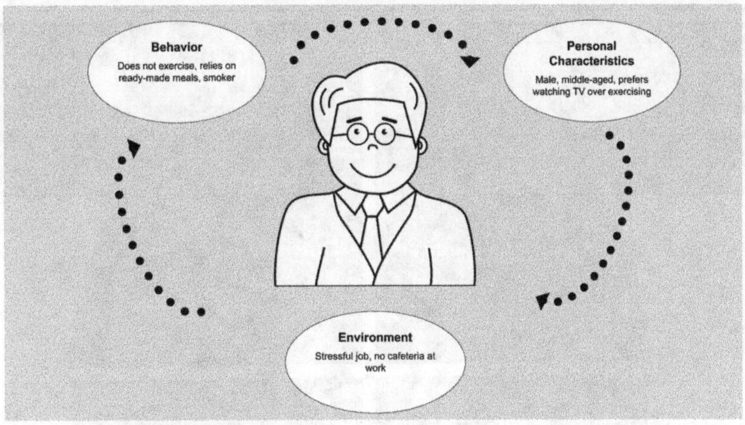

(Bandura, 1977) and dedicated a considerable amount of his writings to the application of SCT in health promotion (Bandura, 1998, 2004, 2005).

Bandura (1978, 1998, 2004) explained that the occurrence of a behavior is the result of the interplay of behavior, personal characteristics, and environmental factors. Personal characteristics such as physical attributes, beliefs, emotions, and cognitions affect how people act and behave. On the other hand, environmental factors that are mostly social, provide modeling, instruction, and social persuasion. Interestingly, Benight and Bandura (2004) argue that people create and select their environments and therefore are producers as well as products of the environments. People's personal characteristics affect the reactions they receive from their social surroundings, shaping their reaction to the environment either by reinforcing or hindering their behaviors (Bandura, 1998).

The Health Educator Diagnosis: From the lens of SCT, the health educator would analyze Ryan's position as follows. Ryan likes his job. The competitive environment drives him to work hard and to put in long hours. So, his working environment drives the hard work but, on the other hand, Ryan enjoys the success he gets from it. Here, he is prioritizing the rewards from his environment that, in turn, are shaping his behavior.

However, analyzing Ryan's position from the lens of SCT is a little more complex than doing so using HBM, because the constructs are layered and interconnected. Bandura (1998) explained that knowledge, the basis for any learning and subsequent behavioral change, is not enough. There are other influences that affect behavior. These are beliefs in self-efficacy, outcome expectations, cognized goals, and barriers preventing behavioral expression.

If Ryan understands his risks for heart disease and knows what he needs to do to quit smoking, start exercising, and follow a healthy diet, what could prevent him from acting? Figure 6 continues the scenario.

Bandura (2004) states that self-efficacy affects one's outcome expectations of a certain behavior, one's goal settings, and one's perceptions of the barriers to behavior adoption. If Ryan believes in his capabilities, he will then be motivated to change, he will have positive expectations, he will be able to set good goals, and he will find ways to overcome the barriers.

The role of the health educator here is to determine Ryan's level of self-efficacy and to help him set goals, address barriers to improve expectations of outcomes. To do so, the health educator will look further into the constructs of STC. Bandura (1998) stated that beliefs of self-efficacy can be strengthened

Figure 6. Analysis of Ryan's health determinants through four SCT constructs

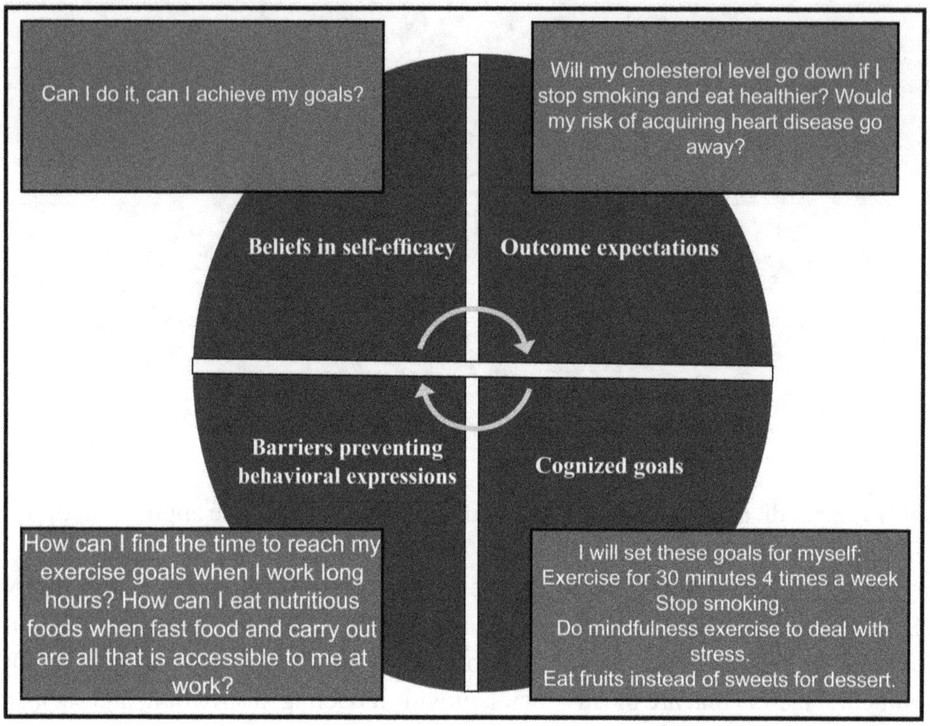

by mastery experience (what is the experience like when mastering a behavior), vicarious experiences (modeling provided from the social environment), social persuasion (such as verbal persuasion), and emotional states that result from all the above experiences (Bandura, 1998). Figure 7 goes further into the scenario.

Based on the analysis guided by SCT, the health educator would then start to design the appropriate intervention accordingly.

Although the models discussed above are widely used, they do have limitations. For example, HBM lacks a description of the process of behavioral change and lacks clarity about the relationship between the constructs that may result in variations in evaluation and intervention studies (Abraham & Sheeran, 2005). Similarly, TRA/TPB does not provide an explanation of the behavioral change to guide behavior modification and does not take into account personal, environmental, and other factors that might impact behavioral intentions (Sharma & Romas, 2012; Boston University School of Public Health, 2019). On the other hand, TTM raises questions on the validity of the self-reported stages of change and the categorization of the change in stages; additionally, the many constructs of TTM limit the practicality of its use in interventions (Sharma & Roams, 2012; Sutton, 2005). Likewise, for SCT, the complexity and the number of its constructs hinder the application of all its constructs in interventions (Glanz & Maddock, 2002; Sharma & Romas, 2012).

Figure 7. Analysis of Ryan's health determinants through additional SCT constructs

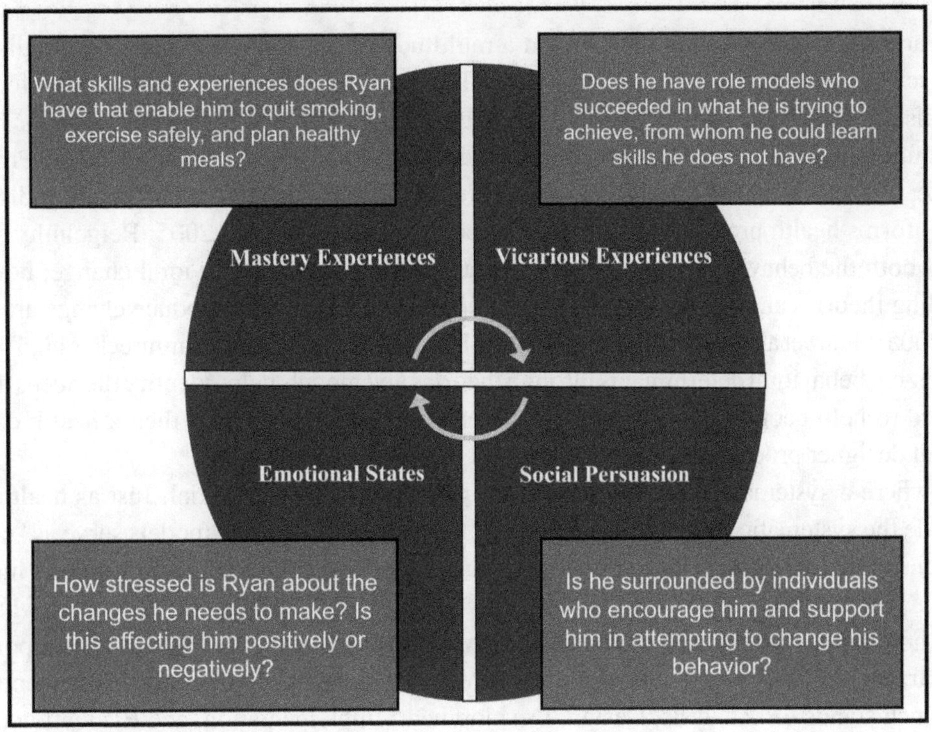

Putting All Together

This is by no means a comprehensive list nor a systematic review. These are just examples of how a health educator, or anyone involved in health education, could analyze the causes of Ryan's behavior to target the constructs with the right intervention. The different models reflect the "different ways of knowing, different lenses for viewing reality and different realities to be known (from the differing perspectives of different beings)" (Green et al. 1994, p. 401).

As stated earlier, the importance of relying on a theory or model to design health education interventions stems from the need to specify the constructs that could be targeted for behavioral change, to facilitate the selection of intervention strategies, and to determine the evaluation process (Michie & Prestwich, 2010). However, Weinstein (2007) posits that health behavior theories "explain the same types of health behaviors and use many of the same social and cognitive constructs" (p. 1). Similarly, Fishbein (2008) argues that although many constructs explain health behavior, only a few are needed to affect change. Principally, constructs comprise cognition, affect, and skills that work in tandem to direct health behavior (Green & Keuter, 2005; Magnan et al. (2017).

Once health determinants are analyzed, the step that follows would be the design of an intervention that targets the educational need and prompts behavioral change. This is where the discipline of education comes into play in health education, and more specifically, instructional design.

INSTRUCTIONAL DESIGN PROCESS

As stated earlier, health education draws from a multitude of disciplines, especially, the discipline of behavioral sciences and the discipline of education. The discipline of behavioral sciences informs health professionals about why people behave the way they do in health and offers guidance for behavioral change through health behavior theories (Bandura, 1978, 1998, 2004; Glanz et al., 2015; Prochaska & DiClemente, 1986; Rosenstock, 1974; Rosenstock et al., 1988). On the other hand, the discipline of education informs health professionals about how people learn (Driscoll, 2005; Reigeluth, 1999). The end goal of both the behavioral sciences and education disciplines is behavioral change; however, the corresponding theories and models describing the approaches on how to produce change are divergent (Driscoll, 2005; Glanz et al., 2008; Reigeluth, 1999; Sharma & Romas, 2011; Timmreck et al., 1988/2010).

Categorizing behavioral determinants through theories and models helps identify the needs that should be addressed to help people move towards healthier behaviors. How would then a health educator or instructional designer proceed to design the health education intervention?

This is where a systematic instructional design process becomes essential. Just as health behavior models guide the systematic design of an intervention, instructional design models serve as "conceptual and communication tools to visualize, direct, and manage processes for creating high quality instruction" (Gustafson & Branch, 2002, p.1). Instructional design models guide designers not only on what to teach but also on how to teach (Reigeluth & An, 2021). Several instructional design models are reported in the literature (Branch & Kopcha, 2014), but all consist of five major steps represented by the generic model ADDIE, which stands for Analysis, Design, Development, Implementation, and Evaluation (Molenda, 2003).

Analysis

The analysis begins with a determination of the need for instruction, in other words, what part of the behavior can be changed through instruction. It also covers the identification of the learner's characteristics and the context in which learning is to occur. In Ryan's case, his knowledge, beliefs, attitudes, skills, and sense of self-efficacy can be targeted through instruction (the learning need). His age, gender, profession, social status, and interests are examples of his characteristics that cannot be changed through instruction, but they might impact the choice of instructional strategies and message design. Next, it is important to determine where and how the instruction is going to be delivered. An intervention meant to be in a face-to-face setting requires a set of instructional strategies different from one intended to be delivered virtually (Dick et al., 2015; Morrison et al., 2013; Reigeluth & An, 2021).

Another essential element in the needs analysis is task analysis. Task analysis is "a process of analyzing and articulating the kind of learning that you expect the learners to know how to perform" (Jonassen et al., 1999, p. 3). This step helps to identify the objectives, decide on the sequence of instruction, and design the evaluation process (Jonassen et al., 1999). Thus, a task analysis determines the facts, concepts, principles, rules, procedures, skills, and attitudes that need to be addressed in the instructional unit. Finally, resources such as time, budget, and accessibility have to be analyzed to determine need and availability (Reigeluth & An, 2021). For example, for Ryan, one of the goals of the intervention is for him to plan healthy meals. To do so, he needs to learn how to include a variety of fruits and vegetables in meals, increase sources of protein, limit the amount of saturated fat, and keep track of calorie intake (Centers for Disease Control 2020). Each of these "tasks" should be broken down further into the corresponding facts, concepts, skills, such as the benefits of fruits and vegetables, what saturated fats are and their harmful effects on the body, etc., to help determine the learning objectives.

Design

Once the instructional needs have been identified, the crucial step that follows is the selection of objectives. Objectives determine the expected learning outcome and the ultimate change in behavior (Popham, 1972/2017). Moreover, objectives guide the selection and organization of instructional material, and they guide assessment and evaluation (Tyler, 1949/2017). However, learning outcomes vary in nature. Educational scholars, such as Benjamin Bloom and Robert Gagné, pioneered the field in classifying types of learning based on behavioral learning outcomes (Reigeluth & Moore, 1999). Bloom et al. (1956) identified three domains of learning: cognitive, affective, and psychomotor. Similarly, Gagné (1984) described five categories of learning: intellectual skills, verbal information, cognitive strategies, attitude, and motor skills. Differentiating the behavioral outcomes as such enables designers to choose suitable teaching and training strategies and types of assessment (Smith & Ragan, 1996).

Many scholars have classified learning outcomes into different taxonomies (Reigeluth & Moore, 1999), but for simplicity purposes, this chapter will focus on the following. In the cognitive domain, Bloom's classified types of cognitive learning from simple to more complex behaviors as follows: knowledge, comprehension, application, analysis, synthesis, and evaluation (Bloom et al, 1956). In 2002, Krathwohl revised it as follows: remembering, understanding, applying, analyzing, evaluating, and creating, adding the cognitive process to levels of knowledge. Additionally, Krathwohl et al. (1964, as cited in Morrison et al., 2013) classified the affective domain into five categories across a continuum of attitudinal change: receiving, responding, valuing, organizing, and characterizing by a value complex. Similarly, Heinich et al., (1993, as cited in Morrison et al., 2013) classified the psychomotor domain on a continuum based on the degree of coordination, from imitation, to manipulation, precision, and articulation. These taxonomies go deep, aiming at the development of precise objectives and evaluation that target the level of desired behavioral change based on the instructional need and meeting the learners where they are. Objectives for Ryan's intervention could be: (1) explain the benefits of fruits and vegetables-cognitive; (2) choose healthy snacks-attitude: and (3) cook a healthy meal-psychomotor.

The design of instructional materials also includes strategic sequencing of the content to maximize comprehension and mastery. For example, content can be sequenced from least difficult to most difficult, or from more familiar to less familiar. It could also follow a temporal, logical, or conceptual sequence (English & Reigeluth, 1996; Posner & Strike, 1976). For Ryan, the health educator would start by introducing him to the benefits of fruits and vegetables and the harmful effects of saturated fats, then guide him into making healthy food choices, then work with him on cooking a healthy meal. Once the content is selected in alignment with the objectives, categorized by types of learning, then sequenced, instructional approaches are then selected, followed by the corresponding instructional strategies.

Instructional approaches are grounded in learning theories. Learning theories explain how people learn, with three main types of theories mapping the terrain: behaviorist, cognitivist, and constructivist learning theory. Behaviorist theorists focus on the observable change in behavior, which results from the interplay of stimuli, responses, and reinforcements, with no interest in the cognitive process behind it (Deubel, 2003; Skinner, 1966; Reigeluth & An, 2021). As a result, the instructional approach is based on reinforcing the desired behavior through feedback and reward (Driscoll, 2005). For example, a behaviorist approach to the design of an intervention would use badges, points, and rewards for goal achievement (Tamim, 2012). In contrast, cognitivist theorists emphasize cognitive load, the mental processing of information, and its storage and retrieval (Driscoll, 2005; Sweller et al., 2011). Here, the instructional approach focuses on structuring, sequencing, and organizing the material to the learner to maximize retention and understanding. Examples of these strategies are stimulating prior knowledge to make connections, rehearsal, chunking the material in small enough pieces, and organizing and sequencing it in a manner that aid retention (Reigeluth & An, 2021; Richey et al. 2011; Sweller et al., 2011). An example of a cognitivist approach would be an incremental release of information and controlling the number of options presented to the learner to avoid learner fatigue (Tamim, 2012). On the other hand, constructivist theorists highlight the construction of knowledge rather than its mere acquisition, through authentic, social, and collaborative learning experiences (Duffy & Cunnigham, 2005; Jonassen et al., 2007). Consequently, the instructional approach follows "a problem, a project, or a question" (Jonassen, 1999, p. 217) with scaffolding and coaching. A constructivist design approach would incorporate problem-solving through games, authentic lived experiences, learning by doing, and goal setting (Tamim, 2012). The question then becomes what learning theory to ground the design in. The choice of learning theories is linked to one's own beliefs about learning (Walker & Mascadri, 2015). However, often, the design of educational interventions combines different theoretical perspectives (Cronjé, 2006) stemming from a combination of beliefs (Schiro, 2013).

Historically, health education has focused on the transmission of knowledge, aligning with behavioral instructional models (Keyser & Broadbear, 1999/2010). However, the need to empower critical thinking and decision-making in behavioral change shifted the learning paradigm of health education towards a cognitivist and constructivist approach, especially with the fast pace of information driven by technology and the advent of ehealth and mhealth interventions (Greenberg, 1978/2010; Keyser & Broadbear, 1999/2010; Welle et al., 1995/2010).

As noted earlier, it is important to categorize the objectives based on the learning domains because learning outcomes vary. Consequently, the selected instructional strategies must also align with the learning domains. What works for cognitive objectives might not work for affective and psychomotor objectives. Additionally, in each of these learning domains, and based on the learner analysis, the design must meet the learners where they are with respect to their prior knowledge, attitudes, and mastery of skills. In particular, the design must incorporate motivational strategies, without which learning is unsuccessful (Reigeluth & An, 2021). Careful planning of instructional strategies provides instruction that is efficient, effective, and appropriate to the learning environment (Morrison et al., 2013).

The instructional design literature is rich in describing instructional strategies best appropriate for each domain and for each level to help learners succeed, making connections between their prior and new knowledge, skills, and affect (Morrison et al., 2013). This is a brief overview of suggested strategies for each learning domain.

For the cognitive domain, linking to prior knowledge, organizing, and elaborating are key. This could be achieved through advance organizers, metaphors, labels, lists, names, images, analogies, graphic organizers, mnemonics, Socratic dialogue, simulations, problem and project-based instruction (Smith & Ragan, 2005; Fiddian-Green et al. 2019).

For the affective domain, motivation, self-efficacy, and emotions in general are targets, to drive relevance, confidence, and satisfaction (Keller, 2009). These could be attained through role-playing, modeling, storytelling, discussion groups, use of multimedia, facilitating the expression of emotions, and skill-building (Bichelemeyer et al., 2009; Driscoll, 2005; Martin & Reigeluth, 1999). In particular, goal setting is an instructional strategy that enhances self-efficacy. As learners advance towards their goals,

Table 5. Alignment between objectives and instructional strategies

Objective	Instructional Strategy
Explain the benefits of fruits and vegetables (Cognitive).	Help Ryan construct a graphic organizer depicting the benefits of fruits and vegetables.
Choose healthy snacks (Attitude).	Ask Ryan to keep a diary of daily snacks to discuss and reflect on with the health educator.
Cook a healthy meal (Psychomotor).	Guide Ryan in cooking a healthy meal in the kitchen.

they gain skills, their motivation increases as does their sense of self-efficacy (Schunk, 1991), especially when they have a choice in setting their goals, accompanied by the development of metacognitive skills and perception of challenge without a threat (Locke & Latham, 2006). As for the psychomotor domain, demonstration, modeling, providing practice opportunities and feedback are strategies that facilitate mastery (Dick et al., 2015; Morrison et al., 2013).

Going back to objectives the health educator might have set for Ryan, the instructional strategies in Table 5 might be used.

Development and Implementation

The development phase includes the production of content and instructional materials adequate to the medium of delivery and technology where needed (York & Ertmer, 2016; Villachica et al., 2010), with alignment with learners' needs and skills (Morrison et al., 2012). However, constraints of time and budget in addition to clear communication with stakeholders need to be considered, starting at the design phase (Ertmer et al., 2009; Smith &Ragan, 2005) in addition to monitoring implementation and providing support (Villachica et al., 2010).

Evaluation

The success of educational interventions cannot be determined without evaluation. "Evaluation involves making judgments about the merit, value, significance, credibility, and utility of whatever is being evaluated" (Patton, 2018, p. 5). However, an evaluation plan must be put in place during the design process because it needs to align with goals and objectives, and it needs to be performed at different intervals during the design and implementation processes. Formative evaluation is done during the development of instruction to ensure its quality, and summative evaluation takes place after implementation to measure the level of achievement of learning outcomes (Morrison et al., 2013; Reigeluth & Ann, 2021). Summative evaluation can be done right after implementation and beyond to ensure the attainment of learning outcomes and long-term behavioral change (Kirkpartrick & Kayser, 2016).

A design process of interest lately linked to evaluation is user-centered design. It involves the user or learner in the design process to address their needs and wants and to ensure its success (Pratt & Nunes, 2012), where the design becomes iterative and multidisciplinary (Mao et al., 2005). It is commonly used in web-based and digital design and in testing for usability to allow for quick evaluation and revisions at each phase of the design process (Lyon & Koerner, 2016).

The instructional design process is systematic and detailed. Although described in a linear fashion, is it not always applied as such. In fact, it is an iterative process (Ertmer et al., 2009) taking the form of rapid prototyping, where incomplete products go through evaluation cycles before finalization, for efficiency in development (Nixon & Lee, 2001).

HEALTH EDUCATION: A SYSTEMS PERSPECTIVE

Circling back to health behavior and health education in particular, the instructional design process targets one level needed for behavioral change, which is the learning that brings behavioral change at the individual level. For each health behavior construct described in the scenario earlier, instructional strategies drawn from the discipline of education can be applied. However, health determinants also act at other levels, forming an "array of factors that affect health" (Simons-Morton et al., 1995, p 32). These health determinants are categorized differently in the literature, but they all depict the impactful effect of the environment on behavior (Sallis & Owen, 2015). For example, Bandura (1978) discussed reciprocal determinism and interactionism to explain the dynamics between behavior, environment, and personal characteristics. In his ecological systems theory, Bronfenbrenner (1981) proposed five levels that affect human development, the microsystem, mesosystem, ecosystem, macrosystem, and chronosystem. More recently, Cleland et al. (2010) talked about the societal, interpersonal, structural, and environmental levels. Similarly, Bartholomew, Parcel, Gottlieb, and Frenàndez (2011) described six systems levels: individual, interpersonal, organization, community, society, and supernation. Although they are classified and labeled differently, these models aim to show the different environmental entities that influence behavior. In addition, they help steer the discourse away from blaming individuals for their health problems (Leroy, et al., 1988). Moreover, they encourage "a broader perspective on planning and practice that might otherwise drift into a reductionist, person-centered or victim-blaming orientation… examin[ing] both the system as a whole and the component subsystems" (Green et al, 1996, p.273), to help prevent health problems (Simons-Morton et al., 1995).

Emphasizing Bandura's (1978) reciprocal determinism, Green et al. (1996) cautioned about the unanticipated effects of health education interventions. They stated that interventions that lead to behavioral change will also result in a change in the environment and vice versa. Furthermore, they reminded health educators that people behave differently in different environments, highlighting the complexity of the dynamics between behavior and environment. Therefore, health determinants are interconnected parts of an environmental whole that form complex and dynamic systems (Trochim et al., 2006). Describing parts and wholes in systems, Cabrera and Cabrera (2019) said that thinking about systems means:

Splitting things into their constituent parts and seeing everything as part of a larger whole, balancing reductionist with holist orientations.... both micro- and macro-level perspectives must be taken. Thus, ideas exist as both parts and wholes simultaneously, allowing for a deep understanding and analysis of any system. (p.13)

Hence, health interventions designed from a systems perspective and directed at more than one level are more effective (Sallis & Owen, 2015). Nonetheless, their scope depends on priorities and resources (Green et al. 1996). How could then health behavior interventions be approached? For this purpose, health education scholars developed planning models to guide health practitioners into thinking and planning interventions at the macrolevel (Sharma & Romas, 2012) while still incorporating constructs from health behavior models at the microlevel (Sallis & Owen, 2015). Specifically, these planning models aim at program design that could embed several interventions (Green & Kreuter, 2005). The most popular planning models are PRECEDE-PROCEED (Green & Kreuter, 2005) and Intervention Mapping (Bartholomew, Parcel, Gottlieb, & Frenàndez, 2011). Below is a brief description of each.

PRECEDE-PROCEDE

Developed in the 1970s by Green and Kreuter, PRECEDE-PROCEED is one of the most widely used planning models (Porter, 2016). PRECEDE is an acronym that stands for "predisposing, reinforcing, and enabling causes in educational diagnosis and evaluation" (Green & Kreuter, 2005, p. 9) while PROCEED stands for policy, regulatory and organizational constructs in educational and environmental development (Green & Kreuter, 2005, p. 9) and it was added later to the model to reflect the growing interest in health promotion (Sharma & Romas, 2012). PRECEDE phases focus on diagnosis and assessments used to design the steps that follow and PROCEED phases focus on implementation and evaluation. The PRECEDE phases are presented below.

- Phase 1, *social assessment*, identifies the problems communities face in terms of quality of life, through multiple sources of information such as morbidity and mortality data, community surveys, focus groups, and others.
- Phase 2, *epidemiological assessment*, is an in-depth analysis of the problems affecting the quality of life to select the health problems, prioritizing them in terms of importance and changeability. Then, health problems are analyzed to specify their determinants, categorizing them as genetic, environmental, or behavioral.
- Phase 3, *educational and ecological assessment*, is an analysis of the behavioral determinants. Green and Kreuter (2005) recommend looking at three types of factors that affect behavior, suggesting that they encompass all factors affecting health behavior: 1) predisposing factors internal to individuals (knowledge, attitudes, beliefs, and values, etc.); 2) enabling factors residing in external environments (availability of resources, accessibility to resources, skills, etc.); and 3) reinforcing factors that influence behavior (family, peers, employers, health providers, etc.). This phase enables practitioners to focus on the factors that, when targeted, would most likely produce the desired change.
- Phase 4, *administrative and policy assessment and intervention alignment*, is where programs are designed, priorities set, policies and regulations identified, and resources and barriers determined in order to ensure alignment between all program components (Green & Kreuter, 2005; Sharma & Romas, 2012).

The PROCEDE phases are presented below.

- Phase 5, *implementation*, programs are implemented with procedures that ensure the most favorable outcomes.
- Phase 6, *process evaluation*, assesses whether the programs were implemented as planned.
- Phase 7, *impact evaluation*, assesses the direct impact of the programs on health behaviors and their predisposing, enabling, and reinforcing factors.

- Phase 8, *outcome evaluation*, assesses the long-term impact of the programs on the health and social problems determined in phase 1 (Green & Kreuter 2005).

Intervention Mapping

In 1998, Bartholomew, Parcel, and Kok proposed a health planning model they called Intervention Mapping to facilitate collaborative planning. They posited that health programs comprise three types of planning activities: needs assessment, development and implementation, and evaluation (Bartholomew, Parcel, & Kok, 1998). Intervention Mapping includes the following six steps:

- Step 1, *needs assessment*, establishes the collaborative group that conducts a needs assessment on the behavioral and environmental causes of the problems, identifies determinants, and sets program goals, using the PRECEDE model as a guide.
- Step 2, *preparing matrices of change objectives*, determines expected outcomes for behavior and environmental change, prioritizes changeable health determinants, and creates a matrix of performance objectives.
- Step 3, *selecting theory-informed interventions methods and practical applications*, design program components and methods based on theory, and specifies the suitable application strategies.
- Step 4, *producing program components and materials*, consults with participants on their preferences, lays down the scope and sequence of the program, delivery channels, and needed materials, and designs, reviews, and develops materials.
- Step 5, *planning program adoption, implementation, and sustainability*, identifies adopters and implementers, and creates a matrix for adoption, implementation, and sustainability objectives, and designs the intervention.
- Step 6, *planning for evaluation*, develops evaluation tools, processes, and indicators and measures, thinking of the intervention system. As in the evaluation phases of PROCEDE, in this step, the health practitioners evaluate the implementation process, the impact on behavior, and the outcome on quality of life (Bartholomew, Parcel, Gottlieb, & Frenàndez, 2011).

Figure 8 summarizes each of these two planning models.

For Ryan, the health educator working with him needs to collaborate with other professionals to have a good understanding of the epidemiological underpinnings of heart disease and to assess the social and environmental factors to support Ryan in changing his behavior.

CONCLUSION

This chapter presented an overview of the groundwork needed for a strong design of health education interventions, drawing from the disciplines of health behavior psychology and education. The complexity of the design stems from the need to consider the health determinants, the theoretical constructs through which health behavior can be examined to create health education interventions, and the instructional design principles that target the underpinnings of health behavior with fitting instruction. As stated earlier, this is by no means a comprehensive analysis because both fields are rich with theories and models. It is an attempt to bridge health education to instructional design for successful behavioral change.

Figure 8. Health education planning models

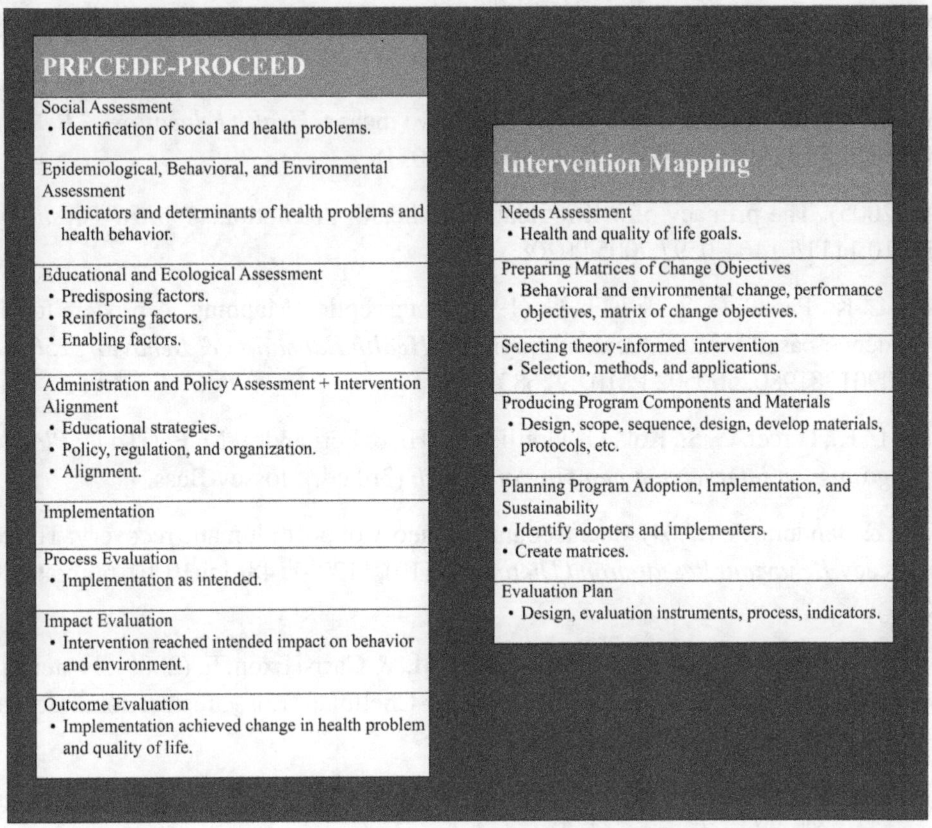

Additionally, the chapter presented a synopsis of two popular health planning models to highlight the importance of a systems view when developing health education interventions. Undoubtedly, program planning is a laborious and complex task. In fact, Green et al. (1996) explained that complexity might bring despair, which might drive health practitioners to wonder "how much is enough" (p. 273). Nevertheless, a collaborative approach to health education interventions that enables addressing the factors that impact health behavior is important for achieving positive outcomes and health improvement (Bartholomew, Parcel, Gottlieb, & Frenàndez, 2011).

This chapter aimed at highlighting the theoretical foundations of health education interventions and the principles of an effective design process, underscoring the importance of a systems perspective that affects the success of these interventions. These fundamentals apply to any setting the interventions are delivered in. While additional considerations are needed for ehealth and mhealth interventions (see Chapter 2), the basic behavioral and educational foundations discussed in the chapter remain the same.

REFERENCES

Bandura, A. (1977). Self-efficacy: Toward a unifying theory of behavioral change. *Psychological Review*, *84*(2), 191–215. doi:10.1037/0033-295X.84.2.191 PMID:847061

Bandura, A. (1978). The self system in reciprocal determinism. *American Psychologist, 33*(4), 344-358.

Bandura, A. (1998). Health promotion from the perspective of social cognitive theory. *Psychology & Health, 13*(4), 623–649. doi:10.1080/08870449808407422

Bandura, A. (2004). Health promotion by social cognitive means. *Health Education & Behavior, 31*(2), 143–164. doi:10.1177/1090198104263660 PMID:15090118

Bandura, A. (2005). The primacy of self-regulation in health promotion. *Applied Psychology, 54*(2), 245–254. doi:10.1111/j.1464-0597.2005.00208.x

Bartholomew, L. K., Parcel, G. S., & Kok, G. (1998). Intervention Mapping: A process for developing theory and evidence-based health education programs. *Health Education & Behavior, 25*(5), 545–563. doi:10.1177/109019819802500502 PMID:9768376

Bartholomew, L. K., Parcel, G. S., Kok, G., Gottlieb, N. H., & Fernandez, M. E. (2011). *Planning health promotion programs: an intervention mapping approach* (3rd ed.). Jossey-Bass.

Benight, C. C., & Bandura, A. (2004). Social cognitive theory of posttraumatic recovery: The role of perceived self-efficacy. *Behaviour Research and Therapy, 42*(10), 1129–1148. doi:10.1016/j.brat.2003.08.008 PMID:15350854

Bichelmeyer, B. A., Marken, J., Harris, T., Misanchuk, M., & Carr-Hixon, E. (2009). Fostering affective development outcomes. In C. M. Reigeluth & A.A. Carr-Chellman (Eds.), Instructional-design theories and models (vol. 3, pp. 249-274). Taylor & Francis.

Bloom, B. S., Engelhart, M. D., Furst, E. J., Hill, W. H., & Krathwohl, D. R. (1956). *Taxonomy of educational objectives: The classification of educational goals*. Longmans.

Boston University School of Public Health. (2019). *The theory of planned behavior*. https://sphweb.bumc.bu.edu/otlt/mph-modules/sb/behavioralchangetheories/BehavioralChangeTheories3.html

Branch, R. M., & Kopcha, T. J. (2014). Instructional design models. In J. M. Spector, M. D. Merrill, J. Elen, & M. J. Bishop (Eds.), *Handbook of research on educational communications and technology* (pp. 77–87). Springer New York. doi:10.1007/978-1-4614-3185-5_7

Centers for Disease Control and Prevention. (2021, April 19). *Healthy eating for a healthy weight*. https://www.cdc.gov/healthyweight/healthy_eating/index.html

Champion, V. L., & Skinner, C. S. (2008). The health belief model. In K. Glanz, B. K., Rimer, & K. Viswanath (Eds.), Health behavior and health education: theory, research, and practice (4th ed., pp. 45-65). Jossey-Bass.

Cleland, V. J., Ball, K., & Crawford, D. (2010). Social and environmental determinants of health behaviors. In A. Steptoe (Ed.), *Handbook of behavioral medicine: Methods and applications* (pp. 3–18). Springer. doi:10.1007/978-0-387-09488-5_1

Coalition of National Health Education Organizations. (2021). 2020 *Health education and promotion terminology report*. http://www.cnheo.org/2020-joint-committee-on-health-education-terminology.html

Crosby, R., & Noar, S. M. (2011). What is a planning model? An introduction to PRECEDE-PROCEED. *Journal of Public Health Dentistry*, *71*(s1), S7–S15. doi:10.1111/j.1752-7325.2011.00235.x PMID:21656942

Deubel, P. (2003). An investigation of behaviorist and cognitive approaches to instructional multimedia design. *Journal of Educational Multimedia and Hypermedia*, *12*(1), 63–90.

Dick, W., Carey, L., & Carey, J. O. (2015). *The systematic design of instruction*. Pearson.

Driscoll, M. P. (2005). *Psychology of learning for instruction* (3rd ed.). Pearson Allyn and Bacon.

Duffy, T. M., & Cunningham, D. J. (2007). Constructivism: Implications for the design and delivery of instruction. In D. H. Jonassen (Ed.), *Handbook of research for educational communications and technology* (pp. 1–31). The Association for Educational Communications and Technology.

Dustin, D. L., Bricker, K. S., & Schwab, K. A. (2009). People and nature: Toward an ecological model of health promotion. *Leisure Sciences*, *32*(1), 3–14. doi:10.1080/01490400903430772

English, R. E., & Reigeluth, C. M. (1996). Formative research on sequencing instruction with the elaboration theory. *Educational Technology Research and Development*, *44*(1), 23–42. doi:10.1007/BF02300324

Ertmer, P. A., York, C. S., & Gedik, N. (2009). Learning from the pros: How experienced designers translate instructional design models into practice. *Educational Technology*, *49*(1), 19–27.

Fiddian-Green, A., Kim, S., Gubrium, A. C., Larkey, L. K., & Peterson, J. C. (2019). Restor(y)ing health: A conceptual model of the effects of digital storytelling. *Health Promotion Practice*, *20*(4), 502–512. doi:10.1177/1524839918825130 PMID:30736703

Fishbein, M. (2008). A reasoned action approach to health promotion. *Medical Decision Making*, *28*(6), 834–844. doi:10.1177/0272989X08326092 PMID:19015289

Fishbein, M., & Ajzen, I. (2010). *Predicting and changing behavior: The reasoned action approach*. ProQuest Ebook Central. https://ebookcentral.proquest.com

Gagné, R. M. (1984). Learning outcomes and their effects: Useful categories of human performance. *The American Psychologist*, *39*(4), 377–385. doi:10.1037/0003-066X.39.4.377

Garrison, D. R. (2000). Theoretical challenges for distance education in the 21st century: A shift from structural to transactional issues. *International Review of Research in Open and Distance Learning*, *1*(1), 6–21. doi:10.19173/irrodl.v1i1.2

Glanz, K., Rimer, B. K., & Viswanath, K. (2008). *Health behavior and health education: theory, research, and practice* (4th ed.). Jossey-Bass.

Glanz, K., Rimer, B. K., & Viswanath, K. (Eds.). (2015). *Health behavior: Theory, research, and practice*. John Wiley & Sons, Incorporated.

Goodson, P. (2010). *Theory in health promotion research and practice: Thinking outside the box*. Jones and Bartlett.

Green, L. W., Glanz, K., Hochbaum, G. M., Kok, G., Kreuter, M. W., Lewis, F. M., Lorig, K., Morisky, D., Rimer, B. K., & Rosenstock, I. M. (1994). Can we build on, or must we replace, the theories and models in health education? *Health Education Research*, *9*(3), 397–404. doi:10.1093/her/9.3.397 PMID:10150456

Green, L. W., & Kreuter, M. W. (2005). *Health program planning: An educational and ecological approach*. McGraw-Hill.

Green, L. W., Richard, L., & Potvin, L. (1996). Ecological foundations of health promotion. *American Journal of Health Promotion*, *10*(4), 270–281. doi:10.4278/0890-1171-10.4.270 PMID:10159708

Greenberg, J. S. (2010). Health education as freeing. In J. M. Black, S. Furney, H. M. Graf, & A. E. Nolte (Eds.), *Philosophical foundations of health education* (pp. 210–205). Jossey-Bass.

Grimley, D., Prochaska, J. O., Velicer, W. F., Blais, L. M., & DiClemente, C. C. (1994). The transtheoretical model of change. In T. M. Brinthaupt & R. P. Lipka (Eds.), *Changing the self: philosophies, techniques, and experiences* (pp. 201–228). SUNY Press. https://books.google.com/books?hl=en&lr=&id=nhrTvXVhBLMC&pgis=1

Gustafson, K. L., & Branch, R. M. (2002). *Survey of instructional development models* (4th ed.). ERIC Clearinghouse on Information & Technology.

Joint Committee on Health Education and Promotion Terminology. (2021). *Joint committee on health education and promotion terminology report.* http://www.cnheo.org/2020-joint-committee-on-health-education-terminology.html

Jonassen, D. (1999). Designing constructivist learning environments. In C. M. Reigeluth (Ed.), Instructional design theories and models (vol. 2, pp. 215-239). Lawrence Erlbaum Associates.

Jonassen, D., Cernusca, D., & Ionas, G. (2007). Constructivism and instructional design: The emergence of the learning sciences and design research. In R. A. Reiser & J. V. Dempsey (Eds.), *Trends and issues in instructional design and technology* (2nd ed., pp. 45–52). Pearson.

Jonassen, D. H., Tessmer, M., & Hannum, W. H. (1999). *Task analysis methods for instructional design*. Lawrence Erlbaum Associates.

Keller, J. M. (2009). *Motivational design for learning and performance: The arcs model approach*. ProQuest Ebook Central. https://ebookcentral.proquest.com

Keyser, B. B., & Broadbear, J. T. (2010). The paradigm shift toward thinking for thinking: Perspectives, barriers, solutions, and accountability. In J. M. Black, S. Furney, H. M. Graf, & A. E. Nolte (Eds.), *Philosophical foundations of health education* (pp. 109–118). Jossey-Bass.

Kirkpatrick, J. D., & Kayser, W. (2016). *Kirkpatrick's four levels of training evaluation*. Association For Talent Development. https://login.pallas2.tcl.sc.edu/login?url=https://search.ebscohost.com/login.aspx?direct=true&db=e025xna&AN=1364594&site=ehost-live

Locke, E. A., & Latham, G. P. (2006). New directions in goal-setting theory. *Current Directions in Psychological Science*, *15*(5), 265–268. doi:10.1111/j.1467-8721.2006.00449.x

Lyon, A. R., & Koerner, K. (2016). User-centered design for psychosocial intervention development and implementation. *Clinical Psychology: Science and Practice*, *23*(2), 180–200. doi:10.1111/cpsp.12154 PMID:29456295

Magnan, R. E., Shorey Fennell, B. R., & Brady, J. M. (2017). Health decision making and behavior: The role of affect-laden constructs. *Social & Personality Psychology Compass*, *11*(8). doi:10.1111/spc3.12333

Maiman, L. A., & Becker, M. H. (1974). The health belief model: Origins and correlates in psychological theory. In M. H. Becker (Ed.), *The health belief model and personal health behavior* (pp. 9–26). Charles B. Slack. doi:10.1177/109019817400200404

Mao, J. Y., Vredenburg, K., Smith, P. W., & Carey, T. (2005). The state of user-centered design practice. *Communications of the ACM*, *48*(3), 105–109. doi:10.1145/1047671.1047677

Martin, B. L., & Reigeluth, C. M. (1999). Affective education and the affective domain: Implications for instructional-design theories and models. In C. M. Reigeluth (Ed.), Instructional design theories and models (vol. 2, pp. 485-509). Lawrence Erlbaum Associates.

McLeroy, K. R., Bibeau, D., Steckler, A., & Glanz, K. (1988). An ecological perspective on health promotion programs. *Health Education Quarterly*, *15*(4), 351–377. doi:10.1177/109019818801500401 PMID:3068205

Michie, S., & Prestwich, A. (2010). Are interventions theory-based? Development of a theory coding scheme. *Health Psychology: Official Journal of the Division of Health Psychology, American Psychological Association*, *29*(1), 1–8. doi:10.1037/a0016939 PMID:20063930

Molenda, M. (2003). In search of the elusive ADDIE model. *Performance Improvement*, *42*(5), 34–36. doi:10.1002/pfi.4930420508

Morrison, G. R., Ross, S. M., Kalman, H. K., & Kemp, J. E. (2013). *Designing effective instruction*. Wiley & Sons, Inc.

Nixon, E. K., & Lee, D. (2001). Rapid prototyping in the instructional design process. *Performance Improvement Quarterly*, *14*(3), 95–116. doi:10.1111/j.1937-8327.2001.tb00220.x

Nutbeam, D. O. N. (1998). Health promotion glossary. *Health Promotion International*, *13*(4), 349–364. doi:10.1093/heapro/13.4.349

Palfrey, C. (2018). The future of health promotion. In *The Future for Health Promotion* (1st ed., pp. 25–54). Bristol University Press., doi:10.2307/j.ctt22rbkdc.6

Popham, W. J. (2017). Objectives. In D. J. Flinders & S. T. Thornton (Eds.), *The curriculum reader* (5th ed., pp. 115–128). Routledge.

Porter, C. M. (2016). Revisiting Precede–Proceed: A leading model for ecological and ethical health promotion. *Health Education Journal*, *75*(6), 753–764. doi:10.1177/0017896915619645

Posner, G. J., & Strike, K. A. (1976). A categorization scheme for principles of sequencing content. *Review of Educational Research*, *46*(4), 665–690. doi:10.3102/00346543046004665

Pratt, A., Nunes, J., & Nunes, J. (2012). *Interactive design: An introduction to the theory and application of user-centered design*. Quarto Publishing Group USA.

Prochaska, J. O., & DiClemente, C. C. (1986). Toward a comprehensive model of change. In N. Miller & R. W. Heather (Eds.), *Treating addictive behaviors* (pp. 3–27). Plenum Publishing Corporation. doi:10.1007/978-1-4613-2191-0_1

Prochaska, J. O., & Norcross, J. C. (2001). Stages of change. *Psychotherapy (Chicago, Ill.), 38*(4), 443–448. doi:10.1037/0033-3204.38.4.443

Prochaska, J. O., Redding, C. A., & Evers, K. E. (2008). The transtheoretical model of stages of change. In K. Glanz, B.K. Rimer, & K. Viswanath (Eds.), Health behavior and health education: theory, research, and practice (4th ed., pp. 45-65). Jossey-Bass. Publications, Inc.

Reigeluth, C. M., & An, Y. (2021). *Merging the instructional design process with learner-centered theory: The holistic 4D model*. Routledge.

Reigeluth, C. M., & Moor, J. (1999). Cognitive education and the cognitive domain. In C. M. Reigeluth (Ed.), Instructional design theories and models (vol. 2, pp. 5-29). Lawrence Erlbaum Associates.

Richey, R. C., Klein, J. D., & Tracey, M. W. (2011). *The instructional design knowledge base: Theory, research, and practice*. Routledge.

Rosenstock, I. M. (1974). The historic origins of the health belief model. In M. H. Becker (Ed.), *The health belief model and personal health behavior* (pp. 1–8). Charles B. Slack.

Rosenstock, I. M., Strecher, V. J., & Becker, M. H. (1988). Social learning theory and the health belief model. *Health Education Quarterly, 15*(2), 175–183. doi:10.1177/109019818801500203 PMID:3378902

Sallis, J. F., & Owen, N. (2015). Ecological models of health behavior. In Health behavior: Theory, research, and practice (5th ed., pp- 43-64). John Wiley & Sons Incorporated.

Schiro, M. (2013). Curriculum theory: Conflicting visions and enduring concerns. *Sage (Atlanta, Ga.)*.

Schunk, D. H. (1991). Self-efficacy and academic motivation. *Educational Psychologist, 26*(3), 207–231. doi:10.120715326985ep2603&4_2

Sharma, M., & Romas, J. A. (2012). *Theoretical foundations of health education and health promotion* (2nd ed.). Jones & Bartlett Learning.

Simoni, J. M., Ronen, K., & Aunon, F. M. (2018). Health behavior theory to enhance ehealth intervention research in HIV: Rationale and review. *Current HIV/AIDS Reports, 15*(6), 423–430. doi:10.100711904-018-0418-8 PMID:30511186

Simons-Morton, B. G., Greene, W. H., & Gottlieb, N. H. (1995). *Introduction to health education and health promotion* (2nd ed.). Waveland Press.

Skinner, B. F. (1966). The phylogeny and ontogeny of behavior. *Science, 153*(3741), 1205–1213. doi:10.1126cience.153.3741.1205 PMID:5918710

Smith, B. J., Tang, K. C., & Nutbeam, D. (2006). WHO health promotion glossary: New terms. *Health Promotion International*, *21*(4), 340–345. doi:10.1093/heapro/dal033 PMID:16963461

Smith, P. L., & Ragan, T. J. (1996). Impact of R.M. Gagné's work on instructional theory. *Proceedings of Selected Research and Development Presentation, National Convention of the Association of Educational Communications and Technology*.

Smith, P. L., & Ragan, T. J. (2005). *Instructional design* (3rd ed.). Wiley & Sons.

Spencer, L. M., Schooley, M. W., Anderson, L. A., Kochtitzky, C. S., DeGroff, A. S., Devlin, H. M., & Mercer, S. L. (2013). Seeking best practices: A conceptual framework for planning and improving evidence-based practices. *Preventing Chronic Disease*, *10*, 130186. doi:10.5888/pcd10.130186 PMID:24331280

Stroebe, W. (2000). *Social psychology and health* (2nd ed.). Open University Press.

Sutton, S. (2001). Back to the drawing board? A review of applications of the transtheoretical model to substance use. *Addiction (Abingdon, England)*, *96*(1), 175–186. doi:10.1046/j.1360-0443.2001.96117513.x PMID:11177528

Sutton, S. (2005). Stage theories of health behavior. In M. Conner & P. Norman (Eds.), Predicting health behaviour: Research and practice with social cognition models (pp. 29-80). Open University Press.

Sweller, J., Ayres, P., Kalyuga, S., Sweller, J., Ayres, P., & Kalyuga, S. (2011). *Cognitive load theory*. Springer. doi:10.1007/978-1-4419-8126-4

Tabak, R. G., Khoong, E. C., Chambers, D. A., & Brownson, R. C. (2012). Bridging Research and Practice. *American Journal of Preventive Medicine*, *43*(3), 337–350. doi:10.1016/j.amepre.2012.05.024 PMID:22898128

Tamim, S. R. (2012). *An exploration of how health professionals create ehealth and mhealth education interventions* (Publication No. 3529980) [Doctoral Dissertation, University of Memphis]. ProQuest Dissertations & Thesis Global.

Timmreck, T. C., Cole, G. E., Gordon, J., & Butterwoth, D. D. (2010). Health education and health promotion: A look at the jungle of supportive fields, philosophies, and theoretical foundations. In J. M. Black, S. Furney, H. M. Graf, & A. E. Nolte (Eds.), *Philosophical foundations of health education* (pp. 67–78). Jossey-Bass.

Trochim, W. M., Cabrera, D. A., Milstein, B., Gallagher, R. S., & Leischow, S. J. (2006). Practical challenges of systems thinking and modeling in public health. *American Journal of Public Health*, *96*(3), 538–546. doi:10.2105/AJPH.2005.066001 PMID:16449581

Tyler, R. W. (2017). Basic principles of curriculum and instruction. In D. J. Flinders & S. T. Thornton (Eds.), *The curriculum reader* (5th ed., pp. 73–82). Routledge.

Villachica, S. W., Marker, A., & Taylor, K. (2010). But what do they really expect? Employer perceptions of the skills of entry-level instructional designers. *Performance Improvement Quarterly*, *22*(4), 33–51. doi:10.1002/piq.20067

Walker, J. L., & Mascardi, J. (2015). Personal epistemologies and teaching. In H. Fives & M. G. Gill (Eds.), *International handbook of research on teachers' beliefs* (pp. 319–335). Routledge.

Weinstein, N. D. (2007). Misleading tests of health behavior theories. *Annals of Behavioral Medicine*, *33*(1), 1–10. doi:10.120715324796abm3301_1 PMID:17291165

Welle, H. M., Russel, R. D., & Kittleson, M. J. (2010). Philosophical trends in health education: Implications for the 21st century. In J. M. Black, S. Furney, H. M. Graf, & A. E. Nolte (Eds.), *Philosophical foundations of health education* (pp. 79–93). Jossey-Bass.

Willgoose, C. E. (2010). Health education as a basic. In J. M. Black, S. Furney, H. M. Graf, & A. E. Nolte (Eds.), *Philosophical foundations of health education* (pp. 17–27). Jossey-Bass.

World Health Organization. (1998). *Health promotion glossary*. https://www.who.int/publications/i/item/WHO-HPR-HEP-98.1

York, C. S., & Ertmer, P. A. (2016). Examining instructional design principles applied by experienced designers in practice. *Performance Improvement Quarterly*, *29*(2), 169–192. doi:10.1002/piq.21220

ADDITIONAL READING

Abraham, C., & Michie, S. (2008). A taxonomy of behavior change techniques used in interventions. *Health Psychology*, *27*(3), 379–387. doi:10.1037/0278-6133.27.3.379 PMID:18624603

Buchanan, D. R. (1994). Reflections on the relationship between theory and practice. *Health Education Research*, *9*(3), 273–283. doi:10.1093/her/9.3.273 PMID:10150450

Campos, M. N. (2007). Ecology of meanings: A critical constructivist communication model. *Communication Theory, 17*(4), 386–410. doi:10.1111/j.1468-2885.2007.00304.x

Carr-Chellman, A., & Savoy, M. (2004). User-design research. In D. H. Jonassen (Ed.), *Handbook of research on educational communications and technology* (pp. 696–711). Routledge.

Gibbons, A. S., Boling, E., & Smith, K. M. (2014). Instructional design models. In J. M. Spector, M. D. Merrill, J. Elen, & M. J. Bishop (Eds.), *Handbook of Research on Educational Communications and Technology* (pp. 607–615). Springer New York. doi:10.1007/978-1-4614-3185-5_48

KEY TERMS AND DEFINITIONS

Health Behavior: The behavior one exhibits with respect to health-related matters.

Health Determinants: The factors that determine one's health status.

Health Education: The field that focuses on health behavior and the needed interventions for change and health improvement.

Health Education Theories and Models: Often used interchangeably, health education theories and models explain the factors directing health behavior and provide guidelines for designing effective interventions.

Health Educator: The practitioner responsible of assessing health education needs and designing appropriate interventions.

Instruction Design: The systematic process of designing instruction valuable in any learning context, including health education.

Instructional Designer: Professional trained in instructional design who collaborate with subject-matter experts and other stakeholders on the creation of instructional interventions that aim at behavioral change.

Chapter 2
eHealth and mHealth– Definitions, Theories, Models, and Applications

Suha R. Tamim
https://orcid.org/0000-0002-1664-747X
University of South Carolina, USA

Hadi Danawi
Walden University, USA

ABSTRACT

The design of ehealth and mhealth interventions is grounded in interconnected fields, mainly education, health, behavioral psychology, communication, and technology. To provide an overview of these interconnections, this chapter begins with a presentation of key concepts and terms related to elearning, mlearning, ehealth, and mhealth, providing an overview of their definitions and understanding. This is followed by a discussion of ehealth and mhealth theories that shed the light on the factors that prompt health behavior. Next, elearning design principles are explained as they play an important role in the design of interventions. The last section of the chapter addresses ehealth and mhealth spread of use, prominent applications, their benefits, and their challenges.

INTRODUCTION

eHealth and mhealth are becoming essential components of the healthcare system (Moss et al., 2019) with many benefits to healthcare and people (Bull, 2011; van Gemert-Pijnen et al., 2018). This includes the area of ehealth and mhealth education that draws from many interconnected fields. The design of such interventions is grounded in education, health, behavioral psychology, communication, and technology, among several others. However, the links between these fields can be ambiguous and complex. The theoretical underpinnings of each as well as the related models expand and shift - a natural phenomenon in all systems. Reigeluth (2019) affirmed, "for a system to be healthy, it must coevolve with

DOI: 10.4018/978-1-7998-9490-2.ch002

its environment: It changes in response to changes in its environment, and its environment changes in response to its changes" (p.2). These changes are driven by changed societal needs. They perturb the system, transform it, and create shifts in thinking (Reigeluth, 2019). These changes are also driven by advancements in the fields, introducing new terms and leading to definitions that are context-dependent (Mil & Henman, 2016; Oh et al., 2005), overlapping, intersecting, and focusing on various factors (Noesgaard & Ørngreen, 2015). Therefore, to clarify the confusion around their use in the literature and in the book, this chapter begins with an overview of key concepts and terms related to ehealth and mhealth, in addition to elearning and mlearning that are fundamental in the design of health education interventions. This is followed by a discussion of select ehealth and mhealth theories that examine the factors that prompt health behavior. Next, elearning design principles that play an important role in the design of interventions are explained. The last section of the chapter addresses ehealth and mhealth uses in the health field, prominent applications, their benefits, and their challenges.

eHealth

Over the years, several terms have been adopted to identify the use of technology in health (Pagliari et al., 2005). Telemedicine was a term commonly accepted earlier to refer to patient-physician interactions through phone calls, covering patient care and patient education. This was followed by telehealth, introduced in 1978, to denote a broader concept, adding a public health perspective to care and education. The availability of the Internet introduced ehealth in 1999 that was later followed by mhealth in 2003, reflecting the mobile technology component (Bashshur et al., 2011).

One of the earliest definitions of ehealth was proposed by Mitchell in 1999. He suggested that ehealth uses the Internet for clinical, administrative, and educational purposes. It is a broad field that subsumes telemedicine and telehealth and one that is becoming an integral part of the healthcare system (Mitchell,1999). Aiming to provide a scholarly definition useful for academic environments, Eysenbach (2001) conceptualized ehealth as:

[A]n emerging field in the intersection of medical informatics, public health and business, referring to health services and information delivered or enhanced through the Internet and related technologies. In a broader sense, the term characterizes not only a technical development, but also a state-of-mind, a way of thinking, an attitude, and a commitment for networked, global thinking, to improve health care locally, regionally, and worldwide by using information and communication technology. (para. 4)

Between 2001 and 2017, the Journal of Medical Internet Research published a range of articles addressing the nature of ehealth, in an attempt to find a common understanding of it and of its challenges. For example, in 2005, Oh et al. identified 41 ehealth definitions that ranged from three to seventy-four words, with the common themes of health and technology. Similarly, Pagliari et al. (2005) identified 36 ehealth definitions with variable scopes, focuses, and theoretical foundations.

In 2006, Ahern et al. reported on ehealth leaders' concerns about the lack of consensus and standardization in the field, challenges in process and outcome evaluation, lack of regulation and quality control, and health disparities due to unequal access to technology. Recently, Otto et al. (2020) proposed an ehealth ontology. Their search yielded a multitude of terms used in this context: telemedicine, telehealth, ehealth, mhealth, digital health, and health IT. Underlying all of them are the concepts of digitization and information and communication technology. However, Bashshur et al. (2011) cautioned that although these terms are related, they are not interchangeable because they differ in attributes.

Inconsistencies in definitions alarm scholars in the field. Showell and Nøhr (2012) report "no clear, common understanding of the scope and boundaries of activities which might be categorized as ehealth" (p.882), expressing concerns about a hindering effect on planning, comparing, and evaluating ehealth initiatives. Likewise, Shaw et al. (2017) attempted to operationalize the term to improve practice, education, and research around it. They interviewed experts in the field of ehealth and identified three conceptual domains: *health in our hands*, *interacting for health*, and *data enabling health*. Accordingly, they proposed a model where these three domains overlap to empower consumers to take charge of their health.

Addressing the different terms used in the field of ehealth, Scott and Mars (2019) wondered about the introduction of yet another term, digital health, and questioned what it means and how it differs from ehealth, predicting the same trajectory of finding a consensus on the elusive definition of ehealth. They argued that even when technology changes, principles do not: "Let us not muddy the waters still further by bringing yet another term to the lexicon. Rather let us finally bring clarity to the field and at least agree on the term eHealth" (p. 2).

In brief, the large-scale integration of technology in the health system imposes a degree of self-organization by understanding the new dynamics, the new nature of the system, and a willingness to grow to adopt a new identity (Reigeluth, 2019). The plethora of research on the nature of ehealth is an indication of this self-organization.

mHealth

With the spread of mobile devices, mhealth branched out from ehealth. It began with simple voice and text-messages to a profusion of complex apps made possible with the growth of smartphones (Cameron et al., 2017; Dicianno, 2015). mHealth is transformative to health care systems and should be viewed as an opportunity to alter the system rather than just an add-on (Steinhub et al., 2015). The World Health Organization (2011) defined mhealth as "medical and public health practice supported by mobile devices, such as mobile phones, patient monitoring devices, personal digital assistants (PDAs), and other wireless devices" (p.6). However, as with ehealth and despite the proliferation of mhealth research, a clear definition is still absent (Cameron et al., 2017). Nacinovich (2011) denoted a learning curve health professionals need to experience when it comes to mhealth "creation, communication, and consumption" (p. 1) before they adopt it. They need to understand the drivers (e.g., smartphone penetration), the barriers (e.g., lack of standardization regulation and market transparency), and the opportunities of mhealth. Moreover, Steinhub et al. (2015) argued that mhealth researchers are challenged by financial obstacles, privacy and security concerns, and data overload, which might hinder adoption due to lack of evidence of the impact of mhealth use on health behavior change.

Different definitions and taxonomies of ehealth and mhealth point to the broadness of the field, the contextual complexities, and the reach of their impact on many healthcare facets (Mil & Henman, 2016; Oh et al., 2005; van Gemert-Pijnen et al., 2018). The search for identity reminds us of a statement by Reigeluth (2019):

[T]o have a powerful influence on the features that emerge in the system undergoing transformation, the core ideas and beliefs must become integral parts of the mindsets or mental models held by a critical

mass of participants in the transformation process, and, therefore, they must collectively compose the culture of the transformation process as a system. (p.10)

Because health education interventions are interconnected with learning, it is important to discuss principles of elearning and mlearning in the context of ehealth and mhealth education interventions. It is important to understand the nature of elearning and mlearning to underscore the theoretical foundation they provide to ehealth and mhealth interventions.

eLearning

The concept of elearning and how it is defined are changing continuously (Singh & Thurman, 2019). Confusion still exists around them due to the perpetual evolution of technology and the varied socio-economic contextual factors in which they reside (Sangrà et al., 2012). Moreover, an overlap of terms and concepts prevails. These are often used interchangeably (e.g., elearning, online learning, online education, and distance education), lumping together varied designs of learning environments (e.g., hybrid, blended, synchronous, and asynchronous) (Singh &Thurman, 2019). Furthermore, new terms keep being introduced. eLearning extended to mlearning with the advent of mobile devices. Lately, d-learning emerged to encompass all learning that takes place digitally (Kumar Basak et al., 2018). Additionally, the entanglement of terminology and definitions is heightened by a paradigm shift in education towards a learner-centered pedagogy (Harasim, 2000). This shift is transformative to learning, causing changes in mental models, mindsets, beliefs, and behaviors (Duffy, 2009) and leading to new views about learning processes and products (Noesgaard, 2015). Singh and Thurman (2019) explored the different ways scholars define online learning. They found 46 definitions that use 18 different terms. They identified three key concepts inherent to all: technology, time (synchronous and asynchronous), and interactivity. Earlier, Sangrà et al. (2012) observed that definitions differ based on different professional perspectives. They categorized them based on their focus: technology-driven, delivery-system oriented, communication-oriented, and educational-paradigm-oriented. Through a Delphi method with experts in the field, they proposed the following definition:

[e-Learning] is an approach to teaching and learning, representing all or part of the educational model applied, that is based on the use of electronic media and devices, as tools for improving access to training, communication and interaction and that facilitates the adoption of new ways of understanding and developing learning. (p.152)

Hubbard (2013) suggested that “elearning is when we use computers and the networks to which these are linked to in some way support the learning process” (p.3). The succinctness of this definition is appealing; however, it is important for educators to remember the organizational mesh that lies beneath elearning and its impact on design and outcomes.

mLearning

After reviewing several definitions of mlearning, Crompton et al. (2013) summarized it as “learning across multiple contexts, through social and content interactions, using personal electronic devices” (p.83). Similar to the work of Sangrà et al. (2012) discussed above, Grant (2019) categorized the definitions of mlearning into four groups. The first group related to distance education; the second focused on the type of devices used in mlearning; the third targeted the "interactions among the learner, the technologies, and the environment" (p. 367); and the fourth centered on the nature of learning in mobile environments. Crompton (2013) conceded that mlearning will continuously be redefined to parallel advancements in technology and the affordances they provide to the paradigm shift towards learner-centered pedagogies.

In summary, eleanring and mlearning definitions are shaped by advancements in technology and educational paradigm shifts. As these fields expand, conceptual organization and clarity of focus are needed to maintain design and research rigor. Strangely, this debate about definitions and terms seems to echo the one discussed earlier on ehealth and mhealth, confirming the natural path for novel fields (Oh et al., 2005).

Select eHealth and mHealth Theories and Models

eHealth interventions, same as all health interventions, draw from several disciplines, theories, and models, resulting in fragmented design, development, and evaluation, with frequent integration of multidisciplinary frameworks (Cruz-Martínez, Noort et al., 2019; Heinsch et al., 2021; Timmreck et al., 2010).

Heinsch et al. (2021) identified 36 theories informing ehealth interventions and classified them based on Sovacool and Hess (2017) typology of sociotechnical change. They found 53% agency-centered theories (focused on the individual and stakeholders), 20% relational (analyzing the dynamics and interactions in social structures), 16% structure-centered (focusing on the environment), and 8% meaning-centered (explaining the co-construction of meaning between individuals and structure). They concluded that most studies "emphasiz[ed] individual factors rather than the broader social and environmental factors impacting implementations" (p. 11). Additionally, they questioned whether the theories used "adequately address the multiple and complex factors that influence implementation" (p.11), reminding us of Intervention Mapping proposed by Bartholomew et al. (2011) and presented in Chapter 1, who call for an ecological approach to program planning taking into consideration the individual, interpersonal, organizational, community, and societal factors.

In that respect, the multitude of theories and models drove scholars to recommend a holistic view of the design of ehealth interventions. van Gemert-Pijnen et al. (2011) proposed a framework that looks at all the components and actors in the system (patients, health care professionals, resources, etc.) to improve the uptake and impact of ehealth technologies. Similarly, Cruz-Martínez, Wentzel et al. (2020) called for addressing not only the theoretical grounding but also all the interconnected parts of ehealth interventions.

In addition to concerns over the fragmented design process that impacts the quality of ehealth interventions, the functionality of the technology is central to these interventions (van Gemert-Pijnen et al., 2018). Understanding users' adoption of technology needs to be inherent to design and evaluation that cannot be solely focused on behavioral change (Cruz-Martínez, Noort et al., 2019). Users need to be persuaded to change their behavior by creating a good fit between user, context, and intervention (van Gemert-Pijnen et al., 2018).

In 1986, Davis proposed the technology acceptance model (TAM) that revolved around the theoretical constructs of intentions, attitudes, and social influence, proposed earlier by Fishbein and Ajzen (1975), which they later developed into the theory of reasoned action and theory of planned behavior discussed in Chapter 1. In his model, Davis argued that the actual use of a system is influenced by users' motivation to use the system, which is determined in turn by the system's features and capabilities. He explained that design features produce a cognitive response of perceived usefulness and perceived ease of use that triggers an affective response to form attitudes that ultimately translate into actual use.

TAM became one of the most widely used models, evolving to elaborate forms (TAM1, TAM2, TAM3) that include a wider range of theoretical models and determinants of technology use (Binyamin & Zafar, 2021; Lee et al., 2003). However, the presence of many forms of technology acceptance models alarmed researchers who were "confronted with a choice among a multitude of models and find that they must "pick and choose" constructs across the models, or choose a "favored model" and largely ignore the contributions from alternative models" (Venkatesh et al., 2003, p.426). Therefore, Venkatesh et al. (2003) compared the research on existing models and introduced the unified theory of acceptance and use of technology (UTAUT). They identified the key components of performance expectancy, effort expectancy, social influence, and facilitating conditions that influence behavioral intention and use behavior, which are all affected by age, gender, experience, and voluntariness of use.

Lately, Nadal et al. (2020) drew attention to the missing temporal dimension in technology acceptance models. They argued that change is a process that takes place over time, mirroring the stages of change of the transtheoretical model of behavioral change (Prochaska & Norcross, 2001) discussed in Chapter 1. As a result, they presented the technology acceptance lifecycle (TAL) model, aimed at clarifying the measurements of technology acceptance. They distinguished between acceptability, acceptance, and adoption, dividing the stages of acceptance between pre-use, initial use, and sustained use (Nadal et al. 2020).

Similarly, addressing the multitude of technology acceptance models and the limitations of each, Binyamin and Zafar (2021) proposed a general model that integrates factors proven to be strong determinants of acceptance such as perceived ease of use, perceived usefulness, attitudes toward behavior, subjective norms (perceptions of others' views of self), and facilitating conditions (availability of resources) that lay the ground for behavioral intention (plan to use intervention) and actual use, finding attitude toward behavior to be the strongest determinant of acceptance and facilitating conditions the weakest.

In short, the presentation above indicates that acceptance of technology in health is determined by enabling and inhibiting factors that affect attitudes that will ultimately drive use and behavioral change (Tsai et al., 2018).

Closely related to technology acceptance is the concept of persuasive technology, pioneered by B.J. Fogg (van Gemert-Pijnen et al., 2018). Persuasive technology is rooted in theories of persuasive communication (van Gemert-Pijnen et al., 2018) defined as "any message that is intended to shape, reinforce, or change the responses of another, or others" (Stiff & Mongeau, 2016, p.4). Persuasive communication is an important factor in achieving effective interventions that aim for changes in attitudes and behaviors (McGuire, 1981). Therefore, going beyond accepting the use of technology, Fogg (2009) stressed the need for designers to understand the factors that drive human behavior in order to be able to persuade them to change their behavior through technology. He called his model Fogg's behavior model and based it on three factors:

1. Motivation: one must be motivated to change behavior. Motivation can take the form of pleasure/pain, hope/fear, or social acceptance/rejection.
2. Ability (or Simplicity): one must perceive an ability to change behavior. Ability is determined by time, money, needed physical effort, brain cycles (or cognitive effort), if the target behavior entails social deviance, or is non-routine.
3. Triggers: one must be triggered to change behavior, a spark for low motivation, a facilitator for high motivation but low ability, or a signal for high motivation and high ability.

Building on Fogg's behavior model, Oinas-Kukkonen and Harjumaa (2013), introduced the persuasive systems design model and defined seven postulates that needed to be considered in the design of persuasive systems aimed at behavioral change. The postulates are:

1. Technology is never neutral. It is always influencing and persuading people.
2. People like their views about the world to be organized and consistent. Inconsistencies (cognitive or affective) might trigger behavioral change.
3. Direct and indirect routes are key to persuasion strategies.
4. Persuasion is often incremental.
5. Persuasion through persuasive systems should always be open. The intent and bias of the designer should be transparent not to weaken the effectiveness of the persuasion.
6. Persuasive systems should aim at unobtrusiveness, not to inconvenience users at inappropriate times.
7. Persuasive systems should aim at being both useful and easy to use. (pp. 487-488)

Additionally, Oinas-Kukkonen and Harjumaa (2009) stressed the importance of analyzing the persuasion context to reveal inconsistencies in the thinking of the user and to determine appropriate times for message delivery. Mainly, they pointed to the need for analyzing the intent behind the persuasion (attitude or behavior change), the persuasion event (user's goals, information processing preferences, and technology context), and the persuasion strategy (the message that would trigger the change).

Recently, user-centered persuasive design that is evidence-based and grounded in theory became the focus of ehealth and mhealth interventions (Cruz-Martínez, Noort et al., 2019). Carr Chellman and Savoy (2003) explained that user design "empowers the users to engage authentically in the decision-making process that is design. In this case, the end users are empowered to play a central role in the creation of their own systems" (p. 702). User-centered design plays an important role in quality and usability improvement (Mao et al., 2005). Additionally, adopting a bottom-up approach to the design and development by involving users and addressing their needs helps to embrace diversity and inclusion (van Hierden, 2021). Table 1 summarizes key features of the select theories discussed above.

eHealth interventions can do more harm than good if not well-designed. The validity of these interventions rests on the credibility of the sources that develop them (Lupton, 2014). Moreover, rapid and efficient development, understanding and promoting engagement, advancing models and theories, evaluating effectiveness, evaluating cost-effectiveness, and ensuring regulatory, ethical, and information governance are essential to the development and evaluation of ehealth interventions (Michie et al., 2017) in addition to timely interaction and dynamic feedback (Riely et al., 2011).

The overview presented above on ehealth, mhealth, elearning, and mlearning reveals the similarities of challenges. Borrowing the acronym VUCA (Volatility, Uncertainty, Complexity, and Ambiguity) from the military, Reeves and Reeves (2015) reminded us that novel things are volatile with unpredictable turns, and concepts are complex and accompanied with ambiguity. As these new fields grow, they co-evolve with the needs of society, they self-organize and transform to create new identities for the new emerging systems (Reigeluth, 2019). The aim of this presentation is to draw attention to the conceptual and theoretical landscape of ehealth and mhealth interventions to highlight the multidisciplinary complexities behind their design and the continuous efforts of scholars to improve the models and the research based on them.

Table 1. Select theories that inform ehealth and nhealth interventions

Model	Key Features
Technology Acceptance	
Technology Acceptance Model (TAM) Davis (1986)	Perceived Usefulness & Perceived Ease of Use ↓ Attitude towards Use ↓ Actual Use *All influenced by design features.
Unified Theory of Acceptance and Use of Technology (UTAUT) Venkatesh et al. (2003)	Performance Expectancy, Effort Expectancy, Social Influence, & Facilitating Conditions ↓ Behavioral Intention ↓ Behavioral Use *All influenced by age, gender, experience, and voluntariness of use.
Technology Acceptance Lifecycle Nada et al. (2020)	Pre-Use Acceptability ↓ Initial Use Acceptance ↓ Sustained Use Adoption
General Model for Mobile Apps Acceptance Binyamin and Zafar (2021)	Perceived Ease of Use, Perceived Usefulness, Attitudes toward Behavior, Subjective Norms & Facilitating Conditions ↓ Behavioral Intention ↓ Actual Use
Persuasive Technology	
Persuasive Technology B.J. Fogg (2009)	Motivation Ability Triggers
Persuasive Systems Design Model Oinas-Kukkonen & Harjumaa (2013)	Seven Postulates: 1. Non-neutrality of technology 2. Consistencies/inconsistencies in world views 3. Direct/indirect routes to persuasion strategies 4. Persuasion is incremental 5. Open persuasion 6. Unobtrusiveness 7. Useful and easy to use *Need to analyze the intent behind the persuasion, the persuasion event, and the persuasion strategy.
User-Centered Persuasive Design	User engagement in design Design aligns with users' needs and wants Embraces diversity and inclusion

General eLearning Design Principles

Besides seeking common definitions and terms for technology integration in education and health, and in addition to the importance of theoretical grounding, designing ehealth and mhealth interventions requires a consideration of yet another angle, which is elearning design principles. For clarity purposes, elearning used in this section is meant to denote all types of learning that use communication technologies, including health education and health promotion. So, successful elearning is not limited to the incorporation of technology in the learning materials. A sound learning design is based on a good understanding of how people learn, creating learning instances that maximize learning and behavioral change, by using the affordances provided by technology (Crompton, 2003; Fee, 2009; Lynch et al., 2012). Moreover, it follows a systematic process as described in Chapter 1. However, additional elearning design characteristics worth considering are collaboration, learner control, navigation, interaction, and the use of multimedia among several others.

Collaboration

Examples of tools that can be used for collaboration are chats, message boards, email, in addition to problem-solving, peer tutoring, gaming, and online communities (Clark & Mayer; 2016; Neuhauser & Kreps, 2010). Collaboration creates a sense of community, allows for exchange of experiences and knowledge, and enhances the social learning experience (Clark & Mayer, 2003; Hill et al., 2004).

Learner Control

Giving learners control over the process of learning results in a shift from an external locus of control to an internal locus of control (Hill et al., 2004; Shapiro & Niederhauser, 2004). Internal locus of control prompts engagement and supports behavioral change (Bennett et al. 2017). Learners can be provided control over content sequence and pace, allowing them to move freely back and forth (Clark & Mayer, 2016).

Navigation

Navigation helps orient the learner who can get lost in hyperspace easily (Alessi & Trollip, 2001; Hill et al., 2004). Navigation tools such as menus, links and buttons must serve a clear purpose, be visible, and be located consistently on the screen (Alessi & Trollip, 2001). New developments have opened the way for voice activated navigation assistants, which lend themselves to a new category of design (Chung et al., 2018).

Interaction

Three types of interactions are identified in the literature: learner-content, learner-expert, and learner-learner (Moore, 1989). The learner-content interaction is the learner's interaction with the materials provided in the elearning environment. The learner-expert interaction is the interaction between the learner and the instructor or health professional who provide feedback, support, and motivation. The learner-learner interaction is the collaborative work between learners to exchange information, construct knowledge, or support each other (Hill et al., 2004; Moore, 1989). These three types of interaction are essential to providing knowledge construction, guidance and support, and active engagement (Hill et al., 2004; Neuhauser & Kreps, 2010).

The Use of Media

Technology allows for the inclusion of several media formats that enhance engagement (Clark & Mayer, 2016). Examples of these formats are text, hypertext, sound, graphics, video, and animation (Alessi &

Trollip, 2001). However, elearning design must follow certain rules on how the media is used in order to support the learning process (Clark & Mayer, 2016). For example, text should be well spaced to increase readability, blinking and moving text should be avoided, and the use of graphics and animations must serve an educational purpose. Clark and Mayer (2016) suggest certain principles for successful use of media that emphasize staying away from using graphics as decorative tools and combining them with words only when they enhance the learning experience, placing words next to the graphics that represent them to facilitate connections, avoiding the use of background music and extraneous pictures and words to avoid distraction and cognitive load.

Therefore, the design of elearning must be systematic, grounded in instructional design principles, and focused on the needs of the learner with a focus on collaboration, learner control, navigation, interaction, and provision of help and practice. Moreover, the use of media can enrich the learning experience. However, if not properly incorporated, its use might hinder the learning process instead of enhancing it.

This first section of the chapter highlighted terms, concepts, theories, models, and principles related to the design of ehealth and mhealth interventions. Moreover, it pointed to the fluctuations and trends shaping the field. Additionally, it showed the interconnectedness of several elements, at multiple levels, (Pieterse et al., 2018) that could challenge health professionals involved in the creation of ehealth and mhealth interventions. Therefore, it is important to "understand how the individuals, processes, and infrastructure interact with one another" (Stefaniak, 2019, p. 202) and to look at these interventions as parts of complex and dynamic systems in which human and contextual elements interact, influence, and depend on each other (Akeel & Mundy, 2019; Kip & van Gemert-Pijnen, 2018; Trochim et al., 2006; van Gemert-Pijnen et al., 2018). The next section presents a practical overview on ehealht and mhealth applications.

Overview of eHealth and mHealth Uses in the Health Field

eHealth has a broad range of applications in various health and health related fields, including healthcare services, health surveillance, health literature, health education, and knowledge and research (World Health Organization, [WHO], 2016a). Additionally, ehealth services have been used widely for chronic disease management (such as cardiovascular and mental health, diabetes, and cancer), promotion of healthy behaviors (such as smoking cessation, healthy eating, and physical activity), and provision of remote access to treatments (Ahern et al., 2006; Ghose et al., 2021). A review conducted in 2021 found that the current uses of ehealth included: (1) monitoring, (2) diagnosis, (3) treatment, (4) rehabilitation, (5) training for professionals, and (6) training for non-professionals (Qureshi et al., 2021). The reviewed ehealth applications targeted a wide range of chronic conditions including, heart-related diseases, obesity, Parkinson disease, diabetes, neuro-psychological disorder, headache, Alzheimers disease, Common Mental Disorder, Chronic Obstructive Pulmonary Disease, and Pre-eclampsia Disorder (Qureshi et al., 2021).

On the other hand, ehealth solutions have been used to expand the limited capacities of healthcare workers, to support systems in healthcare facilities, to support public health in communities, and to provide the data needed to inform management and policy (Ahern et al., 2006; WHO, 2016a). Furthermore, ehealth has provided patients with more access to information about their health. This improved access to information have triggered a paradigm shift in the roles of healthcare workers and patients, facilitating a transition toward a "patient-health care interface", a model which has allowed patients to be fully integrated in their care plan (Ahern et al., 2006; van Gemert-Pijnen et al., 2018). As such, ehealth is now being used to promote a shift to a patient-centered approach to healthcare services (van

Gemert-Pijnen et al., 2018; WHO, 2016b). In addition, the current COVID-19 pandemic has highlighted the importance of ehealth solutions in the healthcare sector. eHealth applications were widely launched and used throughout the world during the pandemic to enable patients to interact with practitioners but, at the same time, limit the spread of the virus (Tebeje & Klein, 2020).

Prominent Uses and Applications

Prominent uses and applications of ehealth include clinical decision support, electronic health records, telehealth, elearning, wireless medical technology, and mhealth.

Clinical Decision Support (CDS)

CDS uses computers to provide healthcare workers evidence-based knowledge alongside patient-specific information that are integrated into the decision-making process. For example, CDS uses computer-based alarms to alert healthcare workers to integrate patient information from the electronic health record (Chaffee & Zimmerman, 2010). CDS also allows the automation of evidence-based data, such as medical recommendations and guidelines, diagnostic algorithms, and other relevant information at point of care (van Rooij & Marsh, 2016). By combining clinical knowledge and patient-specific information, CDS allows for interpretation of information and automated recommendations, which assists healthcare workers to make informed decisions .

Electronic Health Records (EHRs)

Although first introduced in 1991, EHR implementation witnessed a surge about a decade ago when high-speed internet became widely accessible. EHR systems, which is a digital version of a patient's medical history, are a key element in the provision of universal health coverage, as it provides people with insight to healthcare costs, and access to promotional, preventive, curative, rehabilitative and palliative health services (WHO, 2016a). An effective EHR system improves the quality, accuracy, reliability, and timeliness of patient information, reduces costs, supports patient mobility, and can help highlight areas of concerns in the health care sector (Casey et al., 2016; WHO, 2016a).

Telehealth

Telehealth includes a wide range of clinical applications, with the most common being interactive videos (del Carmen Ortega-Navas, 2017). According to WHO (2016a), telehealth disciplines have five specific uses:

1. Teleradiology - using Information and Communications Technology (ICT) to transmit digital radiological images for diagnosis or consultation.
2. Teledermatology - using ICT to transmit medical information related skin conditions for the purpose of diagnosis or consultation.
3. Telepathology - using ICT to transmit digitized pathological results, such as microscopic images of cells, for the purpose of diagnosis or consultation.
4. Telepsychiatry - using ICT to provide mental health service.

5. Remote patient monitoring - where patients, from home, transmit information about their condition to external monitoring centers using sensors and monitoring equipment.

eLearning for Healthcare Providers

eLearning was first developed to provide high-quality, relevant, and up-to-date health science education to scale up the health workforce to attain universal health coverage. eLearning aimed to build knowledge, skills, attitudes, behaviors and core values of healthcare providers (WHO, 2016a). Both the United Nations and WHO recognized the importance of elearning in addressing educational needs of healthcare workers (Frenk et al., 2010; Safie & Aljunid, 2013). eLearning constitutes a wide variety of interventions in terms of tools utilized, content and information delivered, learning objectives, educational approaches and setting of delivery (WHO, 2016a). It can be a blended learning approach (a mix of traditional and ICT based learning) or purely eLearning approach (WHO, 2016a).

Wireless Medical Technologies

The advancement in wireless technologies based on Wi-Fi or mobile access enabled healthcare providers to stay connected to the network while making communication devices mobile (such as smartphones and tablets) (Perera, 2012; van Rooij & Marsh, 2016). mHealth, which will be discussed further in the forthcoming section, was built around this idea. Besides the use of smartphones and tablets, other wireless devices such as wearable technologies were also used in the detection of wide range of medical measurements including blood pressure, heart rate, blood oxygen, or steps taken by patients, in addition to medical sensors that are worn directly on the body (van Rooij & Marsh, 2016). Moreover, advancement in technology has enabled the development of specialized devices that resemble mobile equivalents of large pieces of equipment such as ultrasound scanners, devices for deep venous thrombosis prophylaxis, in addition to devices which interface with smartphones that allows monitoring of conditions, such as blood sugar level (Perera, 2012; Tucker et al., 2010). Advancement of medical technologies also made way for the use of Geographic Information Systems (GIS) with mobile applications which allowed practitioners to capture spatial data of patients' physical activity. These data have allowed healthcare providers to measure social, environmental, and psychological patterns of health activities and to help identify correlations with socio-demographic factors (van Rooij & Marsh, 2016).

mHealth Applications

Smartphone uses in health has been a catalyst for the transition of ehealth to mhealth, whereby smartphones are currently being used for various clinical uses. (Hsieh et al., 2004; Perera, 2012). For example, in its simplest form, smartphones are being used in the diagnosis of wounds using picture messages. Push-email and notifications have also been used to enhance communication between healthcare providers and hospitals, in addition to the use of paging systems with phone notifications (Wu et al., 2010). And with the advancement of application design, a number of applications have been developed to support certain healthcare services and systems, including but not limited to, infectious diseases tracking, health promotion, orthopedic decision support applications, and offsite radiology access (Dala-Ali et al., 2011; Franko, 2011; Oehler et al., 2010). Recent data shows that the number of these tools are increasing, specifically the number of health applications available in the app store currently exceed 318,500 applications and more than 200 new apps added on a daily basis (IQVIA, 2017).

A review conducted in 2013 found that mhealth applications addressed a wide range of conditions including, from most prominent to least, diabetes, obesity/overweight, mental health, tobacco use, HIV, wellbeing, cancer, medication compliance/appointment reminder, sexual health, cardiovascular conditions and tuberculosis (Fiordelli et al., 2013). The strategies employed in these mhealth applications varied from text messaging, add-ons, voice, video and multimedia messaging services, while others applied some features developed ad hoc for a specific condition (Fiordelli et al., 2013). According to this review, the interventions were directed mostly toward health promotion activities and self-management of diseases, and also on communication, remote monitoring, data gathering, improvement of adherence, and training/education (Fiordelli et al., 2013).

According to WHO, there are three overarching categories for mhealth use (WHO, 2016a):

1. Accessing/providing health services: through services such as health call centers, toll-free emergency calls, treatment adherence, appointment reminders, mobile telehealth, and emergencies.
2. Accessing/providing health information: through services such as community mobilization, access to info, resources, databases and tools, decision support systems, electronic patient information/records, and mlearning.
3. Collecting health information: through services such as health surveys, surveillance, and patient monitoring.

Ultimately, the literature discussed above showed that ehealth has become a salient field of practice in the health and health-related field. eHealth services have played an important role in the transition towards a patient-centered healthcare model. The most prominent uses and applications of ehealth listed above, including clinical decision support, electronic health records, telehealth, elearning, and mhealth, have all been used to strengthen the capacities of healthcare workers, support healthcare systems, and widen their reach, advance public health by fully integrating and engaging patients in their care plan, and inform health-related policies and practices.

Benefits of eHealth

According to Ahern et al. (2006), ehealth services offer many benefits: (1) expanding the reach of health services, reaching underserved and marginalized populations, at relatively low cost; (2) scalability; (3) time efficiency; and (4) allowing the personalization and customization of health services for patients to ensure effectiveness of intervention. In addition, the personalization of health services allows tailoring according to participants' attributes such as race/ethnicity, age and gender, which advances the effective uptake of these applications and shows a promise in addressing health disparities (Ahern et al., 2006). As discussed above, one of the most prominent applications of ehealth services is the automation of system data flow (Meier et al., 2013). And although the process of system implementation is challenging, it has proven to achieve measurable results in recent applications (Meier et al., 2013). For example, the Southeast Alabama Medical Center established an Electronic Health Records and Computerized Physician Order Entry in order to standardize and transform all paper-based forms to electronic formats and introduce evidence-based medicine (Hanover & Perry, 2011). In 2011, the medical center reported a 5.05 million USD cumulative benefit over 3 years, 1.3 million USD in annual physician productivity, and 4,572 USD in annual operating profit (Hanover & Perry, 2011). Other benefits achieved were reduction in medical errors, improving the quality of care, while reducing its cost by using evidence-based medicine and enhancing overall patient and staff satisfaction (Meier et al., 2013; Qureshi et al., 2021).

Furthermore, the application of ehealth offers benefits pertaining to public health surveillance (Black et al., 2011; Castillo-Salgado, 2010). With the emergence of pandemics, threats of bioterrorism and newly emerging and reemerging infectious diseases, global health surveillance has been recognized for its importance (Castillo-Salgado, 2010). Thus, there has been an increased interest in the application of ehealth in global surveillance systems to improve its quality, capacity, and effectiveness (Ginsberg et al., 2009). For instance, a new approach was proposed to detect influenza outbreak using data from search engines (Ginsberg et al., 2009). This approach was applied in the United States; researchers analyzed historical data logs of at least 50 million of the most common online web search queries and reported a high correlation between Google queries (influenza-like illness related search queries) and the percentage of doctor visits by patients with influenza-like symptoms (Ginsberg et al., 2009).

Over the past decade, the application of ehealth has played an important role in increasing accessibility to diagnostic services, enhancing the quality of healthcare services, improving coordination between health providers, enhancing patient management and increasing their engagement in their own health and wellbeing, in addition to overcoming physical distances between healthcare providers and patients (van Gemert-Pijnen et al., 2018; WHO, 2016b). ehealth allows patient to have a wider access to medical information using EHRs, which enables them to conduct risk assessments of their own health and enhances interaction with physicians via email (Meier et al., 2013). eHealth also enables online communication between practitioners from different regions and countries which allows them to have an open discussion about medical issues and diagnosis of complicated diseases (Meier et al., 2013).

In addition, ehealth presents a new paradigm that facilitate data collection and mining and accessibility to data by multiple stakeholders (Meier et al., 2013). It promotes evidence-based decision making and builds long-lasting relationships between the patient and healthcare provider, and enhances patient participation (Meier et al., 2013; Qureshi et al., 2021). eHealth also supports the partnering and cooperation of medical practitioners, insurers and patients, and ensures transparency of the process (Rodrigues, 2008). Moreover, ehealth services that address health promotion have also several benefits. The OECD health policy studies reported the following benefits; improved health quality, reduced health costs, and reduced time between diagnosis and treatment to (OECD, 2010). In addition, patients' hospital stays and waiting list are reduced and healthcare providers productivity are enhanced. Health promotion technologies also provides patients with a better understanding of their diseases, more efficient use of health services, enhanced adherence to treatment, and improved participation in health decisions (Vance et al., 2009).

Similarly, several benefits to the use of mhealth, telehealth and elearning have been identified in the literature. According to WHO, mhealth can help achieve universal health coverage by increasing availability and accessibility of health services to reach underserved communities and remote populations, in addition to areas where limited infrastructure is available to support technologies or traditional health services (but areas where infrastructure to manage mobile communication is prioritized (WHO, 2016a). Telehealth also offers various benefits including improved access to healthcare by increasing the speed of access and reducing the associated cost. Other benefits include increasing the uniformity of practice, thus contributing to higher quality of care. Telehealth may also provide enhanced support for rural healthcare providers. Avoiding travel of the patient or healthcare provider to access specialized services also increases the speed of access to services, particularly in rural areas (Matsumoto et al., 2015). It also supports equitable access to healthcare, as patients, wherever they are located, have the same accessibility as other (WHO, 2016a). This is particularly important in low-resource setting. On the other hand, elearning provides access to learning for people who are geographically isolated or those who live in areas with limited training facilities (WHO, 2016a). eLearning can improve the quality of education, convey information to a broader audience and promote collaborations (Ruggeri et al., 2013). It also provides an opportunity for healthcare workers to expand their knowledge and skills in an efficient, flexible and personalized way, without the need for travel or commuting (Safie & Aljunid, 2013). eLearning can also help health systems in accomplishing reforms by increasing training and effective dissemination of information, which are needed to redesign the responsibilities and roles of healthcare professionals. By providing efficient and effective access to training and education, it can improve essential and people-centered health services and support in achieving universal health coverage (WHO, 2016a).

Based on the above, ehealth offers various benefits that improve all aspects of patient care including quality, effectiveness, efficiency, communication, education, equity, affordability and accessibility, and ultimately plays an important role in achieving universal health coverage.

Challenges in eHealth

As e-health creates new opportunities and offers a multitude of benefits for traditional healthcare services, it also produces new challenges and is faced with various barriers to implementation. At a first glance, the adoption of ehealth services by both healthcare providers and patients is dependent on two main factors (1) the cost and availability of information technology and (2) the individual's technology literacy level (Rudolph M et al., 2008). According to a set of interviews conducted with key stakeholders in the e-health services sector, the following challenges associated with the utilization of e-health services were identified (Ahern et al., 2006; Qureshi et al., 2021):

- *Lack of standardization and comparability within the field of ehealth*: Researchers and purchasers need a set of criteria that allows for the identification of quality information, sharing and comparing findings, and building upon current evidence in order to move ehealth forward.
- *Questionable quality of information*: Concerns over the quality of information that are obtained from patients online
- *Patient's data inter-operability among different settings such hospitals, private clinics, medical laboratories*: Due to lack of interoperability, the data collected from patients remain fragmented and thus data analysis cannot be conducted. In addition, the exchange of data between different systems also presents a challenge.
- *Detection of disease at early stage*: For certain diseases such as cancer, early detection is key to a good prognosis. However, currently there is no infrastructure available for the detection of a disease at its early stage in ehealth solutions.
- *Complexity of healthcare infrastructure*: Infrastructure to support ehealth services is currently insufficient and poorly distributed. Availability of basic infrastructure, mainly Internet access and electricity, are indispensable for successful adoption of ehealth services (Qureshi et al., 2013). Although one of the objectives of ehealth is to provide equal access to healthcare services among all population, this proved to be difficult in situations where Internet access is not available, poor internet connections, and inability to afford to buy a suitable device (Jokinen et al., 2021). For instance, in rural areas and some developing countries, there is insufficient electricity, and unavailability or poor-quality internet access which hinders patients' ability to use ehealth services.

- *Barriers to healthcare provider adoption:* For health care providers, several barriers exist that hinder the adoption of ehealth solution, including: the costs associated with purchasing and installing required systems, the disruption incurred to office workflow, and the absence of reimbursement for networking and engaging with patients electronically via messages and emails or online consultations.
- *Limited Regulations:* The limited number of quality control entities regulating ehealth
- *Lack of policies*: eHealth friendly policies are not developed in most part of the world.

In addition, several methodological concerns in ehealth service evaluation were identified (Ahern et al., 2006; Qureshi et al., 2021; WHO, 2016a):

- Although randomized controlled trials were considered to be the "gold standard" for clinical evaluation, their application in evaluating e-health services has been questioned, as it may produce results that are not accurate nor credible, which could affect the outcomes of the perceived effectiveness, and, ultimately, the uptake of these technologies.
- Limited evaluation methods are available to measure usage, including traffic and utilization. Current data collection methods do not distinguish among usage behaviors. For example, a usage tracker may be able to track the period of time a webpage is being viewed, but not how long the user is interacting with the page.
- Evaluating changes in behavioral outcomes addressed by e-Health services is another major challenge. Instruments that are widely used to measure behavior change have not been validated for the evaluation of online interventions.
- Although one of the key benefits that ehealth offers is that it enables the personalization of material to individuals, however this poses challenges during evaluation. Achieving comparable samples when evaluating an intervention becomes a challenge, as the participants are receiving tailored intervention and not the same messaging programs, which makes comparison difficult.
- Users' access and technological literacy limits the recruitment of a representative population of interest without selection bias.
- Controlling for unknown confounders is difficult when measuring the effectiveness of discrete ehealth interventions. Many study designs, such as quasi-experimental designs, case-control studies, and field trials may provide inaccurate and unreliable results.
- Health care and technology are constantly and rapidly changing, which may change a patient's experience during the course of an evaluation trial.
- With the fast proliferation of ehealth programs, it has become more challenging to recruit an unexposed control population.

Ethical consideration is another main concern that accompanies ehealth applications, as presented by the increased flow of information and the issue of privacy (Qureshi et al., 2021; WHO, 2016a) – this is one of the main concerns expressed by consumers of ehealth. The two issues related to privacy concerns are (1) concerns about inappropriate patient data exchange between organizations (such as unauthorized access/dissemination of information); and (2) concerns about the systemic flow of patient data throughout the health care system and related industries (information flow between providers, payers, secondary users, etc.) – which refers to invading patient's privacy by disclosing information that identifies the patient to parties that may act against the patient's interest (National Research Council, 1997; Liu and Wassyng,

2012). In some jurisdictions, the information available in medical patient records are a property of the patients. In other cases, such as those in the United States, healthcare providers are in control of the information and access to patient is provided by the health workers. This presents challenges with the globalization of ehealth (Kluge, 2011; Qureshi et al., 2021). In addition, when working with patients as co-deliverers of health services, ehealth also presents the challenge of liability (WHO, 2016a). In most developed countries, healthcare decision-making data and data gathering and manipulation are developed and controlled by healthcare providers and thus any mistake is a reflection of the quality of professional care and competence of the providers. However, with ehealth and particularly when automation processes are not adopted, patients may play an important role in data generation processes, which allows for patient error in measuring or reporting of data (Kluge, 2011). Liability apportionment also take on a new dimension that is more complicated when significant others are involved and the issue of their co-responsibility arises.

Similar to ehealth services, other segments of ehealth such as mhealth, telehealth and elearning have their own set of barriers. According to the WHO 2015 global survey on ehealth, there are barriers to the implementation of mhealth services including, by order of importance, lack of funding and lack of legal regulation covering mhealth programmes. Similarly, common barriers to the adoption of telehealth included lack of funding to develop and support telehealth programmes, a lack of infrastructure, competing health system priorities, and a lack of regulations and legislation relevant to telehealth programmes. As for the implementation of elearning, it requires significant human and financial resources (WHO, 2016a). In addition, the cost-effectiveness of elearning is yet to be proven (Frehywot et al., 2013; Hersh et al., 2010). Similar to other ehealth services, lack of a robust and comprehensive evaluation standards is another main challenge (Bernard et al., 2004). Other barriers for the implementation of elearning services include lack of capacity, lack of availability of suitable eLearning courses, and lack of funding (WHO, 2016a).

In summary, although ehealth solutions have provided good opportunities for the advancement of healthcare services in various applications, one cannot deny the ample challenges and barriers that often hinder their uptake and implementation. With the globalization of ehealth services, ethical considerations are one of the main challenges, in addition to the lack of policies and regulations governing the field. Another main challenge discussed in the literature is the methodological concerns in evaluating ehealth services, which have considerably affected the uptake of these technologies. Rigorous evaluation of ehealth services is thus essential to effective and successful implementation.

REFERENCES

Ahern, D. K., Kreslake, J. M., Phalen, J. M., & Bock, B. (2006). What is ehealth (6): Perspectives on the evolution of ehealth research. *Journal of Medical Internet Research*, *8*(1), e4. doi:10.2196/jmir.8.1.e4 PMID:16585029

Akeel, A. U., & Mundy, D. (2019). Re-thinking technology and its growing role in enabling patient empowerment. *Health Informatics Journal*, *25*(4), 1278–1289. doi:10.1177/1460458217751013 PMID:29366367

Alessi, S. M., & Trollip, S. R. (2001). *Multimedia for learning: methods and development* (3rd ed.). Allyn and Bacon.

Bashshur, R., Shannon, G., Krupinski, E., & Grigsby, J. (2011). The taxonomy of telemedicine. *Telemedicine Journal and e-Health, 17*(6), 484–494. doi:10.1089/tmj.2011.0103 PMID:21718114

Bernard, R. M., Abrami, P. C., Lou, Y., Borokhovski, E., Wade, A., Wozney, L., Wallet, P. A., Fiset, M., & Huang, B. (2004). How does distance education compare with classroom instruction? A meta-analysis of the empirical literature. *Review of Educational Research, 74*(3), 379–439. doi:10.3102/00346543074003379

Binyamin, S. S., & Zafar, B. A. (2021). Proposing a mobile apps acceptance model for users in the health area: A systematic literature review and meta-analysis. *Health Informatics Journal, 27*(1). Advance online publication. doi:10.1177/1460458220976737 PMID:33438494

Black, A. D., Car, J., Pagliari, C., Anandan, C., Cresswell, K., Bokun, T., McKinstry, B., Procter, R., Majeed, A., & Sheikh, A. (2011). The impact of ehealth on the quality and safety of health care: A systematic overview. *PLoS Medicine, 8*(1), e1000387. doi:10.1371/journal.pmed.1000387 PMID:21267058

Bull, S. (2011). *Technology-based health promotion*. SAGE Publications, Inc.

Cameron, J. D., Ramaprasad, A., & Syn, T. (2017). An ontology of and roadmap for mHealth research. *International Journal of Medical Informatics, 100*, 16–25. doi:10.1016/j.ijmedinf.2017.01.007

Casey, J. A., Schwartz, B. S., Stewart, W. F., & Adler, N. E. (2016). Using electronic health records for population health research: A review of methods and applications. *Annual Review of Public Health, 37*(1), 61–81. doi:10.1146/annurev-publhealth-032315-021353 PMID:26667605

Castillo-Salgado, C. (2010). Trends and directions of global public health surveillance. *Epidemiologic Reviews, 32*(1), 93–109. doi:10.1093/epirev/mxq008 PMID:20534776

Chaffee, B. W., & Zimmerman, C. R. (2010). Developing and implementing clinical decision support for use in a computerized prescriber-order-entry system. *American Journal of Health-System Pharmacy, 67*(5), 391–400. doi:10.2146/ajhp090153 PMID:20172991

Clark, R. C., & Mayer, R. E. (2016). *e-Learning and the science of instruction: Proven guidelines for consumers and designers of multimedia learning*. John Wiley & Sons, Incorporated.

Cruz-Martínez, R. R., Noort, P. D., Asbjornsen, R. A., Van Niekerk, J. M., Wentzel, J., Sanderman, R., & Van Gemert-Pijnen, L. (2019). Frameworks, models, and theories used in electronic health research and development to support self-management of cardiovascular diseases through remote monitoring technologies: Protocol for a metaethnography review. *JMIR Research Protocols, 8*(7), e13334. Advance online publication. doi:10.2196/13334 PMID:31313659

Cruz-Martínez, R. R., Wentzel, J., Asbjørnsen, R. A., Noort, P. D., van Niekerk, J. M., Sanderman, R., & van Gemert-Pijnen, J. E. (2020). Supporting self-management of cardiovascular diseases through remote monitoring technologies: Metaethnography review of frameworks, models, and theories used in research and development. *Journal of Medical Internet Research, 22*(5), e16157. doi:10.2196/16157 PMID:32436852

Dala-Ali, B. M., Lloyd, M. A., & Al-Abed, Y. (2011). The uses of the iPhone for surgeons. *The Surgeon, 9*(1), 44–48. doi:10.1016/j.surge.2010.07.014 PMID:21195331 del Carmen Ortega-Navas, M. (2017). The use of new technologies as a tool for the promotion of health education. *Procedia: Social and Behavioral Sciences, 237*, 23–29. doi:10.1016/j.sbspro.2017.02.006

Dicianno, B. E., Parmanto, B., Fairman, A. D., Crytzer, T. M., Yu, D. X., Pramana, G., Coughenour, D., & Petrazzi, A. A. (2015). Perspectives on the evolution of mobile (mHealth) technologies and application to rehabilitation. *Physical Therapy, 95*(3), 397–405. doi:10.2522/ptj.20130534 PMID:24925075

Duffy, F. M. (2009). Paradigms, mental models, and mindsets: Triple barriers to transformational change in school systems. *Journal of Educational Leadership Preparation, 4*(3), 357–376.

Eysenbach, G. (2001). What is e-health? *Journal of Medical Internet Research, 3*(2), e20. doi:10.2196/jmir.3.2.e20 PMID:11720962

Fiordelli, M., Diviani, N., & Schulz, P. J. (2013). Mapping mHealth research: A decade of evolution. *Journal of Medical Internet Research, 15*(5), e95–e95. doi:10.2196/jmir.2430 PMID:23697600

Fogg, B. (2009). A behavior model for persuasive design. *Proceedings of the 4th International Conference on Persuasive Technology (Persuasive '09).* 10.1145/1541948.1541999

Franko, O. I. (2011). Smartphone apps for orthopaedic surgeons. *Clinical Orthopaedics and Related Research, 469*(7), 2042–2048. doi:10.100711999-011-1904-0 PMID:21547414

Frehywot, S., Vovides, Y., Talib, Z., Mikhail, N., Ross, H., Wohltjen, H., Bedada, S., Korhumel, K., Koumare, A. K., & Scott, J. (2013). E-learning in medical education in resource constrained low-and middle-income countries. *Human Resources for Health, 11*(1), 1–15. doi:10.1186/1478-4491-11-4 PMID:23379467

Frenk, J., Chen, L., Bhutta, Z. A., Cohen, J., Crisp, N., Evans, T., Fineberg, H., Garcia, P., Ke, Y., Kelley, P., Kistnasamy, B., Meleis, A., Naylor, D., Pablos-Mendez, A., Reddy, S., Scrimshaw, S., Sepulveda, J., Serwadda, D., & Zurayk, H. (2010). Health professionals for a new century: Transforming education to strengthen health systems in an interdependent world. *Lancet, 376*(9756), 1923–1958. doi:10.1016/S0140-6736(10)61854-5 PMID:21112623

GhoseA.GuoX.LiB.DangY. (2021). *Empowering patients using smart mobile health platforms: Evidence from a randomized field experiment. Forthcoming at MIS Quarterly, NYU Stern School of Business Forthcoming.* https://ssrn.com/abstract=377318

Ginsberg, J., Mohebbi, M. H., Patel, R. S., Brammer, L., Smolinski, M. S., & Brilliant, L. (2009). Detecting influenza epidemics using search engine query data. *Nature, 457*(7232), 1012–1014. doi:10.1038/nature07634 PMID:19020500

Grant, M. M. (2019). Difficulties in defining mobile learning: Analysis, design characteristics, and implications. *Educational Technology Research and Development, 67*(2), 361–388. doi:10.100711423-018-09641-4

Hanover, J., & Perry, R. (2011). The business value of automating evidence-based medicine: Southeast Alabama Medical Center. *IDC Health Insights,* 1–9.

Heinsch, M., Wyllie, J., Carlson, J., Wells, H., Tickner, C., & Kay-Lambkin, F. (2021). Theories informing ehealth implementation: Systematic review and typology classification. *Journal of Medical Internet Research, 23*(5), e18500. Advance online publication. doi:10.2196/18500 PMID:34057427

Hersh, W., Margolis, A., Quirós, F., & Otero, P. (2010). Building a health informatics workforce in developing countries. *Health Affairs, 29*(2), 274–277. doi:10.1377/hlthaff.2009.0883 PMID:20348073

Hill, J. R., Wiley, D., Nelson, L. M., & Han, S. (2004). Exploring research on Internet-based learning: From infrastructure to interactions. In D. H. Jonassen (Ed.), *Handbook of research on educational communications and technology* (2nd ed., pp. 433–460). Lawrence Erlbaum Associates.

Hsieh, C.-H., Tsai, H.-H., Yin, J.-W., Chen, C.-Y., Yang, J. C.-S., & Jeng, S.-F. (2004). Teleconsultation with the mobile camera-phone in digital soft-tissue injury: A feasibility study. *Plastic and Reconstructive Surgery, 114*(7), 1776–1782. doi:10.1097/01.PRS.0000142402.07896.21 PMID:15577348

IQVIA. (2017). *Grows as Innovation, Evidence and Adoption of Mobile Health Apps Accelerate*. https://www.iqvia.com/newsroom/2017/11/impact-of-digital-health-grows-as-innovation-evidence-and-adoption-of-mobile-health-apps-accelerate

Jokinen, A., Stolt, M., & Suhonen, R. (2021). Ethical issues related to eHealth: An integrative review. *Nursing Ethics, 28*(2), 253–271. doi:10.1177/0969733020945765 PMID:32930041

Kip, H., & van Gemert-Pijnen, L. J. (2018). Holistic development of eheatlh technology. In eHealth research, theory and development (pp. 131-166). Routledge.

Kluge, E.-H. W. (2011). e-Health promises and challenges: Some ethical considerations. *Studies in Health Technology and Informatics, 164*, 148–153. PMID:21335703

Kumar Basak, S., Wotto, M., & Bélanger, P. (2018). e-Learning, m-learning and d-learning: Conceptual definition and comparative analysis. *E-Learning and Digital Media, 15*(4), 191–216. doi:10.1177/2042753018785180

Lee, Y., Kozar, K. A., & Larsen, K. R. T. (2003). The technology acceptance model: Past, present, and future. *Communications of the Association for Information Systems, 12*, 50. Advance online publication. doi:10.17705/1CAIS.01250

Liu, Z., & Wassyng, A. (Eds.). (2012). *Foundations of Health Informatics Engineering and Systems: First International Symposium, FHIES 2011, Johannesburg, South Africa, August 29-30, 2011. Revised Selected Papers* (*Vol. 7151*). Springer. 10.1007/978-3-642-32355-3

Lupton, D. (2014). Apps as artefacts: Towards a critical perspective on mobile health and medical apps. *Societies (Basel, Switzerland), 4*(4), 606–622. doi:10.3390oc4040606

Mao, J.-Y., Vredenburg, K., Smith, P. W., & Carey, T. (2005). The state of user-centered design practice. *Communications of the ACM, 48*(3), 105–109. doi:10.1145/1047671.1047677

Matsumoto, M., Koike, S., Kashima, S., & Awai, K. (2015). Geographic distribution of radiologists and utilization of teleradiology in Japan: A longitudinal analysis based on National Census Data. *PLoS One, 10*(9), e0139723. doi:10.1371/journal.pone.0139723 PMID:26421721

McGuire, W. J. (1981). Behavioral medicine, public health and communication theories. *Health Education, 12*(3), 8–13. doi:10.1080/00970050.1981.10618148 PMID:6792134

Meier, C. A., Fitzgerald, M. C., & Smith, J. M. (2013). eHealth: Extending, enhancing, and evolving health care. *Annual Review of Biomedical Engineering, 15*(1), 359–382. doi:10.1146/annurev-bioeng-071812-152350 PMID:23683088

Michie, S., Yardley, L., West, R., Patrick, K., & Greaves, F. (2017). Developing and evaluating digital interventions to promote behavior change in health and health care: Recommendations resulting from an international workshop. *Journal of Medical Internet Research, 19*(6), e232. doi:10.2196/jmir.7126 PMID:28663162

Moss, R. J., Süle, A., & Kohl, S. (2019). eHealth and mHealth. *European Journal of Hospital Pharmacy. Science and Practice, 26*(1), 57–58. doi:10.1136/ejhpharm-2018-001819 PMID:31157099

Nacinovich, M. (2011). Defining mhealth. *Journal of Communication in Healthcare, 4*(1), 1–3. doi:10.1179/175380611X12950033990296

Nadal, C., Sas, C., & Doherty, G. (2020). Technology acceptance in mobile health: Scoping review of definitions, models, and measurement. *Journal of Medical Internet Research, 22*(7), e17256. doi:10.2196/17256 PMID:32628122

National Research Council. (1997). Privacy and Security Concerns Regarding Electronic Health Information. In *For the Record Protecting Electronic Health Information*. National Academies Press.

Noesgaard, S.S., & Ørngreen, R. (2015). The effectiveness of e-learning: An explorative and integrative review of the definitions, methodologies and factors that promote e-Learning effectiveness. *Electronic Journal of e-Learning, 13*(4), 278-290.

OECD. (2010). *Improving health sector efficiency, the role of information and communication technologies*. OECD.

Oehler, R. L., Smith, K., & Toney, J. F. (2010). Infectious diseases resources for the iPhone. *Clinical Infectious Diseases, 50*(9), 1268–1274. doi:10.1086/651602 PMID:20233061

Oh, H., Rizo, C., Enkin, M., Jadad, A., Powell, J., & Pagliari, C. (2005). What is ehealth (3): A Systematic review of published definitions. *Journal of Medical Internet Research, 7*(1), e1. doi:10.2196/jmir.7.1.e1 PMID:15829471

Oinas-Kukkonen, H., & Harjumaa, M. (2009). Persuasive systems design: Key issues, process model, and system features. *Communications of the Association for Information Systems, 24*. Advance online publication. doi:10.17705/1CAIS.02428

Otto, L., Harst, L., Timpel, P., Wollschlaeger, B., Richter, P., & Schlieter, H. (2020). Defining and delimitating telemedicine and related terms - An ontology-based classification. *Studies in Health Technology and Informatics, 268*, 113–122. https://doi-org.pallas2.tcl.sc.edu/10.3233/SHTI200010 PMID:32141883

Pagliari, C., Sloan, D., Gregor, P., Sullivan, F., Detmer, D., Kahan, J. P., Oortwijn, W., & MacGillivray, S. (2005). What Is eHealth (4): A scoping exercise to map the field. *Journal of Medical Internet Research, 7*(1), e9. doi:10.2196/jmir.7.1.e9 PMID:15829481

Perera, C. (2012). The evolution of e-health–mobile technology and m-health. *Journal of Mobile Technology in Medicine, 1*(1), 1–2. doi:10.7309/jmtm.1

Pieterse, M., Kip, H., & Cruz-Martínez, R. R. (2018). The complexity of ehealth implemetation: A theoretical and pracitcal perspective. In eHealth research, theory and development (pp. 247-270). Routledge.

Prochaska, J. O., & Norcross, J. C. (2001). Stages of change. *Psychotherapy (Chicago, Ill.), 38*(4), 443–448. doi:10.1037/0033-3204.38.4.443

Qureshi, M., Farooq, A., & Qureshi, M. (2021). *Current ehealth challenges and recent trends in ehealth applications*. https://arxiv.org/ftp/arxiv/papers/2103/2103.01756.pdf

Qureshi, Q. A., Shah, B., Kundi, G. M., Nawaz, A., Miankhel, A. K., Chishti, K. A., & Qureshi, N. A. (2013). Infrastructural barriers to e-health implementation in developing countries. *European Journal of Sustainable Development, 2*(1), 163–163.

Riley, W. T., Rivera, D. E., Atienza, A. A., Nilsen, W., Allison, S. M., & Mermelstein, R. (2011). Health behavior models in the age of mobile interventions: Are our theories up to the task? *Translational Behavioral Medicine, 1*(1), 53–71. doi:10.100713142-011-0021-7 PMID:21796270

Rodrigues, R. J. (2008). *Compelling issues for adoption of e-health. In The Commonwealth Health Ministers Reference Book.* Henley Media Group Ltd.

Rudolph, M., Barr, M. S., Kuhn, T., Hersh, W. R., & McDonald, C. J. (2008). *e-Health and its impact on medical practice*. https://www.acponline.org/advocacy/where_we_stand/policy/ehealth.pdf

Ruggeri, K., Farrington, C., & Brayne, C. (2013). A global model for effective use and evaluation of e-learning in health. *Telemedicine Journal and e-Health, 19*(4), 312–321. doi:10.1089/tmj.2012.0175 PMID:23472702

Safie, N., & Aljunid, S. (2013). E-learning initiative capacity building for healthcare workforce of developing countries. *Journal of Computational Science, 9*(5), 583–591. doi:10.3844/jcssp.2013.583.591

Sangrà, A., Vlachopoulos, D., & Cabrera, N. (2012). Building an inclusive definition of e-learning: An approach to the conceptual framework. *The International Review of Research in Open and Distributed Learning, 13*(2), 145. doi:10.19173/irrodl.v13i2.1161

Scott, R., & Mars, M. (2019). Here we go again—'Digital health'. *Journal of the International Society for Telemedicine and EHealth, 7*, e1. doi:10.29086/JISfTeH.7.e1

Shaw, T., McGregor, D., Brunner, M., Keep, M., Janssen, A., & Barnet, S. (2017). What is ehealth (6)? Development of a conceptual model for ehealth: Qualitative study with key informants. *Journal of Medical Internet Research, 19*(10), e324. doi:10.2196/jmir.8106 PMID:29066429

Showell, C., & Nøhr, C. (2012). How should we define ehealth, and does the definition matter? *Studies in Health Technology and Informatics, 180*, 881–884. PMID:22874319

Singh, V., & Thurman, A. (2019). How many ways can we define online learning? A systematic literature review of definitions of online learning (1988-2018). *American Journal of Distance Education, 33*(4), 289–306. doi:10.1080/08923647.2019.1663082

Sovacool, B. K., & Hess, D. J. (2017). Ordering theories: Typologies and conceptual frameworks for sociotechnical change. *Social Studies of Science*, *47*(5), 703–750. doi:10.1177/0306312717709363 PMID:28641502

Stefaniak, J. (2020). The utility of design thinking to promote systemic instructional design practices in the workplace. *TechTrends*, *64*(2), 202–210. doi:10.100711528-019-00453-8

Steinhubl, S. R., Muse, E. D., & Topol, E. J. (2015). The emerging field of mobile health. *Science Translational Medicine*, *7*(283), 283rv3. Advance online publication. doi:10.1126citranslmed.aaa3487 PMID:25877894

Stiff, J. B., & Mongeau, P. A. (2016). *Persuasive communication* (3rd ed.). Guilford Publications

Tebeje, T. H., & Klein, J. (2020). 2021/02/01). Applications of e-health to support person-centered health care at the time of COVID-19 pandemic. *Telemedicine Journal and e-Health*, *27*(2), 150–158. doi:10.1089/tmj.2020.0201 PMID:32746750

Trochim, W. M., Cabrera, D. A., Milstein, B., Gallagher, R. S., & Leischow, S. J. (2006). Practical challenges of systems thinking and modeling in public health. *American Journal of Public Health*, *96*(3), 538–546. doi:10.2105/AJPH.2005.066001 PMID:16449581

Tsai, J.-M., Cheng, M.-J., Tsai, H.-H., Hung, S.-W., & Chen, Y.-L. (2019). Acceptance and resistance of telehealth: The perspective of dual-factor concepts in technology adoption. *International Journal of Information Management*, *49*, 34–44. doi:10.1016/j.ijinfomgt.2019.03.003

Tucker, A., Maass, A., Bain, D., Chen, L., Azzam, M., Dawson, H., & Johnston, A. (2010). Augmentation of venous, arterial and microvascular blood supply in the leg by isometric neuromuscular stimulation via the peroneal nerve. *The International Journal of Angiology*, *19*(01), e31–e37. doi:10.1055-0031-1278361 PMID:22477572

van Gemert-Pijnen, J. E., Nijland, N., van Limburg, M., Ossebaard, H. C., Kelders, S. M., Eysenbach, G., & Seydel, E. R. (2011). A holistic framework to improve the uptake and impact of ehealth technologies. *Journal of Medical Internet Research*, *13*(4), e111. doi:10.2196/jmir.1672 PMID:22155738

van Gemert-Pijnen, L. J., Kip, H., Kelders, S. M., & Sanderman, R. (2018). Introducing ehealth. In eHealth research, theory and development (pp. 3-26). Routledge. doi:10.4324/9781315385907-1

van Rooij, T., & Marsh, S. (2016). eHealth: Past and future perspectives. *Personalized Medicine*, *13*(1), 57–70. doi:10.2217/pme.15.40 PMID:29749870

Vance, K., Howe, W., & Dellavalle, R. P. (2009). Social internet sites as a source of public health information. *Dermatologic Clinics*, *27*(2), 133–136. doi:10.1016/j.det.2008.11.010 PMID:19254656

Venkatesh, M., Morris, Davis, & Davis. (2003). User acceptance of information technology: Toward a unified view. *Management Information Systems Quarterly*, *27*(3), 425. doi:10.2307/30036540

World Health Organization. (2016a). *Global difusion of ehealth: Making universal health coverage achievable. Report of the third global survey on eHealth*. World Health Organization.

World Health Organization. (2016b). *From innovation to implementation: eHealth in the WHO European region*. World Health Organization.

Wu, R. C., Morra, D., Quan, S., Lai, S., Zanjani, S., Abrams, H., & Rossos, P. G. (2010). The use of smartphones for clinical communication on internal medicine wards. *Journal of Hospital Medicine*, *5*(9), 553–559. doi:10.1002/jhm.775 PMID:20690190

ADDITIONAL READING

Ahern, D. K. (2007). Challenges and opportunities of ehealth research. *American Journal of Preventive Medicine*, *32*(5), S75–S82. doi:10.1016/j.amepre.2007.01.016 PMID:17466822

Andrews, R. (2011). Does e-learning require a new theory of learning? Some initial thoughts. *Journal for Educational Research Online*, *3*(1), 104–121.

Doarn, C. R., Pruitt, S., Jacobs, J., Harris, Y., Bott, D. M., Riley, W., Lamer, C., & Oliver, A. L. (2014). Federal efforts to define and advance telehealth—A work in progress. *Telemedicine Journal and e-Health*, *20*(5), 409–418. doi:10.1089/tmj.2013.0336 PMID:24502793

Erlingsdottir, G., & Sandberg, H. (Eds.). (2016). eHealth opportunities and challenges: A white paper. The Pufendorf Institute of Advanced Studies, Lund University.

Fateh, F., Samadbeik, M., & Kazemi, A. (2020). What is digital health? Review of definitions. *Studies in Health Technology and Informatics*, *275*. Advance online publication. doi:10.3233/SHTI200696 PMID:33227742

Noesgaard, S. S., & Ørngreen, R. (2015). The effectiveness of e-learning: An explorative and integrative review of the definitions, methodologies and factors that promote e-learning effectiveness. *Electronic Journal of E-Learning*, *13*(4), 278–290.

Perakslis, E., & Ginsburg, G. S. (2021). Digital health—The need to assess benefits, risks, and value. *Journal of the American Medical Association*, *325*(2), 127–128. doi:10.1001/jama.2020.22919 PMID:33369627

Perakslis, E. D., & Stanley, M. (2021). *Digital health: Understanding the benefit-risk patient-provider framework*. Oxford University Press. doi:10.1093/oso/9780197503133.001.0001

Rogers, Y. (2004). New theoretical approaches for human-computer interaction. *Annual Review of Information Science & Technology*, *38*(1), 87–143. doi:10.1002/aris.1440380103

van Mil, J. W. F., & Henman, M. (2016). Terminology, the importance of defining. *International Journal of Clinical Pharmacy*. Advance online publication. doi:10.100711096-016-0294-5 PMID:27073076

KEY TERMS AND DEFINITIONS

Digital Health: A discipline where healthcare services and digital technologies intersect.

eHealth: All types of health interactions taking place digitally.

eLearning: All learning that takes place digitally.

mHealth: A form of ehealth focused on mobile applications.

mLearning: A form of elearning focused on mobile applications.

Patient-Centered Healthcare Model: A model that uses patient preferences to guide the provision of healthcare services.

Telehealth: Remote healthcare services utilizing digital technologies.

Chapter 3
Framing eHealth Design on Critical Race Theory to Mitigate Barriers in Access to Healthcare

Christina B. Gunther
Sacred Heart University, USA

Bronwyn Cross-Denny
Sacred Heart University, USA

Melanie M. Reyes
Sacred Heart University, USA

Danielle Provenzano
Sacred Heart University, USA

ABSTRACT

The importance of telehealth applications reached a critical nature during the COVID-19 pandemic of 2020. Telehealth allowed for a continuum of care while maintaining patient satisfaction during times of complete lockdown, quarantine, or isolation. The likelihood of a full audio-video telehealth visit for Black patients or those on Medicaid, however, was reduced. In fact, the Black patient population experienced two-times the rate of incomplete visits or telephone only visits compared to non-Hispanic White patients. Rivera et al. identified several significant barriers. Platform and portal designers must consider these barriers when creating telehealth tools. Framing the design on critical race theory can work towards equity in access to telehealth services.

INTRODUCTION

eHealth, or telehealth, platforms have been in use in healthcare since the 1970s (Westby et al., 2021). In 2017, the American Hospital Association (AHA) annual survey showed that 76% of hospitals were using telehealth services. The initial purpose of the ehealth or telehealth platforms was to reach communities

DOI: 10.4018/978-1-7998-9490-2.ch003

that had limited access to healthcare, for example, people living in very rural areas in the United States. Unfortunately, barriers to telehealth adoption grew, which included financial and government regulations limiting telehealth usage to communities that already had relative ease in accessing healthcare services (Westby et al., 2021). When the COVID-19 pandemic forced many healthcare services to limit in-person visits, telehealth services exploded (Berg et al., 2020; Bitar & Alismail, 2021; Seivert & Badowski, 2021). Many of the barriers in employing telehealth services persisted; however, for marginalized communities expanded the gap in inequity of healthcare services.

This chapter describes the barriers in using eHealth, or telehealth, platforms for marginalized communities and how applying a Critical Race Theory (CRT) framework can provide more equitable and inclusive access. A widening of the digital divide along with increasing insurance costs, data use concerns, and persisting language barriers will be detailed in reference to telehealth. Limited access to telehealth platform use can be mitigated by centering the needs of marginalized communities during development and implementation of the platforms. Critical Race Theory is suggested as a guiding framework for telehealth access and service provision.

For the purposes of this chapter, inclusive language and sensitive terminology is used with the intent to consider preferred identity labels of all people within all groups. According to Cross-Denny et. al.'s 2015 article on dismantling systemic racism, "language… has meaning and develops over time within a sociocultural, historical, and political context and is a social practice… it can also be a distraction from the intent being communicated in writing" (p. 10). Vulnerable populations included in this chapter are marginalized communities in the scope of race and socioeconomic status, and communicating the issues effectively requires respectful language for how one may self-identify. The following sections will consider the term Latinx in addition to Hispanic communities to avoid negative stereotypes and inclusion for LGBTQ+ communities that prefer the newer term and consider it inclusive of all gender types (Cardemil, Millan & Aranda, 2019; Salinas & Lozano, 2017; Salinas, 2020). The term Black/African American will also be used rather than African American to include all Black racial groups who do not culturally identify as African or American.

BACKGROUND

In order to frame solutions through a CRT lens to address the digital divide in ehealth for vulnerable, marginalized populations, a background is offered to understand these various components. A brief description of CRT is important, especially given the controversy that surrounds it in current political circles (Gibbons & Ray, 2021). Understanding the advantages of ehealth access as well as the structural barriers for vulnerable communities provides a foundation for envisioning and implementing solutions to increase access to healthcare. Populations that are most impacted are discussed: Native Americans, rural communities, Black/Latino communities, lower socioeconomic status, and global communities.

CRT began in the 1970s as Critical Legal Studies, a legal movement that challenged liberalism, denying that law was neutral (Brown & Jackson, 2013). Supporters of the CLS movement were marginalized, causing frustration and dissatisfaction which led to the creation of CRT. CRT evolved out of the CLS movement by scholars who believed CLS did not adequately address the issues and concerns of Blacks/African Americans and other groups of people of color (Brown & Jackson, 2013; Hartlep, 2009). Ladson-Billings and Tate (1995) recognized that race should be theorized as gender and class had been in the field of education, and pushed forward ideas of racial salience and perspective. Although CRT initially focused on issues of race and racism in the law, it has evolved to be more interdisciplinary. CRT has now grown to be an expansive and credible movement that is inner and cross-disciplinary (Hartlep, 2009). CRT attempts to demystify racial stereotypes, racial inequities, sexism, classism, xenophobic practices, and advances opportunities for groups that are not of White European descent (Brown & Jackson, 2013; Hartlep, 2009; Ladson-Billings & Tate, 1995; Tate, 1997). Telehealth platforms are typically developed using digital systems and structures based on White colonial designs (Hamilton, 2020). Applying principles of CRT to the design and application phases of telehealth, specifically the use of "counter-stories" (Mills & Godley, 2017), will open access to underserved populations and promote health equity (Ford & Airhihenbuwa, 2018).

eHealth

eHealth is often referred to as telehealth, telemedicine, or telecare in the healthcare field. For the purposes of this chapter, the term "telehealth" is used and refers to the United States Department of Health Resources and Services Administration's definition, "the use of electronic information and telecommunication technologies to support long-distance clinical health care, patient and professional health-related education, health administration, and public health" (HRSA, 2021, para. 1). Simply, telehealth refers to virtual patient-provider interactions using a video platform (Berg et al., 2020; Bitar & Alismail, 2021; Westby et al., 2021). Since the COVID-19 pandemic was declared, telehealth services have become increasingly more important for healthcare delivery.

The World Health Organization (WHO) declared the COVID-19 pandemic on March 11, 2020, three months after the viral outbreak in Wuhan, China, and by September 10, 2020, there were 27.7 million confirmed cases and deaths reached 899,000 globally (Bhaskar et al., 2020). As businesses closed and individuals across the world were asked to stay home, telehealth became necessary to provide healthcare services while protecting the general public from further spread of the disease (Bhaskar et al., 2020; Berg et al., 2020; Chunara et al., 2021). Despite the increase in telehealth to broaden access to healthcare, the lack of Internet connection and access to technology caused an expansion of the digital divide affecting vulnerable populations including people of color, immigrants, older adults, people who are homeless and poor, or people living in rural areas (Farrish, 2020, para. 8; Garfan et al., 2021; Sanders & Scanlon, 2021). The Federal Communications Commission (FCC) reported that 15 million Americans that rely on Medicare lack access to a computer with high-speed Internet and smartphones with wireless data, tools essential for successful telehealth visits. Hospitalization rates during the COVID-19 pandemic disproportionately impacted certain racial and ethnic minority groups (Centers for Disease Control and Prevention [CDC], 2022). Hispanic/Latino, Black, American Indian or Alaskan Native had higher hospitalization rates due to COVID-19 related illness than non-Hispanic Asian/Pacific Islander or non-Hispanic Whites (CDC, 2022). These vulnerable populations have been disproportionately impacted by the COVID-19 pandemic due to significant barriers to accessing healthcare, self-isolating, social distancing, and following public health directives (Chunara et al., 2021; Kazevman et al., 2021).

Native Americans on Reservations

Native American communities face challenges accessing healthcare and the use of telehealth services is cost effective and overall improves access to medical services, but many barriers remain (Graves et al., 2021; Hays et al, 2014; Kruse et al., 2016; Lee et al., 2016). Tribal reservations were formed in the U.S.

between the 1850s and the end of the century in a scheme of land allotments in a consolidation effort for government monitoring and control (Dippel, 2014). When the U.S. government redistributed land back to Native Americans, it was land that had very little value in terms of basic resources (International Work Group for Indigenous Affairs [IWGIA], 2021). The result of this is still felt in modern day tribal reservations. Because of the remote locations and inequities in healthcare funding, tribal members must travel a minimum of 30 minutes for basic healthcare (IWGIA, 2021). Prevalence of health conditions and chronic disease include diabetes, cardiovascular disease, substance abuse, and suicide, with exacerbating factors of lack of access to nutritious food and unemployment (IWGIA, 2021; Jetty et al., 2016; Kruse et al., 2021).

Across the United States, only 67% of tribal lands have access to broadband Internet and the FCC has determined that these broadband speeds are considered less than "minimally acceptable" (Edelman, 2021). Even though broadband Internet on reservations is slow, inconsistent, unreliable, and spotty, the cost is high and presumably the reason that less than half of the residents subscribe to services. At least 60% of the tribal residents have no fixed Internet access and during the COVID-19 pandemic, the digital divide became glaringly apparent in telehealth access (Edelman, 2021).

The digital divide in Native American nations is growing and reducing the gap has many barriers including "the isolation of reservations in rural areas, low population densities, a shortage of basic infrastructures such as electricity and telephones, and the complex relationship between the federal government and Native American Nations" (Bissell, 2004, p.139). Although improving technological development on Native American reservations is important to increasing healthcare access via telehealth, information technology can possibly impede on Native American traditions and history.

Native Americans have experienced years of federal policies specifically designed to eliminate cultural habits and history, as well as eliminate them as a people (Hagen et al., 2012; Rushing & Stephens, 2011; Tingey et al., 2021). To increase access to telehealth for Native American reservations, a strong balance between developing technology and preserving Native American beliefs and traditions is critical to success (Bissell, 2004; Schelbert, 2003; Tingey et al., 2021). As with other populations with cultural difference, any response to increase healthcare access must incorporate a culturally sensitive and competent practice (Kruse et al., 2021).

Rural Communities

People living in rural areas in the U.S. who had access to telehealth services reported better health status than those without access (Lee et al., 2019). Travel distance and shortage of healthcare workers are two major barriers rural communities face when seeking healthcare (Hirko et al., 2020; Jetty et al., 2016). Rural communities have greater health disparities in comparison to urban communities, including higher prevalence of diabetes, heart disease, and obesity, as well as risky health behaviors such as smoking, drinking alcohol, and lower exercise rates (Honeycutt et al., 2015). Much of this has to do with lack of resources and health literacy (Chunara et al., 2021; Honeycutt et al., 2015). Individuals living in rural communities also have higher costs for healthcare due to travel requirements (Garfan et al., 2021). The higher rates of chronic disease and barriers in access to healthcare often lead to disability and death (Jetty et al., 2016). Although adoption rates of telehealth services in rural communities have expanded overall, barriers include low awareness of reimbursement and restrictions with Medicare, lack of participating physicians, poor financial support, limited technological equipment, and lack of secure connections (Jetty et al., 2016). The COVID-19 pandemic exposed the need for online medical services as well as the inequities in telehealth access and use (Garfan et al., 2021). The rapid expansion of telehealth services increased access in rural communities, but broadband difficulties still need to be addressed to improve the effectiveness of telehealth in these areas (Garfan et al., 2021; Hirko et al., 2020).

Black/African American and Hispanic/Latinx Communities

During the COVID-19 pandemic, disproportionate morbidity and mortality rates among Black/African American and Hispanic/Latinx populations emphasized racial and ethnic disparities in healthcare throughout the United States (Van Dyke et al., 2021). In comparison to White patients, Black/African American patients experienced a higher risk of hospitalization due to COVID-19 because of previously higher rates of comorbidities, including hypertension and diabetes (Ogedegbe et al., 2020). Chunara et al. (2021) found that although the use of telehealth services had increased for Black/African American patients since the beginning of the COVID-19 pandemic, Black/African American patients were less likely to use telehealth services than White patients. Research also found that Black/African American patients were more likely to test positive for COVID-19 than White patients (Chunara et al., 2021). Despite the growing use of telehealth for Black patients during the pandemic, barriers still need to be addressed as the population lacks access to telehealth in comparison to majority populations.

Similar data exists for Hispanic/Latinx population COVID-19 rates and use of telehealth services. The Hispanic/Latinx community experienced higher death rates than White communities from COVID-19 due to frontline jobs as essential workers and previous increased rates of comorbidities compounding illness severity (Riley et al., 2021). Hispanic/Latinx communities also experience barriers in access to healthcare including telehealth services. Excess deaths in COVID-19 caused increased overall deaths by race and ethnicity in 2019 to 2020 (Shiels et al., 2021). The magnitude in disparities in health were exposed during this time period, particularly in access to telehealth. Many in the Hispanic/Latinx community lack access to Internet services and experience language barriers to English-only telehealth platforms (Silvaet al., 2020).

Intersectionality of Race and Socioeconomic Status

Higher socioeconomic status (SES) and digital literacy correspond directly to positive health status and access to telehealth. Poverty and race represent a prevailing intersection in the U.S. that stems from historical legacies of slavery and modern-day racism against immigration status of Hispanic/Latinx community members (Rose, 2020). Individuals living in poverty are more likely to be Black/African American or Hispanic/Latino due to these systemic issues. Rivera et al. (2021) note that the intersection of poverty and race create a double barrier to accessing telehealth services. The first barrier surrounds accessing Internet services, computers, and smart phones because of inability to meet the high cost. The second barrier surrounds language and health literacy, or illiteracy stemming from lack of education, avoidance of healthcare facilities out of fear of deportation, and systemic racism in the structure of healthcare. Patients with low SES backgrounds who are Black/African American or Hispanic/Latinx are less likely to use telehealth services than individuals with high SES backgrounds who are White creating a wider gap in health disparities between racial groups (Rivera et al., 2021).

Prior to the COVID-19 pandemic, the use of telehealth services was low for urban Medicaid beneficiaries. Talbot et al. (2018) concluded that broadband access, system licensure rules, and payment for telehealth services all limited Medicaid beneficiaries' use of online health services. By 2017, the United

States offered coverage of telehealth services through Medicaid across all 50 states (Talbot et al., 2018). Overall, Medicaid beneficiaries most often used online health services for mood disorders (Talbot et al., 2018). Racial and ethnic disparities are also prominent in Medicaid beneficiaries that use telehealth services. In comparison to White, non-Hispanic individuals, Black, non-Hispanic individuals used telehealth services at least three times less, and Hispanics/Latinx used telehealth services at least two times less (Talbot et al., 2018). The populations needing telehealth services the most are receiving them least.

Global Communities

Throughout nations across the globe, the health disparities gap has become wider during the COVID-19 pandemic with the adoption of telehealth (Kazevman et al., 2021). For example, without access to cellphones and/or Internet connection, vulnerable populations throughout Canada were unable to utilize telehealth. Vulnerable populations, including those experiencing homelessness and poverty, were more likely to become infected with COVID-19 and have overall worse health outcomes than those with access to telehealth (Kazevman et al., 2021). Improved access to technology allowed vulnerable populations to have improved overall health, as they had access to suicide hotlines, emergency medical services, and were able to strengthen their social networks. As the COVID-19 pandemic continues, the need for phone connectivity will also increase. If the digital divide is not addressed, the need for digital health equity will become vital, and will continue to grow (Kazevman et al., 2021).

Several low-income Asian countries are experiencing drastic increases in telehealth platforms as a result of COVID-19 (Bhaskar et al., 2020). According to a multi-country study by Suzuki et al. (2016) many countries, such as Thailand, have a shortage of physicians which limits their ability to adopt telehealth. In comparison, some countries (e.g., India, China) have experienced digital disparities between urban and rural areas which reduce the effectiveness of telehealth, similar to the issues in the U.S.

Notably, many countries had already begun adopting telehealth pre-COVID-19 such as countries in Central Asia, China, Singapore, India, countries in Latin America, Australia, New Zealand, Canada, U.S., United Kingdom, Italy, and Spain. Some regions of the world needed telehealth support from the World Health Organization (WHO) during the COVID-19 pandemic, such as countries in Africa. In comparison, in other countries, such as Italy, many hospitals became overwhelmed with COVID-19 patients. Some hospitals were able to effectively use telehealth and shared their experiences and encouraged adaptation to its use for other healthcare facilities (Bhaskar et al., 2020). Despite many areas in the world already having telehealth services prior to COVID-19, telehealth use in many countries has not been broadly studied presenting an opportunity for further research.

Disparities in telehealth are prominent throughout many nations and are dependent on various regional and structural factors, as well as governmental policies (Basu et al., 2021). Regionally, gaps exist in the current telehealth framework and communication barriers, educational needs, and professional development requirements need to be addressed to improve telehealth (Bhaskar et al., 2020). COVID-19 has illuminated the need for telehealth throughout the world, and is predicted to be sustained beyond the pandemic. To address the telehealth adoption disparities, public health and international efforts are important to ensure effective and equitable care for populations across nations. Growing evidence suggests that telehealth can have a positive impact on health systems and outcomes across nations once barriers to equitable access are determined and solutions are in place (Kruse et al., 2018).

MAIN FOCUS OF THE CHAPTER

Issues, Controversies, Problems

The potential to create accessible healthcare for vulnerable groups is a perceived strength of telehealth systems. However, this innovation in healthcare does not eliminate all barriers; in fact, many disparities are still highlighted with telehealth use (Rivera et al., 2021). The digital nature of telehealth can pose tedious demands on both providers and patients compared to an in-person clinical visit. Providers express frustration in limitations and navigation of telehealth, and patient abilities vary in health and digital literacy, which can interfere with successful communication (as cited in Becevic, et al., 2015; Wang, et al., 2020). Additionally, the following sections will address the inequities in access to technology and years of mistrust in the US healthcare system by marginalized groups. All issues, controversies, and problems related to telehealth can deter efficient healthcare delivery from treating the most vulnerable populations.

Patient Skepticism and Historic Mistrust

For certain groups and patient demographics, telehealth contributes to preexisting skepticism and historic mistrust in healthcare systems. Patients who lack familiarity with technology such as senior citizens or immigrants are already at a disadvantage when navigating telehealth systems. In addition to reduced physical visibility in an unfamiliar setting, there may be difficulty establishing trust between providers and a new patient (Breton, 2021). The nature of telehealth eliminates human interaction from the visit, where subtle cues such as body language and touch contribute to a patient's comfort level with the provider. Additionally, certain sensitive topics may not be disclosed due to perceived lack of privacy. The virtual aspect of a telehealth visit and the constant influx of new telehealth systems contribute to one's risk of exposure to fraud or data breaches (Garfan et al., 2021). These perceived barriers may deter skeptical patients from embracing telehealth as a feasible option to care.

Disadvantaged groups struggle with systemic and social barriers that are further amplified with the implementation of telehealth. In particular, racial minority patients may present with bias against the United States healthcare system and struggle to trust qualified providers. Substantial research has explored the effects of systemic racism and adverse healthcareexperiences, as minority patients experience severe health disparities compared to White patients (Feagin & Bennefield, 2014). This 2014 systematic review by Feagin and Bennefield verifies several health disparities: "African-American women are more likely to die of breast cancer than women of any other racial or ethnic group; American Indians are nearly three times as likely to be diagnosed with diabetes as White Americans; Eighty-two percent of the pediatric AIDS cases consisted of African-American and Latino children" (p. 10).

Black/African American patients struggle with the history of highly unethical research studies such as the Tuskegee Syphilis study. In 1932 the Tuskegee Institute was permitted by the U.S. Public Health Service to study the effects of untreated syphilis in Black patients; White physicians withheld the known cure so Black/African American participants died or passed on the disease to others (Jones & Tuskegee Institute, 1981). Further, Scharff et. al. (2010) assert that, "More than four centuries of a biomedical enterprise designed to exploit African Americans is a principal contributor to current mistrust" (p. 880).

Similarly, Hispanic/Latinx groups struggle with mistrust in the healthcare system due to historic exploitation. One specific study that is often cited as representative of Hispanic/Latinx population are the Puerto Rico Pill Trials held in 1956. Clinical trials for the synthetic estrogen, mestranol, were held in Puerto Rico because it was not yet legal to distribute contraceptives in the United States (Chadwick et. al., 2012; Keating, 2020). The scientists assumed that Puerto Rican women would be easily exploited for clinical trials purposes due to lack of education and low socioeconomic status, and they marketed the drug as pregnancy prevention without disclosing the clinical trial (Keating, 2020; Gibber, 2021). While the developers of the oral contraceptive believed it was safe and effective, more than 26 women suffered blood clots, including six women who died during the trials (Vargas, 2017). Pharmaceutical companies were eventually pressured to sponsor research into adverse effects and found that the high synthetic estrogen content was unsafe (Gibber, 2021). This exploitation of vulnerable women in the Puerto Rican Pill Trials contribute to the skepticism and mistrust for Hispanic/Latinx communities.

From the Tuskegee study to the Puerto Rico Pill Trials, minority groups in the United States contend with perhaps the most severe skepticism and mistrust due to historic exploitation for medicine. Minority patients are subject to implicit biases in a healthcare system that consists of predominantly White providers, therefore adding present-day layers of mistrust in addition to historic exploitation. The issue of healthcare access becomes complex for Black/African American and Hispanic/Latinx patients with low socioeconomic status. In the scope of telehealth, Black/African American and Hispanic/Latinx patients and patients of lower socioeconomic status tend to have similar challenges in access to technology.

Digital Divides in Telehealth

Despite advancements in technology, Internet and sufficient broadband access remains an issue for several groups. Patients who reside in rural areas suffer from reduced access and proximity to a hospital, in addition to poor broadband access and coverage (Hirko et al., 2020). Patients who have physical limitations or transportation issues may be drawn to the convenience of telehealth but may lack technological skills for a successful virtual visit; patient satisfaction with telehealth is positively correlated with user knowledge of current technology and applications (Koivunen & Saranto, 2018). The following section will explore the divides in technology access and education in further detail.

Health Literacy

A patient's health literacy positively correlates with the quality of a telehealth consultation. Berkman et al. (2010) noted that there are varying definitions of the term health literacy; however, it can generally be noted as an individual's ability to obtain and understand health information to make choices regarding healthcare services. A high level of health literacy indicates that a patient has a high capacity to access and comprehend medical information to make informed decisions. Lower health literacy creates more risk of error on behalf of the provider if they do not carefully navigate the patient to the proper terminology. To begin, the patient must present their chief complaints to the provider alone, without the aid of a medical scribe, medical assistant, or nurse to communicate the symptoms and history of present illness. Obtaining pertinent medical information and past medical history is placed solely on the provider. If the patient has difficulty in understanding medical terminology, the provider must also guide the patient towards the correct plan of care. Extra care must be given towards patients with low literacy or limited English capabilities. A review on hybrid telehealth systems conducted by Raj Westwood (2021) states that "[we] risk miscommunication of symptoms, prognosis, or prescriptions amongst patients with literacy challenges" (p.2). If a patient's health literacy is challenging for the provider, the perceived risk of malpractice may contribute to defensive medicine because telehealth limits the ability of providers to conduct a complete physical examination or obtain specimens remotely (Lieneck et al., 2021). Defensive medicine occurs when often unwarranted treatments or procedures are ordered by the provider in the interest of protection from malpractice lawsuits (Sekhar & Vyas, 2013).

Limitations in a Physical Examination

Although telehealth connects patients to healthcare providers, there are physical limitations that impede the quality of an initial examination. In a typical telehealth consultation, the provider completes a review of systems, obtains the history of present illness and pertinent medical history (Pierce & Stevermer, 2020). However, the provider is unable to perform urgent medical interventions or physical treatments (Raj Westwood, 2021). If the patient lacks the technological tools or health literacy to complete the plan of care virtually, they are often referred to the nearest clinic to complete the examination (Breton, 2021). This poses additional stress on those who reside in areas with sparse clinics or hospitals, or those with limited transportation options.

Various degrees of patient capabilities or lack of access to technology tools also contribute to a higher risk of error in telehealth practices (Berg et al., 2020). Some patients may have multiple cameras to conduct the visit, whereas others may have no camera at all. Because physical signs such as gait, general state, or face may not be clear in a virtual visit, the provider may have trouble obtaining a clear diagnosis or root cause of the health issue (Breton, 2021). Additionally, the supporting healthcare staff must also adapt to the workflow of telemedicine (Berg et al., 2020), causing further pressure for the provider to practice defensive medicine (Parimbelli et al., 2018). While access to care is improved, there is a significant potential for higher costs of care for patient compliance in defensive medicine. There may be additional spending on behalf of the patient for transportation, work schedule coordination, and lag time between obtaining a patient's specimen and the result. Conversely when follow-up telehealthcareis advised, the issues of scheduling contribute to patient and provider stress more significantly (Garfan et al., 2021). Provider schedules can quickly become overwhelmed as a commonly cited barrier to telehealth is time consumption; many medical professionals request a more seamless transition throughout the patient encounter from scheduling procedures to specimen collections (Lieneck et al., 2021).

Broadband Access

Patient populations living in rural areas with lower socioeconomic status are subject to barriers in telehealth access due to inadequate broadband, as Raj Westwood (2021) notes in her report, "Telehealth programs often require adequate broadband access, which is often limited in rural and under-served settings…There is a risk that telehealth can further increase health disparities, especially among low-income populations" (p. 324). Indeed, the lack of access becomes amplified when there are differences in Internet speed, quality, and bandwidth between neighborhoods. According to the Fourteenth Broadband and Deployment Report of the United States, there is an estimated 14 million Americans who lack access to reliable broadband or Internet service and the majority are likely to be Black, Hispanic, over the age of 65, lower-income, or live in rural or urban areas (FCC, 2021). There has been progress during the COVID-19 pandemic to address these disparities in healthcare access; however, technological access in rural communities continue to lag. The FCC aims to motivate broadband companies to improve access in rural areas where "more than 17% of Americans lack access" and on Tribal lands "almost 21% lack access" (FCC, 2021). The remaining gaps in technology infrastructure further push these vulnerable patient populations towards more disparate health outcomes.

Differences in broadband quality and speed also disrupt telemedicine consultations. While there is marked progress in the deployment of broadband access itself, the speed tests for these connections lag in all tiers for Tribal and rural areas (FCC, 2021). Video and sound quality is often suboptimal in these regions, contributing to patient and provider frustration in a telehealth visit. Alternatives to poor Internet quality include a telephone call, rescheduling the appointment, or transferring the patient to another clinic or higher level of care (Breton, 2021). Although these strategies are viable, they do not guarantee an effective solution to the differences in Internet access and interrupt patient-provider trust building and quality of care.

Other Considerations

The individual differences in healthcare access can vary depending on technical and physical ability, insurance provider coverage, and telehealth applications (Lee et al., 2019). Persons with disabilities may be physically unable to perform the necessary tasks to conduct a telehealth visit, or there may be a need for translators for patients who have visual or hearing impairments. Private insurance providers can differ in coverage and fees per health visit, and coverage can differ between states and provider networks such as Health Maintenance Organizations (HMOs) or Preferred Provider Organizations (PPOs). "Insurance status was found to be a significant predictor of telehealth service use. This finding likely relates to previous research indicating the challenges associated with access to and use of healthcarefor individuals without insurance" (Lee et. al., 2019, p.1265). These differences should be regulated as telehealth establishes its permanence and effectiveness in the US healthcare system.

Although telehealth has been in development and use for years, the COVID-19 pandemic brought an abundance of new telehealth applications. Some examples of online telehealth consultation platforms include Babylon Health, MDLIVE, LiveHealth, and Express Care Virtual (Wang et. al., 2020). The app-based platforms were developed and offered by commercial companies interested in advancing telehealth services. They provide secure online video consultations with providers, and in some instances, incorporate the use of artificial intelligence (AI). A quick review of the company's website suggests that the incorporation of AI increases efficiency of administrative healthcare functioning (Babylon, 2021). The differences in the applications' functionality, user-friendly interfaces, and support lines can vary significantly. These differences also bring about new challenges in interoperability and accuracy in the healthcare system. Wang et al. (2020) explains in their review on telemedicine barriers:

Another barrier to integrating telehealth is the [lack of] interoperability of patient data; namely, the ability to access, use, and change data across various platforms...As people use more diversified telehealth resources instead of one central health provider's services, communication and standardization of data across different platforms, service providers, and payer organizations are necessary to protect the integrity of patient data. (p. 679)

These considerations, controversies, and problems must be considered in telehealth.

SOLUTIONS AND RECOMMENDATIONS

To mitigate the disparities in telehealth use, the barriers of marginalized communities must be placed at the center of telehealth design and implementation. Framing the design around Critical Race Theory (CRT) can guide designers to develop platforms that are more easily accessed and navigated. Healthcare providers implementing the use of telehealth services must consider barriers to unequal access by understanding what limits successful telehealth visits with marginalized populations on an individual level.

Critical Race Theory (CRT) was initially developed in the field of law as a racial approach to social justice (Ladson-Billings & Tate, 2016). CRT scholars refuted the idea that race is biological, which was proven by geneticists involved in the Human Genome Project in 2003 (NHGRI, 2020). Further, CRT states that legal structures in the United States are inherently based on the White majority, disadvantaging the Black minority. The theory expounds upon the notion that race is a social construct that was invented to maintain inequitable access to resources, thereby, creating a mono- perspective benefiting the White majority population that is allowed to continue (Ladson-Billings & Tate, 2016) .

The theory has evolved to advocate for other oppressed groups such as LGBTQ+, immigrants, and non-native language speakers (Treviño et al., 2008). CRT places the marginalized at the center of social issues so that additional perspectives can be considered. Doing so helps to make social policies, institutions, and structures more equitable for all groups of people (Ford & Airhihenbuwa, 2010). As telehealth design and implementation evolves to address access barriers and increasing demand, patient requirements must be considered from multiple perspectives (Law & Wason, 2014; Wang et al, 2020) Grounding telehealth design on CRT is essential for telehealth equity to focus on the needs of all end users of telehealth tools with a multi-perspective lens.

Noting the barriers in telehealth access and use for immigrants, rural populations, senior citizens, low SES (including people of color) will help mitigate the deep digital divide currently dissecting equitable access to good health. Westby et al. (2021) noted that telehealth has "held the promise of equity in access to care since its implementation in the United States in the 1970s" (p. S29). Unfortunately, that equity has not been realized. Designers and developers have not circumvented the barriers that prevent telehealth from becoming the great equalizer yet. CRT can provide a framework to do that by placing the marginalized person's perspective at the center of the design process.

Several steps during telehealth system design and development must take place for equal access for all patients. These steps include developing systems that are user friendly and simple to use (Kim, 2017). Developers might consider the perspective of seniors who may not be technologically literate and may also have physical barriers to device use due to arthritis or other limitations such as macular degeneration. Built in translation services to telehealth systems could ease barriers in language. Privacy concerns and trust in telehealth use could be addressed during development that speaks directly to concerns of people of color and past health system failures. The point is, CRT places the marginalized at the center of development. Noting their barriers to access and use will assist developers in creating telehealth systems that are equitable to all patients.

Recognizing differences in technological and language ability by focusing on the end user rather than focusing on the development of a "software tool" will assist with equitable access (Kim, 2017). Including photos, videos, and translation options, as well as voice control and voice access circumvents many end user barriers (Lyles et al., 2021). Patients must be able to easily access the tools to access telehealth services, particularly those patients with language barriers. Telehealth tools designed for the English-speaking population adds further to the digital divide (Craig et al., 2021).

Addressing barriers to telehealth access in rural areas will require a more structural level focus. Demand for telehealth in rural areas has already been established, yet barriers in Internet infrastructure persist (Cortelyou-Ward et al., 2020). Rural residents either do not have access to minimum speed broadband services (broadband at a speed of "25 megabytes per second Mbps download/ 3Mbps upload according to the FCC") (as cited in Cortelyou-Ward, et al., 2020, p.1547), or the cost for service is unaffordable. Designers and developers will need to collaborate with broadband service companies, and perhaps townships, to expand infrastructure to areas without access. An example of that occurred in Chattanooga, TN. The publicly owned electric utility became an ISP to expand low-cost broadband service to over 56,000 area customers (Fung, 2013). The U.S. Department of Health Resources and Services Administration is also piloting a three-year program in Alaska, Texas, Michigan, and West Virginia that links communities to available funding to increase broadband access (HRSAb, 2021). If the FCC is encouraging expansion of broadband access, corporations will need to invest resources into the expansion through corporate social responsibility programs or other funding. Alternatively, municipalities will have to take it upon themselves.

Understanding the barriers in access and use to telehealth by marginalized populations is a critical step in design and development. Conducting needs assessments within the marginalized communities on access limitations will provide necessary data. Westby et al. (2021) determined from their clinical experience that telehealth can indeed improve equity in healthcare. They suggest several areas of improvement are needed first so that all populations of patients can access appropriate care. Speaking directly to these populations is the most direct path to equitable telehealth system development using data from all perspectives.

FUTURE RESEARCH DIRECTIONS

The COVID-19 pandemic provided the healthcare industry with an opportunity to implement a full-scale, worldwide telehealth response across the globe. A rapid implementation was required for medical procedures and services that included urgent care, surgery, non-urgent care, and mental health (Garfan et al., 2021; Goddard et al., 2021; Kaplan, 2020; Madigan et al., 2021). The challenges of implementation illustrate areas for modification and continued evaluation from insurance coverage, contracting, and reimbursement to technology training needs, platform constraints, and expenses (Berg et al., 2020; Garfan et al., 2021). High patient satisfaction for telehealth services was reported in neurosurgery, other advanced practice providers, and pediatric surgery indicating continued support and demand for telemedicine beyond the COVID-19 pandemic (Garfan et al., 2021; Lakshin et al., 2021; Zobair et al., 2021).

The challenges encountered in the swift telehealth response provide an opportunity to consider areas for improvement and to make shifts based upon lessons learned (Garfan et al., 2021). Vulnerable and minoritized populations, including those in rural areas and older adults, may have less access to technology including equipment, broadband, training, and comfort with technology. Different countries have varying infrastructure including Internet availability, reliable electricity, and specific equipment needs. The speedy implementation in conjunction with the volume of patients receiving care warrants the evaluation of risks in data privacy, security breaches, and medical legal issues (Garfan et al., 2021; Kaplan, 2020). Some examinations and medical services need to be provided in person such as collecting blood for diagnostic testing or a physical exam as well as the accuracy of health monitoring systems.

The use of School-Based Health Centers (SBHC) has provided an increase in access to healthcare services for children and adolescents from vulnerable populations providing a primary access point to services (Goddard et al., 2021). With the closure of schools, SBHCs also pivoted to telehealth services meeting both physical and mental healthcare needs. It is anticipated that SBHCs will continue to see a rise in mental health issues as a result of the pandemic and ongoing support will be needed with the inclusion of routine screenings of depression, anxiety, and substance abuse. SBHCs will require support by local, state, and federal resources to meet the telehealth needs of children and adolescents, especially those from vulnerable groups who have high utilization of SBHC services.

The future direction of telehealth, and telemental health services was magnified during the COVID-19 pandemic. The implementation of telehealth services and the associated barriers can provide a road map for the next steps in providing and creating new, innovative healthcare delivery, ongoing revisions to service provision, and evaluating efficacy and areas for needed change.

CONCLUSION

Critical Race Theory can provide a framework for creating and implementing solutions to mitigate barriers to healthcare. Creating a telehealth system that is supported by a sound infrastructure can improve access for marginalized and vulnerable populations, including Black/African American and Hispanic/Latinx populations, Indigenous people, older adults, and those in rural settings. CRT provides a framework that centers design and implementation of telehealth on those who are most at risk of health access inequities. Directly involving these populations can provide their valuable first-hand experience and understanding of the barriers they face. Technology platforms that are user-friendly and simple to use increase healthcare access for those who are challenged by technology literacy, physical and communication barriers, and historical issues of privacy and trust. Telehealth provides an opportunity to close the access gap in healthcare and using Critical Race Theory to frame innovative solutions can move the needle closer to achieving equitable service provision.

REFERENCES

American Hospital Association (AHA). (2019, Feb). *Factsheet: Telehealth*. https://www.aha.org/system/files/2019-02/fact-sheet-telehealth-2-4-19.pdf

Babylon. (2021). *About us*. https://www.babylonhealth.com/en-us/about

Basu, A., Kuziemsky, C., de Araújo Novaes, M., Kleber, A., Sales, F., Al-Shorbaji, N., Flórez-Arango, J. F., Gogia, S. B., Ho, K., Hunter, I., Iyengar, S., John, O., John, S., Kulatunga, G., Rajput, V. K., Ranatunga, P., & Udayasankaran, J. G. (2021). Telehealth and the COVID-19 pandemic: International perspectives and a health systems framework for telehealth implementation to support critical response. *Yearbook of Medical Informatics*, *30*(01), 126–133. doi:10.1055-0041-1726484 PMID:33882598

Becevic, M., Boren, S., Mutrux, R., Shah, Z., & Banerjee, S. (2015). User satisfaction with telehealth: Study of patients, providers, and coordinators. *The HealthcareManager*, *34*(4), 337–349. doi:10.1097/HCM.0000000000000081 PMID:26506296

Berg, E. A., Picoraro, J. A., Miller, S. D., Srinath, A., Franciosi, J. P., Hayes, C. E., Farrell, P. R., Cole, C. R., & LeLeiko, N. S. (2020). COVID-19—A guide to rapid implementation of telehealth services: A playbook for the pediatric gastroenterologist. *Journal of Pediatric Gastroenterology and Nutrition, 70*(6), 734–740. doi:10.1097/MPG.0000000000002749 PMID:32443021

Berkman, N. D., Davis, T. C., & McCormack, L. (2010). Health literacy: What is it? *Journal of Health Communication, 15*(sup2, S2), 9–19. doi:10.1080/10810730.2010.499985 PMID:20845189

Bhaskar, S., Bradley, S., Chattu, V. K., Adisesh, A., Nurtazina, A., Kyrykbayeva, S., Sakhamuri, S., Yaya, S., Sunil, T., Thomas, P., Mucci, V., Moguilner, S., Israel-Korn, S., Alacapa, J., Mishra, A., Pandya, S., Schroeder, S., Atreja, A., Banah, M., & Ray, D. (2020). Telemedicine across the globe-position paper from the COVID-19 pandemic health system resilience program (reprogram) international consortium (part 1). *Frontiers in Public Health, 8*(556720), 1–15. doi:10.3389/fpubh.2020.556720 PMID:33178656

Bissell, T. (2004). The digital divide dilemma: Preserving Native American culture while increasing access to information technology on reservations. *University of Illinois Journal of Law, Technology & Policy, 2004*(1), 129–150.

Bitar, H., & Alismail, S. (2021). The role of ehealth, telehealth, and telemedicine for chronic disease patients during COVID-19 pandemic: A rapid systematic review. *Digital Health, 7*. doi:10.1177/20552076211009396 PMID:33959378

Breton, M., Deville-Stoetzel, N., Gaboury, I., Smithman, M. A., Kaczorowski, J., Lussier, M.-T., Haggerty, J., Motulsky, A., Nugus, P., Layani, G., Paré, G., Evoy, G., Arsenault, M., Paquette, J.-S., Quinty, J., Authier, M., Mokraoui, N., Luc, M., & Lavoie, M.-E. (2021). Telehealth in primary healthcare: A portrait of its rapid implementation during the COVID-19 pandemic. *Healthcare Policy, 17*(1), 73–90. doi:10.12927/hcpol.2021.26576 PMID:34543178

Cardemil, E. V., Millán, F., & Aranda, E. (2019). A new, more inclusive name: The Journal of Latinx Psychology. *Journal of Latina/o Psychology, 7*(1), 1–5. doi:10.1037/lat0000129

Centers for Disease Control and Prevention (CDC). (2022). *Disparities in hospitalizations: Racial and ethnic health disparities*. U.S. Department of Health and Human Services. https://www.cdc.gov/coronavirus/2019-ncov/community/health-equity/racial-ethnic-disparities/disparities-hospitalization.html

Chunara, R., Zhao, Y., Lawrence, K., Testa, P. A., Nov, O., & Mann, D. M. (2021). Telemedicine and healthcare disparities: A cohort study in a large healthcare system in New York City during COVID-19. *Journal of the American Medical Informatics Association, 28*(1), 33–41. doi:10.1093/jamia/ocaa217 PMID:32866264

Cortelyou-Ward, K., Atkins, D. N., Noblin, A., Rotarius, T., White, P., & Carey, C. (2020). Navigating the digital divide: Barriers to telehealth in rural areas. *Journal of Healthcarefor the Poor and Underserved, 31*(4), 1546–1556. doi:10.1353/hpu.2020.0116 PMID:33416736

Cross-Denny, B., Betso, A., Cusick, E., Doyle, C., Marbot, M., & Santos-Dempsey, S. (2015). Constructing a deconstruction: Reflections on dismantling racism. *Reflections: Narratives of Professional Helping, 21*(3), 10-17.

Dippel, C. (2014). Forced coexistence and economic development: Evidence from NativeAmerican reservations. *Econometrica, 82*(6), 2131–2165. doi:10.3982/ECTA11423

Edelman, A. (2021, May 23). *Congress could spend big on broadband. Tribal nations say it can't come soon enough.* NBC Universal News Group. https://www.nbcnews.com/politics/joe-biden/congress-could-spend-big-broadband-tribal-nations-say-it-can-n1267923

Farrish, K. (2020). *Healthcareand education suffer when there's no internet access.* Connecticut Investigative Team. http://c-hit.org/2020/08/14/health-care-and-education-suffer-when-theres-no-internet-access/

Federal Communications Commission (FCC). (2021, Feb 1). *Fourteenth broadband deployment report.* https://www.fcc.gov/reports-research/reports/broadband-progress-reports/fourteenth-broadband-deployment-report

Ford, C. L., & Airhihenbuwa, C. O. (2010). Critical race theory, race equity, and public health: Toward antiracism praxis. *American Journal of Public Health, 100*(S1), S30–S35. doi:10.2105/AJPH.2009.171058 PMID:20147679

Ford, C. L., & Airhihenbuwa, C. O. (2018). Commentary: Just what is critical race theory and what's it doing in a progressive field like public health? *Ethnicity & Disease, 28*(Suppl 1), 223. doi:10.18865/ed.28.S1.223 PMID:30116090

Fung, B. (2013). *How Chattanooga beat Google Fiber by half a decade.* https://www.washingtonpost.com/news/the-switch/wp/2013/09/17/how-chattanooga-beat-google-fiber-by-half-a-decade/

Garfan, S., Alamoodi, A. H., Zaidan, B. B., Al-Zobbi, M., Hamid, R. A., Alwan, J. K., Ahmaro, I. Y. Y., Khalid, E. T., Jumaah, F. M., Albahri, O. S., Zaidan, A. A., Albahri, A. S., Al-qaysi, Z T., Ahmed, M. A., Shuwandy, M. L., Salih, M. M., Zughoul, O., Mohammed, K. I., & Momani, F. (2021). Telehealth utilization during the COVID-19 pandemic: A systematic review. *Computers in Biology and Medicine, 138.* doi:10.1016/j.compbiomed.2021.104878

Goddard, A., Sullivan, E., Fields, P., & Mackey, S. (2021). The future of telehealth in school- based health centers: Lessons from COVID-19. *Journal of Pediatric Health Care, 35*(3), 304–309. https://doi.org/10.1016/j.pedhc.2020.11.008

Hagen, J. W., Skenandore, A. H., Scow, B. M., Schanen, J. G., & Clary, F. H. (2012). Adolescent pregnancy prevention in a rural Native American community. *Journal of Family Social Work, 15*(1), 19–33.

Hamilton, A. M. (2020). A genealogy of critical race and digital studies: Past, present, and future. *Sociology of Race and Ethnicity (Thousand Oaks, Calif.), 6*(3), 292–301.

Hartlep, N. D. (2009). *Critical Race Theory an examination of its past, present, and future implications.* https://files.eric.ed.gov/fulltext/ED506735.pdf

Hays, H., Carroll, M., Ferguson, S., Fore, C., & Horton, M. (2014). The success of telehealthcarein the Indian Health Service. *AMA Journal of Ethics, 16*(12), 986–996. https://doi.org/10.1001/virtualmentor.2014.16.12.stas1-1412

Health Resources & Services Administration (HRSA). (2021a, Sept). *What is telehealth?* https://www.hrsa.gov/rural-health/telehealth/what-is-telehealth

Health Resources & Services Administration (HRSA). (2021b, Oct). *Telehealth programs*. https://www.hrsa.gov/rural-health/telehealth

Hirko, K. A., Kerver, J. M., Ford, S., Szafranski, C., Beckett, J., Kitchen, C., & Wendling, A. L. (2020). Telehealth in response to the COVID-19 pandemic: Implications for rural health disparities. *Journal of the American Medical Informatics Association*, *27*(11), 1816–1818. https://doi.org/10.1093/jamia/ocaa156

Honeycutt, A. A., Wile, K., Dove, C., Hawkins, J., & Orenstein, D. (2015). Strategic planning for chronic disease prevention in rural America: Looking through a PRISM lens. *Journal of Public Health Management and Practice*, *21*(4), 392–399.

International Work Group for Indigenous Affairs (IWGIA). (2021, Mar 18). *The indigenous world 2021: The United States of America*. https://www.iwgia.org/en/usa/4253-iw-2021-usa.html

Jetty, A., Moore, M. A., Coffman, M., Petterson, S., & Bazemore, A. (2018). Rural family physicians are twice as likely to use telehealth as urban family physicians. *Telemedicine and eHealth, 24*(4), 268-276.

Kaplan, B. (2020). Revisiting health information technology ethical, legal, and social issues and evaluation: Telehealth/telemedicine and COVID-19. *International Journal of Medical Informatics, 143*. doi:10.1016/j.ijmedinf.2020.104239

Kazevman, G., Mercado, M., Hulme, J., & Somers, A. (2021). Prescribing phones to address health equity needs in the COVID-19 era: The phone-connect program. *Journal of Medical Internet Research*, *23*(4), e23914. https://doi.org/10.2196/23914

Keating, A. (2020). The history of the birth control pill. *Journal of Undergraduate Social Work Research*, *4*(2), 13–23.

Koivunen, M., & Saranto, K. (2018). Nursing professionals' experiences of the facilitators and barriers to the use of telehealth applications: A systematic review of qualitative studies. *Scandinavian Journal of Caring Sciences*, *32*(1), 24–44. https://doi.org/10.1111/scs.12445

Kruse, C. S., Bouffard, S., Dougherty, M., & Parro, J. S. (2016). Telemedicine use in rural Native American communities in the era of the ACA: A systematic literature review. *Journal of Medical Systems*, *40*(6). https://doi.org/10.1007/s10916-016-0503-8

Kruse, C. S., Karem, P., Shifflett, K., Vegi, L., Ravi, K., & Brooks, M. (2018). Evaluating barriers to adopting telemedicine worldwide: A systematic review. *Journal of Telemedicine and Telecare*, *24*(1), 4–12.

Ladson-Billings, G., & Tate, W. F. (2016). Toward a Critical Race Theory of education. In *Critical Race Theory in Education* (pp. 10–31). Routledge.

Lakshin, G., Banek, S., Keese, D., Rolle, U., & Schmedding, A. (2021). Telemedicine in pediatric surgery in Germany during the COVID-19 pandemic. *Pediatric Surgery International*, *37*(3), 389–395. https://doi.org/10.1007/s00383-020-04822-w

Law, L. M., & Wason, J. M. (2014). Design of telehealth trials–introducing adaptive approaches. *International Journal of Medical Informatics*, *83*(12), 870–880.

Lee, S., Black, D., & Held, M. L. (2019). Factors associated with telehealth service utilization among rural populations. *Journal of Healthcarefor the Poor and Underserved, 30*(4), 1259–1272. https://doi.org/10.1353/hpu.2019.0104

Lieneck, C., Weaver, E., & Maryon, T. (2021). Outpatient telehealth implementation in the United States during the COVID-19 global pandemic: A systematic review. *Medicina, 57*(5), 462. doi:10.3390/medicina57050462

Lyles, C. R., Wachter, R. M., & Sarkar, U. (2021). Focusing on digital health equity. *Journal of the American Medical Association, 326*(18), 1795–1796.

Madigan, S., Racine, N., Cooke, J. E., & Korczak, D. J. (2021). COVID-19 and telemental health: Benefits, challenges, and future directions. *Canadian Psychology, 62*(1), 5–11. doi:10.1037/cap0000259

Mills, K. A., & Godley, A. (2017). Race and racism in digital media: What can Critical Race Theory contribute to research on techno-cultures? In *Handbook of writing, literacies, and education in digital cultures*. Routledge. https://acuresearchbank.acu.edu.au/download/301a941263cff02cedb052d909d0ef4cdb109b0549084c9102e2f5c49cd7d221/152464/AM_Mills_2017_Race_and_racism_in_digital_media.pdf

National Human Genome Research Institute (NHGRI). (2020, Dec 22). *The human genome project.* https://www.genome.gov/human-genome-project

Ogedegbe, G., Ravenell, J., Adhikari, S., Butler, M., Cook, T., Francois, F., ... Horwitz, L. I. (2020). Assessment of racial/ethnic disparities in hospitalization and mortality in patients with COVID-19 in New York City. *JAMA Network Open, 3*(12), e2026881–e2026881.

Parimbelli, E., Bottalico, B., Losiouk, E., Tomasi, M., Santosuosso, A., Lanzola, G., Quaglini, S., & Bellazzi, R. (2018). Trusting telemedicine: A discussion on risks, safety, legal implications and liability of involved stakeholders. *International Journal of Medical Informatics, 112*, 90–98. https://doi.org/10.1016/j.ijmedinf.2018.01.012

Pierce, R. P., & Stevermer, J. J. (2020). Disparities in use of telehealth at the onset of the COVID-19 public health emergency. *Journal of Telemedicine and Telecare.*

Raj Westwood, A. (2021). Is hybrid telehealth model the next step for private healthcare in India? *Health Services Insights*, 1–4. doi:10.1177/11786329211043301

Ray, R., & Gibbons, A. (2021, November). *Why are states banning Critical Race Theory?* Brookings. https://www.brookings.edu/blog/fixgov/2021/07/02/why-are-states-banning-critical-race-theory/

Riley, A. R., Chen, Y. H., Matthay, E. C., Glymour, M. M., Torres, J. M., Fernandez, A., & Bibbins-Domingo, K. (2020). Excess death among Latino people in California during the COVID-19 pandemic. *SSM Population Health, 15.* doi:10.1016/j.ssmph.2021.100860

Rivera, V., Aldridge, M. D., Ornstein, K., Moody, K. A., & Chun, A. (2021). Racial and socioeconomic disparities in access to telehealth. *Journal of the American Geriatrics Society, 69*(1), 44–45. https://doi.org/10.1111/jgs.16904

Rose, P. R. (2020). *Health equity, diversity, and inclusion: Context, controversies, and solutions.* Jones & Bartlett Learning.

Rushing, S. C., & Stephens, D. (2011). Use of media technologies by Native American teens and young adults in the Pacific Northwest: Exploring their utility for designing culturally appropriate technology-based health interventions. *The Journal of Primary Prevention, 32*(3), 135–145.

Salinas, C. Jr. (2020). The complexity of the "x" in Latinx: How Latinx/a/o students relate to, identify with, and understand the term Latinx. *Journal of Hispanic Higher Education, 19*(2), 149–168.

Salinas, C. Jr, & Lozano, A. (2019). Mapping and recontextualizing the evolution of the term Latinx: An environmental scanning in higher education. *Journal of Latinos and Education, 18*(4), 302–315.

Sanders, C. K., & Scanlon, E. (2021). The digital divide is a human rights issue: Advancing social inclusion through social work advocacy. *Journal of Human Rights and Social Work*, 1–14. Advance Online Publication. doi:10.1007/s41134-020-00147-9

Scharff, D. P., Mathews, K. J., Jackson, P., Hoffsuemmer, J., Martin, E., & Edwards, D. (2010). More than Tuskegee: Understanding mistrust about research participation. *Journal of Healthcarefor the Poor and Underserved, 21*(3), 879–897. https://doi.org/10.1353/hpu.0.0323

Schelbert, L. (2003). Pathways of human understanding: An inquiry into Western and North American Indian worldview structures. *American Indian Culture and Research Journal, 27*(1), 61–75.

Sekhar, M. S., & Vyas, N. (2013). Defensive medicine: A Bane to Healthcare. *Annals of Medical and Health Sciences Research, 3*(2), 295–296. 9248.113688 doi:10.4103/2141-

Shiels, M. S., Haque, A. T., Haozous, E. A., Albert, P. S., Almeida, J. S., García-Closas, M., . . . de González, A. B. (2021). Racial and ethnic disparities in excess deaths during the COVID-19 pandemic, March to December 2020. *Annals of Internal Medicine.* doi:10.7326/M21-2134

Silva, M. A., Perez, O. F. R., Añez, L. M., & Paris, M. (2021). Telehealth treatment engagement with Latinx populations during the COVID-19 pandemic. *The Lancet. Psychiatry, 8*(3), 176–178.

Talbot, J. A., Burgess, A. R., Thayer, D., Parenteau, L., Paluso, N., & Coburn, A. F. (2018). Patterns of telehealth use among rural Medicaid beneficiaries. *The Journal of Rural Health.* doi:10.1111/jrh.12324

Van Dyke, M. E., Mendoza, M. C., Li, W., Parker, E. M., Belay, B., Davis, E. M., ... Clarke, K. E. (2021). Racial and ethnic disparities in COVID-19 incidence by age, sex, and period among persons aged< 25 years—16 US jurisdictions, January 1–December 31, 2020. *Morbidity and Mortality Weekly Report, 70*(11), 382.

Vargas, T. (2017, May 15). Guinea pigs or pioneers? How Puerto Rican women were used to test the birth control pill. *Washington Post.* https://link.gale.com/apps/doc/A491755323/ITOF?u=24034&sid=bookmark-ITOF&xid=4ad4241c

Wang, C. J., Liu, T. T., Car, J., & Zuckerman, B. (2020). Design, adoption, implementation, scalability, and sustainability of telehealth programs. *Pediatric Clinics of North America, 67*(4), 675–682.

Wegermann, K., Wilder, J. M., Parish, A., Niedzwiecki, D., Gellad, Z. F., Muir, A. J., & Patel, Y. A. (2021). Racial and socioeconomic disparities in utilization of telehealth in patients with liver disease during COVID-19. *Digestive Diseases and Sciences*, 1–7.

Westby, A., Nissly, T., Gieseker, R., Timmins, K., & Justesen, K. (2021). Achieving equity in telehealth: "centering at the margins" in access, provision, and reimbursement. *Journal of the American Board of Family Medicine*, *34*(Supplement), S29–S32.

Westwood, A. R. (2021). Telehealth and maternity: Has the onset of the pandemic changed the way we utilise telemedicine forever? *British Journal of Midwifery*, *29*(6), 352–355. https://doi.org/10.12968/bjom.2021.29.6.352

Zobair, K. M., Sanzogni, L., Houghton, L., & Islam, M. Z. (2021). Forecasting care seekers satisfaction with telemedicine using machine learning and structural equation modeling. *PLoS One*, *16*(9), 1–31. https://doi.org/https://doi.org/10.1371/journal.pone.0257300

ADDITIONAL READING

Adkins-Jackson, P. B., Chantarat, T., Bailey, Z. D., & Ponce, N. A. (2021). Measuring structural racism: A guide for epidemiologists and other health researchers. *American Journal of Epidemiology*, kwab239. Advance online publication. doi:10.1093/aje/kwab239 PMID:34564723

Al-Thani, D., Monteiro, S., & Tamil, L. S. (2020). Design for ehealth and telehealth. In *Design for Health* (pp. 67–86). Academic Press. doi:10.1016/B978-0-12-816427-3.00004-X

Demiris, G., Charness, N., Krupinski, E., Ben-Arieh, D., Washington, K., Wu, J., & Farberow, B. (2010). The role of human factors in telehealth. *Telemedicine Journal and e-Health*, *16*(4), 446–453. doi:10.1089/tmj.2009.0114 PMID:20420540

Ervin, K., Weller-Newton, J., & Phillips, J. (2021). Primary healthcare clinicians' positive perceptions of the implementation of telehealth during the COVID-19 pandemic using normalisation process theory. *Australian Journal of Primary Health*, *27*(2), 158–162. doi:10.1071/PY20182

Ford, C. L., & Airhihenbuwa, C. O. (2018). Commentary: Just what is Critical Race Theory and what's it doing in a progressive field like public health? *Ethnicity & Disease*, *28*(Suppl 1), 223. doi:10.18865/ed.28.S1.223 PMID:30116090

Kreps, G. L., & Neuhauser, L. (2010). New directions in ehealth communication: Opportunities and challenges. *Patient Education and Counseling*, *78*(3), 329–336. doi:10.1016/j.pec.2010.01.013 PMID:20202779

Mills, K. A., & Godley, A. (2017). Race and racism in digital media: What can Critical Race Theory contribute to research on techno-cultures? In *Handbook of writing, literacies, and education in digital cultures*. Routledge. doi:10.4324/9781315465258-12

Morland, L. A., Greene, C. J., Rosen, C. S., Kuhn, E., Hoffman, J., & Sloan, D. M. (2017, April). Telehealth and ehealth interventions for posttraumatic stress disorder. *Current Opinion in Psychology*, *14*, 102–108. doi:10.1016/j.copsyc.2016.12.003 PMID:28813306

KEY TERMS AND DEFINITIONS

Critical Race Theory: A theory and social movement that provides a multi-perspective racial approach to social structures and services.

Digital Divide: The gap between individuals who have access to computers, broadband service, and other technologies and those who do not.

Equity: Addressing imbalances in equality so that all populations have the resources needed to reach equal access to healthcare.

Technology Gap: Differences between individuals who use computers and other technology and those who do not.

Telehealth: The delivery of healthcare services in a virtual or remote manner most typically via video conferencing.

Telemedicine: The act of a healthcare provider diagnosing and treating a patient virtually or remotely.

Chapter 4
Determining Needs to Support mHealth Interventions

Jill Erin Stefaniak
University of Georgia, USA

ABSTRACT

Needs assessment and analyses allow for organizations and individuals to identify any gaps or discrepancies between a current state of performance and a desired state. In regards to m-health technology, needs assessment can be used to help healthcare providers identify specific gaps or areas that could benefit from m-health technologies such as reducing the cancellation of appointments, improving health records, consolidating paperwork, and improving patient education efforts. The purpose of this chapter is to explore how needs assessment strategies can be leveraged to support healthcare providers' abilities to identify, select, and in implement m-health technologies into their patient plans. This chapter will review the types of needs healthcare providers must consider when implementing m-health technologies, as well as strategies that can support their decisions.

INTRODUCTION

In recent years, technological advances in healthcare, informatics, and mobile education have led the medical field to explore ways in which they can reach patients outside of the typical healthcare system. In an attempt to improve upon the efficiencies of healthcare communication and record keeping, mobile-health (m-health) has emerged as a viable strategy (Diao & Kvedar, 2021; Martínez-Pérez et al., 2013; Qudah & Luetsch, 2019).

M-health is defined by the World Health Organization as "medical public health practices supported by mobile devices, such as mobile phones, patient monitoring devices, personal digital assistants (PDAs), and other wireless devices (2011, p. 6). To date, there is a growing body of definitions to describe e-health and m-health initiatives (Silva et al, 2015; Steinhubl et al., 2013). Despite advances with the technological capabilities, mobile-health (m-health) can be described as health interventions that use the Internet for administrative, clinical, and educational practices (Mitchell, 1999). Such interventions provide patients with opportunities to connect to their healthcare providers remotely.

DOI: 10.4018/978-1-7998-9490-2.ch004

M-health technology provides several benefits to patients and healthcare providers. It provides patients with direct access to their providers and electronic health records, allows for patients living in remote and desolate areas to connect with healthcare professionals without having to travel to a facility, improves patient safety by sharing healthcare records among providers, pharmacies, and patients, and provides a platform for improving communication and the planning of routine visits (Ganasegeran et al., 2017; Nisha et al., 2019).

While m-health technologies have the potential to increase efficiencies and improve communication and patient safety, there are challenges associated with increasing the rate of adoption of m-health technologies. It is important that healthcare professionals take into consideration the role that m-health technologies will have in their practice. It is important that m-health technologies do not substitute interactions with patients that need to occur in medical facilities. Another challenge is ensuring patient compliance and ability to use m-health technologies (Leung & Chen, 2019). If there is an expectation that patients are to use m-health technologies to communicate with their providers, challenges exist with ensuring patients are using the technological applications correctly, accessing data as needed, and monitoring their health vitals per the instructions of their healthcare providers (Fatehi et al., 2017; Hashemi et al., 2018; Hoque & Sorwar, 2017; Hwabamungu & Willilams, 2010; Liew et al., 2019; Triantafyllidis et al., 2019). There is a growing concern with supporting elderly patients in the adoption of m-health technologies (Guo et al., 2013; Hoque & Sorwar, 2017; Quaosar et a., 2018; Safdari et a., 2018).

Additional challenges exist with determining what technological factors may impede the implementation of m-health technologies. While m-health has the potential to support patients living in developing countries and rural locations, these interventions will only be successful if there is an adequate infrastructure in place to support patients' ability to access information (Aamir et al., 2018; Alaiad et al., 2019; Alam et al., 2020; Crib et al., 2015; Dwivedi et a., 2016; Gleason, 2015).

Over the past decade, there has been an increase in mobile education where individuals have used their phones and other devices to use the Internet to connect to educational opportunities. As mobile education has continued to evolve, m-health has also expanded to include additional resources to support patient education. Examples include the use of educational videos to support patients with chronic health issues. Videos provide opportunities for healthcare professionals to explain health conditions and associated medical procedures as well as demonstrate proper exercise, monitoring, and medical care (Lee et al., 2018; Salvi et al., 2018; Yang & Korvarik, 2021).

Through the development of various mobile applications that can be downloaded directly to a phone or mobile device, patients are now able to track their vitals and other important health information. Examples of things that patients can track in real-time include glucose levels, oxygen levels, pulse rates, nutrition, and medicine. Resources for how to improve adherence to medical health plans are also available through mobile instruction in addition to providing patients with medical alerts and reminders (Free et al., 2010).

With the growing number of options available to healthcare providers interested in integrating m-health technology into their practices, it is of the utmost importance that they select technologies and platforms that align with their provider needs in addition to the needs of their patients. Needs assessment and analyses allow for organizations and individuals to identify any gaps or discrepancies between a current state of performance and a desired state (Altschuld & Kumar, 2010). Needs assessment can be used to help healthcare providers identify specific gaps or areas that could benefit from m-health technologies such as reducing the cancellation of appointments, improving health records, consolidating paperwork, and improving patient education efforts. The purpose of this chapter is to explore how needs assessment strategies can be leveraged to support healthcare providers' abilities to identify, select, and in implement m-health technologies into their patient plans. This chapter will introduce the purpose of needs assessment and analyses and theories that guide and influence needs assessment. In addition, it will review the types of needs healthcare providers must consider when implementing m-health technologies, as well as strategies that can support their decisions.

PURPOSE OF A NEEDS ASSESSMENT IN M-HEALTH

Prior to developing a m-health intervention, educators and community health partners should conduct a needs analysis to ensure adequate alignment between the community audience's needs and the features being included in the m-health intervention. The purpose of a needs assessment is to identify any gaps or discrepancies between the current state of affairs and the desired state of affairs. When conducting needs assessments pertaining to the development and implementation of a m-health resource, most needs assessments will fall under the broad category of community needs assessments. These types of assessments provide an overview of the community's needs from a public health standpoint.

Community needs assessments may identify specific topics of information that members of a population (or community) may benefit from receiving additional resources, trainings, or consultations. If a community has a large subset of a population that is experiencing particular health issues (e.g., heart disease, diabetes, obesity, lack of prenatal care), then the results of the needs assessment will identify the prevalence that needs may exist within a community.

Keeping in mind that the purpose of a needs assessment is to identify that a need exists and warrants an intervention in order to reach a desired state of affairs, educators and community health professionals must extend beyond identifying that a gap exists and conduct a needs analysis to determine what is causing that gap to exist. By identifying factors that are contributing to a gap, those involved in the development and implementation of a m-health intervention are positioned to design sustainable solutions to mitigate existing challenges members of the community may be experiencing.

THEORIES THAT SUPPORT NEEDS ASSESSMENTS AND ANALYSES

When conducting a needs assessment, it is important to recognize the theoretical foundations that are guiding and supporting needs assessment activities. Regardless of the purpose for conducting a needs assessment, there are three theoretical constructs that often contribute to needs assessment. These are human needs theory and general systems, theory (Stefaniak, 2021). While there may be additional theoretical constructs related to the specific context of the needs assessment, these three constructs will inevitably contribute to the structure of the project.

Human Needs Theory

Needs can be classified according to various types. Bradshaw (1972) developed a taxonomy of social needs that categorizes needs in four groups: 1) normative, 2) felt, 3) expressed, and 4) comparative. Normative needs are often defined by a standard that has been set by experts or a governing entity (Labonté, 2016; Watson, 2002). Examples of normative needs in healthcare may include, but are not limited to, determining how frequently patients should visit their healthcare provider (i.e., annual health check) and comparing one's body mass index (BMI) to a normative standard pertaining to height and weight.

Felt needs consist of what an individual wants (Bradshaw, 1972). It is important to note that these are needs that have been identified by the individual and may not be a need in actuality. For example, an individual may seek medical care and receive a diagnosis from their healthcare provider. Upon receiving their physician's recommendations, the individual may feel that their needs have not been addressed and may seek additional resources or a second opinion. While the healthcare provider may have run the necessary diagnostics to make an appropriate diagnosis and recommendations, the individual's (the patient's) perception is that their needs have not been met (Stefaniak, 2021).

It is important to proceed with caution when addressing felt needs during health-related needs assessments. These needs should not be disregarded; however, it is important that sufficient data is gathered to support those needs that are brought forth by individuals. It is also important to take into consideration any discrepancies that may exist between felt needs and actual needs as these differences in opinion may impact individuals' abilities to adopt m-health technologies for their intended purposes (Han et al., 2019).

Expressed needs are defined by Bradshaw (1972) as needs turned into action. Examples of expressed needs may include patients requesting additional instructions for their plan of care, a legal guardian or caregiver asking for an appointment to ensure a patient's medication has been regulated.

Comparative needs consist of comparing the needs of an individual or group to other individuals and groups that may have similar needs or health conditions. Examples may include comparing cancer patients living in rural areas to other cancer patients living in similar rural areas. Comparative needs may include comparing health needs across different demographics such as race, ethnicity, gender, age, and geographical location (Lucchini et al., 2017; Milsom et al., 2009; Woltmann et al., 2012). Exploring comparative needs during a m-health needs assessment may help determine if different resources should be provided or marketed with different populations.

Additional needs that are often explored during needs assessment include future needs, critical needs, and maintenance needs (Altschuld & Kumar, 2010). Future needs entail preparing for things that are not currently needed but will be in the near future. Examples of future needs may include preparing for an increase in health facilities required by a large aging population in a community. Maintenance needs may include improving upon or updating resources that currently exist. A local health organization may have a number of patient education materials that they disseminate routinely but need to update per changes in standards related to patient care. Critical needs are needs that must be addressed immediately. These needs typically take prioritization over other needs as they are often linked to severe consequences if left ignored. Examples may include a population requiring medical treatment after a natural disaster (Chan & Kim, 2011; Lillibridge et al., 1993; Schonfeld & Gurwitch, 2009).

General Systems Theory

General systems theory provides a framework for viewing an organization or environment as a system. Within a systems lens, a needs assessor will examine the components that make up the system. This includes, but is not limited to, the individuals, objects, processes, and interactions (Skyttner, 2001). Taking a systems view recognizes the systemic nature of needs assessment. This is also applicable to m-health interventions.

It is important to note that the term *systems* is scalable. Systems come in all shapes and sizes. A healthcare organization can be considered a large system. Individual departments or units within that system could also be considered their own system. A community organization or healthcare provider's office who uses m-health applications could be considered individual systems. Regardless of whether a group or individual is considered a system or a subsystem of a much larger system, it is important to identify the reach of the system that is being considered for the needs assessment. This will help the needs assessor recognize the systemic relationships that may exist between various objects and processes within a given system.

The following are examples of the types of questions a needs assessor may consider when conducting a needs assessment pertaining to m-health:

- Are the processes or instructions provided in the m-health application suitable for all patients/patrons?
  - To what extent do processes outlined in the m-health intervention need to be customized for different audiences or types of patients?
- What types of technological support are needed for individuals to access the application?
- How can information documented in the application be shared with multiple healthcare providers?
- Are there means for patients to track information offline in the application?
  - What happens if a patient does not have continuous access to the Internet?
- How are individuals expected to use the m-health application?
  - Is this a substitute for other interventions and/or resources that have been made available in the past?

It is especially important that the needs assessor embraces a systems view when conducting needs assessments related to m-health as there are many elements comprising the *system* to be impacted. This includes the individuals designing and implementing the interventions and/or resources across the m-health platform, the technology needed to support the m-health platform, health care providers, patients, and any other individuals who may be responsible for assisting patients and individuals with accessing and using the m-health applications appropriately. Throughout this chapter, examples are given regarding the types of environmental affordances needs assessors should be aware of when conducting a needs assessment.

AN OVERVIEW OF THE NEEDS ASSESSMENT PROCESS

While there are several resources that have been written that outline the process of conducting a needs assessment, they all follow a similar approach to gathering sufficient data to inform what types of interventions may be needed. Needs assessment can be broken down broadly into six steps (Stefaniak, 2021):

1. Identifying the problem
2. Identification and verification of needs
3. Identification of data sources
4. Data collection
5. Data analysis
6. Recommendations

Table 1. Examples of needs assessments to support medical initiatives

Purpose of Needs Assessment	Context	Reference
Explore how cultural factors impact health and illness.	Community health in medical education	Dowell et al. (2001)
To seek a better understanding of how nonprofit hospitals are fulfilling health needs assessment provisions.	Nonprofit hospitals	Pennel et al. (2015)
To identify patient education and resource needs among homeless populations.	Homeless shelters	Stefaniak, J. E., Mi, M., & Afonso, N. (2015). Triangulating perspectives: A needs assessment to develop an outreach program for vulnerable and underserved populations. *Performance Improvement Quarterly*, *28*(1), 49-68.
Exploring how libraries can support the health needs of their communities.	Libraries	Rubenstein, E. (2016). Knowing how to help: providing health information in public libraries. *Journal of Consumer Health on the Internet*, *20*(3), 114-129.

When conducting a needs assessment, the first step is to identify the problem. The term *problem* is broadly used to describe the situation that is warranting a change. When conducting a needs assessment, the individual(s) responsible will determine what are the parameters of a project. During this phase, they must identify the purpose of the project. When conducting a needs assessment specific to mobile health technologies, this is the phase where they will identify what they hope to explore or target with the needs assessment to inform the implementation and adoption of a specific m-health intervention. Problem identification consists of an individual or group expressing a need for a solution. The needs that are expressed initially will later be explored in further detail and verified as a part of the needs assessment process. Examples of needs that may be expressed pertaining to m-health interventions could be the following:

- A local health clinic expressing a need to improve communication with patients in between visits;
- A network of healthcare providers wanting to ensure that each provider and the patient have up to date records for treatment plans;
- An interest in patients monitoring their glucose levels to record and establish a pattern; and
- Providing opportunities for disseminating information to communities.

Table 1 provides examples of community-based needs assessments that were conducted to support medical initiatives.

Identifying and Verifying Needs

Once the scope and purpose have been identified, the needs assessment team will begin identifying and verifying that the needs initially presented in the problem identification phase are actual needs.

In addition to various types of needs, Altschuld and Witkin (2000) classified needs according to three levels: primary, secondary, and tertiary. Level one primary needs consist of individuals who will receive products or services to address their needs. Level two secondary needs consist of the needs belonging to the individuals or groups responsible for delivering services. Examples of secondary needs may be training for healthcare providers on how to use m-health applications, how to design and deliver instruction across a m-health platform, and the process of troubleshooting interventions pertaining to patient support.

Level three tertiary needs consist of the infrastructural needs required to support level one and two needs. Level three tertiary needs should be considered foundational to the success of subsequent needs in the systems at both the primary and secondary levels. Examples of tertiary needs could include determining if a healthcare facility has the appropriate information technology infrastructure to support electronic health records and medical informatics that may be supported by m-health technologies.

While scholarship on designing m-health interventions has continued to grow over the past few years, little has been written about how to effectively conduct needs assessments and analyses to support the design of such interventions. When conducting a needs assessment pertaining to a m-health project, educators, healthcare providers, and community partners must gather data across four domains: patient affordances, provider affordances, technology affordances, and environmental affordances.

Identification of Data Sources and Data Collection

Once the needs to be explored have been determined, the needs assessment team will begin to identify data sources that will provide sufficient and adequate data to support or refute those needs. During the selection of data sources, it is most helpful to gather data from multiple sources to ensure that different perspectives have been included. To determine optimal data sources to inform the needs assessment and analysis, Cavanagh and Chadwick (2005) recommend that the project team consist of the *right* people. They describe the *right* people as being individuals who know about the issues, care about the issues, and are in a position of authority to help implement change.

When selecting data sources for a needs assessment, it is important that the individual(s) involved are able to gather data that provides an accurate portrayal of the environment. This entails gathering data that informs the perspectives of all constituents associated with the problem. For example, in a needs assessment that explored topics for an educational outreach program to support homeless and underserved populations, Stefaniak et al. (2015) gathered data through surveys, interviews, and existing documents from patrons of a homeless shelter, case workers of the homeless shelter, medical professionals, and local libraries to determine appropriate topics to be included in the educational program. By gathering data from multiple constituents, the research team was able to get insights from a number of individuals and compare them to see if certain topics were identified by all groups as priorities for the program. The data collected from the patrons also yielded insightful information as to their prioritized needs.

Common forms of data collection for needs assessments include, but are not limited to, one-on-one interviews with constituents, focus groups, surveys, direct observations, and document analyses. It is important to consider how much time has been allocated for the needs assessment as well as resources, money, and any other constraints that may hinder data collection. These factors will significantly impact data sources that are selected. Table 2 provides an overview of the advantages and disadvantages of various data collection techniques.

Needs assessments that are conducted to support m-health projects should be structured in a way that gathers information across four domains: patient affordances, provider affordances, technology affordances, and environmental affordances. Similar to the three levels of needs suggested by Altschuld and Witkin (2000), there is a need for alignment in order to design and implement a m-health intervention that is adopted by members of a patient community.

Table 2. Advantages and disadvantages of data collection techniques

Data Collection Technique	Advantages	Disadvantages
One-on-one interviews	Provides an opportunity for individuals to share their concerns and opinions pertaining to the situation.	Individuals may not feel comfortable disclosing information. Takes additional time.
Focus groups	Provides an opportunity for discussion with a group of individuals (approximately 6-8 at a time). Individuals often feel heard.	Individuals may not feel comfortable discussing their opinions in a group if the subject matter is sensitive. Facilitator needs to be mindful of dominant individuals in focus group sessions.
Surveys	Can gather data from a large group of individuals in a relatively short about of time.	Individuals may be limited on what information they can share based on how the survey is structured. May lead to generalized results.
Direct observations	Provides an opportunity to see events and behaviors occurring in real-time.	Individuals may behave differently while being watched.
Document analyses	Provides background information pertaining to the situation. Provides a record of process and decision-making that has taken place within an organization or among a group.	Can be time-consuming to review documents relevant to the needs assessment.

Patient Affordances

Affordances are defined as perceivable actions possible (Norman, 2013). When designing learning interventions, learner affordances take into account the realities of what the learners are capable of doing as the end-users of a learning experience. Considering that m-health interventions may or may not consist of educational resources, the term patient affordances is used in this chapter to reference the end-user. Patient affordances account for the perceivable actions that are possible in terms of how the patient will use the resources and tools provided through the m-health platform (Alam et al., 2020; Kaium et al., 2019; O'Connor, 2020). This may include their abilities to access and understand educational resources as well as use the m-health tools as they were intended to be used. The following are examples of the types of questions needs assessors may ask regarding patient affordances. The types of questions that are asked will help identify appropriate data sources:

- What are the patients' preconceptions regarding the resource?
- What value does the m-health application offer patients?
- What challenges have patients experienced regarding the topic and/or services that are being offered through the m-heath platform?
- What is the likelihood of the patient adopting the resources and services offered by the m-health platform?

The role of context is of particular importance when determining patients' affordances as they relate to m-health technologies. Tessmer and Richey (1997) described three categories of context that influence learning and instructional design: orienting context, instructional context, and transfer context.

The orienting context takes into account learners demographic information and preconceived notions. From an instructional perspective, the orienting context looks at what prior knowledge and experience learners may bring to the learning environment. It is important to consider the orienting context to customize instruction, meet the learners needs, and work with them to set achievable learning goals.

The instructional context accounts for the environment where learning will take place (e.g., classroom, online platform, blended platform, mobile platform). When designing instruction, this particular context, tasks instructional designers with addressing learner role and task perceptions (Tessmer & Richey, 1997). It also considers the necessary supports that learners and teachers may need in the instructional environment space.

The transfer context is where information acquired through instruction will be applied. When designing instruction, it is beneficial for instructional designers to understand the realities of the transfer context. What factors may inhibit an individual's ability to transfer and apply what they have learned? Consideration of any cultural or political factors may impact successful transfer.

Stefaniak (2021) suggests that these same contextual domains should be considered when gathering data during a needs assessment to better understand an organizational system or environment. This supports m-health initiatives by exploring patients' affordances, determining the extent of training they may need, and considering how they will use the m-health resource independently. Asking questions across these three contextual domains helps ensure alignment and increase the likelihood of adoption.

The orienting context should be considered in the design of an m-health platform and its corresponding applications. While not all m-health interventions are instructional, orienting factors of the learner or end-user are similar. Healthcare professionals and m-health developers should be considerate of their familiarity with using technology, perceptions and preconceived notions about m-health technologies and the health information they intend to access through the platform.

When designing and developing m-health resources, the individuals involved should consider what training and guides may be needed for the end-user (i.e., patient, learner, caretaker) to access and navigate the m-health platform. If individuals have caretakers or family members assisting them with using the m-health application, consideration should go into protecting their privacy, use of language, and ability to interpret or translate information.

The transfer context encompasses *where* and *how* individuals will use the m-health platform. Instructional designers and healthcare professionals need to consider the impact that the orienting and transfer contexts may pose for the other. Consideration should be given to whether or not there are adequate resources to ensure the patient or end user uses the m-health application properly if required to track personal health information. Technological infrastructure also needs to be considered for rural or developing areas that may not have strong internet connections.

Provider Affordances

Provider affordances consist of the abilities and potential for action of those individuals responsible for providing services. Regarding the development of m-health interventions, this would consist of healthcare providers, community partners, and other individuals who would have a role in designing, developing, and disseminating information across a m-health platform. During a needs assessment, provider needs would be considered secondary level two needs. These needs must be explored in order to minimize any discrepancies in patient versus provider expectations of resources and services to be shared and communicated in a m-health platform. Examples of provider affordances may include their ability to navigate the m-health application, communicate with their patients and communities through the platform, and identify any necessary training they may be required to support the m-health functions. Questions that needs assessors may ask when conducting a needs assessment include:

- What training have the healthcare providers had regarding the use (and navigation) of the m-health platform?
- Do the providers understand how to share and communicate through the m-health platform?
- Do the providers understand security challenges and concerns associated with m-health interventions?
- Have the providers identified roles and responsibilities within their team regarding who will update and monitor information on the m-health platform?

Technology Affordances

Technology affordances are the capabilities of the technology, itself. Every m-health application or platform has its own capacity and limitations for distributing resources and services. When conducting a needs assessment, it is important that the technological affordances associated with a given technology are aligned to support the provider and patient affordances (Bakdash & Drews, 2012; Houben et al., 2015; Mao et al., 2020). It is also important that alignment occurs between these various domains to inform the identification and selection of m-health technologies that will address the patients' and communities' healthcare needs.

As previously mentioned, technological and environmental affordances should be explored when considering the tertiary needs specific to a m-health needs assessment. These last two domains address the foundational infrastructure needed to support the design of instruction and other supportive interventions that may be distributed through a m-health platform. Examples of questions that may be considered include the following:

- How are services accessed across the platform?
- What are the limitations to the m-health platform under consideration?
- What are the application's capabilities for sharing and distributing health information across a patient's healthcare team?
- How do patients and providers interact with the platform?
- What resources are needed to install and establish the m-health platform under consideration?
- What resources are needed ongoingly to maintain the m-health platform under consideration?

Environmental Affordances

Environmental affordances are often coupled with technological affordances to address a learning environment in literature that is focused on instructional design. This often entails the capabilities of the classroom or online learning space (e.g., the location where learning will take place). When examining affordances for m-health interventions, technological and environmental affordances have been decoupled as environmental affordances may include other factors that pose significant implications for the patient and provider affordances and needs.

A benefit of m-health interventions is that they provide opportunities for connectivity between patients and their healthcare team regardless of their geographical location. The geographical location and living environments may also impact patients' abilities to participate and use the m-health intervention as designed. There are certain factors that may hinder or preclude a patient from full participation that are exclusive from a patient's desire or willingness to participate (Choi et al., 2013).

Examples of environmental factors that may impact the implementation and adoption of m-health resources and services may include undeveloped areas (Chib et al., 2013; Lee et al., 2016; Humble et al., 2016; Van Wyk et al., 2019). These are areas that may not be equipped to support technology needed for m-health services such as access to electricity or the Internet. Other examples of environmental conditions may include areas that have been impacted by natural disasters or other emergencies that have contributed to an increase in particular illnesses. These types of situations will greatly impact the types of resources that may be provided and suggested by providers.

Data Analysis and Making Recommendations

Upon completion of data collection, individuals responsible for conducting the needs assessment must begin to make sense of the data. Results from the various data sources should be triangulated to identify if there are recurring themes and patterns that are emerging from the data. If data from multiple sources are yielding similar results, that is a good indicator that the information is providing an accurate portrayal of the current situation and the needs of members within the system.

When situations occur where data from the various sources are not in agreement, the needs assessment team should consider exploring additional data sources if it is not clear why there may be discrepancies between the current data sources. Sometimes there will be differences depending on the types of data that were collected or different individuals (i.e., patients versus providers) sharing different opinions based on their experiences and role within a healthcare system.

As the needs assessment team begins identifying patterns among the data and verifying that needs initially presented at the beginning of the needs assessment are indeed actual needs, they must then begin prioritizing which needs should be addressed and in what order. When prioritizing needs to be addressed, it is important that the team consider the four types of affordances (patient, provider, technological, and environmental) to determine feasible solutions.

Lack of alignment between the four types of affordances may limit the types of services that may be offered via a m-health platform. When this occurs, additional attention may be placed on addressing the technological and environmental affordances to ensure that adequate infrastructure is in place to support ongoing initiatives.

Needs should also be prioritized in terms of safety. The individuals conducting the needs assessment must differentiate between needs that may lead to significant problems if left unaddressed (Kaufman & Guerra-Lopez, 2013). Other factors that should be considered include the time needed to design, develop, and implement specific services, money associated with these activities and solutions, and any additional resources that be acquired before implementing resolutions.

CONCLUSION

Needs assessments provide individuals and organizations with opportunities to gather information that can inform future action. When exploring the possibilities of m-health platforms and services, data collected from needs assessments can support healthcare providers with the necessary information they need to establish an appropriate technological infrastructure to support m-health services that align with environmental conditions experienced by the patient populations they support. Needs assessments provide healthcare providers with opportunities to align patients' health and education needs, account for what training providers may require in order to support m-health services and ensure that infrastructure is in place.

REFERENCES

Aamir, J., Ali, S. M., Boulos, M. N. K., Anjum, N., & Ishaq, M. (2018). Enablers and inhibitors: A review of the situation regarding mHealth adoption in low-and middle-income countries. *Health Policy and Technology*, *7*(1), 88–97. doi:10.1016/j.hlpt.2017.11.005

Alaiad, A., Alsharo, M., & Alnsour, Y. (2019). The determinants of m-health adoption in developing countries: An empirical investigation. *Applied Clinical Informatics*, *10*(05), 820–840. doi:10.1055-0039-1697906 PMID:31667819

Alam, M. Z., Hoque, M. R., Hu, W., & Barua, Z. (2020). Factors influencing the adoption of mHealth services in a developing country: A patient-centric study. *International Journal of Information Management*, *50*, 128–143. doi:10.1016/j.ijinfomgt.2019.04.016

Alam, M. Z., Hoque, M. R., Hu, W., & Barua, Z. (2020). Factors influencing the adoption of mHealth services in a developing country: A patient-centric study. *International Journal of Information Management*, *50*, 128–143. doi:10.1016/j.ijinfomgt.2019.04.016

Altschuld, J. W., & Kumar, D. D. (2010). Needs assessment: An overview. *Sage (Atlanta, Ga.)*.

Altschuld, J. W., & Witkin, B. R. (2000). From needs assessment to action: Transforming needs into solution strategies. *Sage (Atlanta, Ga.)*.

Bakdash, J. Z., & Drews, F. A. (2012). Using knowledge in the world to improve patient safety: Designing affordances in health care equipment to specify a sequential "Checklist". *Human Factors and Ergonomics in Manufacturing & Service Industries*, *22*(1), 7–20. doi:10.1002/hfm.20289

Bradshaw, J. (1972). Taxonomy of social need. In G. McLachlan (Ed.), *Problems and progress in medical care: Essays son current research* (pp. 71–82). Oxford University Press.

Cavanagh, S., & Chadwick, K. (2005). *Health needs assessment: A practical guide*. Health Development Agency.

Chan, E. Y., & Kim, J. (2011). Chronic health needs immediately after natural disasters in middle-income countries: The case of the 2008 Sichuan, China earthquake. *European Journal of Emergency Medicine*, *18*(2), 111–114. doi:10.1097/MEJ.0b013e32833dba19 PMID:20679898

Chib, A., van Velthoven, M. H., & Car, J. (2015). mHealth adoption in low-resource environments: A review of the use of mobile healthcare in developing countries. *Journal of Health Communication*, *20*(1), 4–34. doi:10.1080/10810730.2013.864735 PMID:24673171

Chib, A., Wilkin, H., & Hoefman, B. (2013). Vulnerabilities in mHealth implementation: A Ugandan HIV/AIDS SMS campaign. *Global Health Promotion*, *20*(1, suppl), 26–32. doi:10.1177/1757975912462419 PMID:23549699

Choi, Y. S., & Bosch, S. J. (2013). Environmental affordances: Designing for family presence and involvement in patient care. *HERD: Health Environments Research & Design Journal*, *6*(4), 53–75. doi:10.1177/193758671300600404 PMID:24089181

Diao, J. A., & Kvedar, J. (2021). *Mobile health technology for diverse populations: challenges and opportunities*. Academic Press.

Dowell, A., Crampton, P., & Parkin, C. (2001). The first sunrise: An experience of cultural immersion and community health needs assessment by undergraduate medical students in New Zealand. *Medical Education*, *35*(3), 242–249. doi:10.1046/j.1365-2923.2001.00772.x PMID:11260447

Dwivedi, Y. K., Shareef, M. A., Simintiras, A. C., Lal, B., & Weerakkody, V. (2016). A generalised adoption model for services: A cross-country comparison of mobile health (m-health). *Government Information Quarterly*, *33*(1), 174–187. doi:10.1016/j.giq.2015.06.003

Fatehi, F., Gray, L. C., & Russell, A. W. (2017). Mobile health (mHealth) for diabetes care: Opportunities and challenges. *Diabetes Technology & Therapeutics*, *19*(1), 1–3. doi:10.1089/dia.2016.0430 PMID:28099051

Free, C., Phillips, G., Felix, L., Galli, L., Patel, V., & Edwards, P. (2010). The effectiveness of M-health technologies for improving health and health services: A systematic review protocol. *BMC Research Notes*, *3*(1), 1–7. doi:10.1186/1756-0500-3-250 PMID:20925916

Ganasegeran, K., Renganathan, P., Rashid, A., & Al-Dubai, S. A. R. (2017). The m-Health revolution: Exploring perceived benefits of WhatsApp use in clinical practice. *International Journal of Medical Informatics*, *97*, 145–151. doi:10.1016/j.ijmedinf.2016.10.013 PMID:27919374

Gleason, A. W. (2015). mHealth—Opportunities for transforming global health care and barriers to adoption. *Journal of Electronic Resources in Medical Libraries*, *12*(2), 114–125. doi:10.1080/15424065.2015.1035565

Guo, X., Sun, Y., Wang, N., Peng, Z., & Yan, Z. (2013). The dark side of elderly acceptance of preventive mobile health services in China. *Electronic Markets*, *23*(1), 49–61. doi:10.100712525-012-0112-4

Han, K. J., Subramanian, R., & Cameron, G. T. (2019). Listen before you leap: Sri Lankan health professionals' perspectives on m-health. *Health Informatics Journal*, *25*(3), 858–866. doi:10.1177/1460458217725903 PMID:28825329

Hashemi, A., Nourbakhsh, S., Tehrani, P., & Karimi, A. (2018). Remote telemonitoring of cardiovascular patients: Benefits, barriers, new suggestions. *Artery Research*, *22*(C), 57–63. doi:10.1016/j.artres.2018.04.001

Hoque, R., & Sorwar, G. (2017). Understanding factors influencing the adoption of mHealth by the elderly: An extension of the UTAUT model. *International Journal of Medical Informatics*, *101*, 75–84. doi:10.1016/j.ijmedinf.2017.02.002 PMID:28347450

Houben, S., Frost, M., & Bardram, J. E. (2015, February). Collaborative affordances of hybrid patient record technologies in medical work. In *Proceedings of the 18th ACM Conference on Computer Supported Cooperative Work & Social Computing* (pp. 785-797). 10.1145/2675133.2675164

Humble, J. R., Tolley, E. A., Krukowski, R. A., Womack, C. R., Motley, T. S., & Bailey, J. E. (2016). Use of and interest in mobile health for diabetes self-care in vulnerable populations. *Journal of Telemedicine and Telecare*, *22*(1), 32–38. doi:10.1177/1357633X15586641 PMID:26026179

Hwabamungu, B., & Williams, Q. (2010, October). m-Health adoption and sustainability prognosis from a care givers' and patients' perspective. In *Proceedings of the 2010 Annual Research Conference of the South African Institute of Computer Scientists and Information Technologists* (pp. 123-131). 10.1145/1899503.1899517

Kaium, M. A., Bao, Y., Alam, M. Z., Hasan, N., & Hoque, M. R. (2019). Understanding the insight of factors affecting mHealth adoption: A systematic review. *International Journal of Research in Business and Social Science, 8*(6), 181-200.

Kaufman, R., & Guerra-Lopez, I. (2013). *Needs assessment for organizational success*. ASTD Press.

Labonté, R. (2016). Health promotion in an age of normative equity and rampant inequality. *International Journal of Health Policy and Management*, *5*(12), 675–682. doi:10.15171/ijhpm.2016.95 PMID:28005546

Lee, M. H., Wu, H. C., Tseng, C. M., Ko, T. L., Weng, T. J., & Chen, Y. F. (2018). Health education and symptom flare management using a video-based m-health system for caring women with IC/BPS. *Urology*, *119*, 62–69. doi:10.1016/j.urology.2018.05.027 PMID:29894774

Lee, S. H., Nurmatov, U. B., Nwaru, B. I., Mukherjee, M., Grant, L., & Pagliari, C. (2016). Effectiveness of mHealth interventions for maternal, newborn and child health in low–and middle–income countries: Systematic review and meta–analysis. *Journal of Global Health*, *6*(1), 010401. doi:10.7189/jogh.06.010401 PMID:26649177

Leung, L., & Chen, C. (2019). E-health/m-health adoption and lifestyle improvements: Exploring the roles of technology readiness, the expectation-confirmation model, and health-related information activities. *Telecommunications Policy*, *43*(6), 563–575. doi:10.1016/j.telpol.2019.01.005

Liew, M. S., Zhang, J., See, J., & Ong, Y. L. (2019). Usability challenges for health and wellness mobile apps: Mixed-methods study among mHealth experts and consumers. *JMIR mHealth and uHealth*, *7*(1), e12160. doi:10.2196/12160 PMID:30698528

Lillibridge, S. R., Noji, E. K., & Burkle, F. M. Jr. (1993). Disaster assessment: The emergency health evaluation of a population affected by a disaster. *Annals of Emergency Medicine*, *22*(11), 1715–1720. doi:10.1016/S0196-0644(05)81311-3 PMID:8214862

Lucchini, R. G., Hashim, D., Acquilla, S., Basanets, A., Bertazzi, P. A., Bushmanov, A., Crane, M., Harrison, D. J., Holden, W., Landrigan, P. J., Luft, B. J., Mocarelli, P., Mazitova, N., Melius, J., Moline, J. M., Mori, K., Prezant, D., Reibman, J., Reissman, D. B., ... Todd, A. C. (2017). A comparative assessment of major international disasters: The need for exposure assessment, systematic emergency preparedness, and lifetime health care. *BMC Public Health*, *17*(1), 1–12. doi:10.118612889-016-3939-3 PMID:28061835

Mao, C. M., & Hovick, S. R. (2020). Adding Affordances and Communication Efficacy to the Technology Acceptance Model to Study the Messaging Features of Online Patient Portals among Young Adults. *Health Communication*, 1–9. PMID:33243017

Martínez-Pérez, B., De La Torre-Díez, I., & López-Coronado, M. (2013). Mobile health applications for the most prevalent conditions by the World Health Organization: Review and analysis. *Journal of Medical Internet Research*, *15*(6), e2600. doi:10.2196/jmir.2600 PMID:23770578

Milsom, K. M., Jones, C., Kearney-Mitchell, P., & Tickle, M. (2009). A comparative needs assessment of the dental health of adults attending dental access centres and general dental practices in Halton & St Helens and Warrington PCTs 2007. *British Dental Journal*, *206*(5), 257–261. doi:10.1038j.bdj.2009.165 PMID:19287420

Nisha, N., Iqbal, M., & Rifat, A. (2019). The changing paradigm of health and mobile phones: An innovation in the health care system. *Journal of Global Information Management*, *27*(1), 19–46. doi:10.4018/JGIM.2019010102

Norman, D. (2013). *The design of everyday things*. Basic books.

O'Connor, S. M. (2020). *Exploring eHealth implementation: understanding factors affecting engagement and enrolment in consumer digital health* (Doctoral dissertation). University of Glasgow.

Pennel, C. L., McLeroy, K. R., Burdine, J. N., & Matarrita-Cascante, D. (2015). Nonprofit hospitals' approach to community health needs assessment. *American Journal of Public Health*, *105*(3), e103–e113. doi:10.2105/AJPH.2014.302286 PMID:25602862

Quaosar, G. A. A., Hoque, M. R., & Bao, Y. (2018). Investigating factors affecting elderly's intention to use m-health services: An empirical study. *Telemedicine Journal and e-Health*, *24*(4), 309–314. doi:10.1089/tmj.2017.0111 PMID:28976824

Qudah, B., & Luetsch, K. (2019). The influence of mobile health applications on patient-healthcare provider relationships: A systematic, narrative review. *Patient Education and Counseling*, *102*(6), 1080–1089. doi:10.1016/j.pec.2019.01.021 PMID:30745178

Rubenstein, E. (2016). Knowing how to help: Providing health information in public libraries. *Journal of Consumer Health on the Internet*, *20*(3), 114–129. doi:10.1080/15398285.2016.1198111

Safdari, R., Shams Abadi, A. R., & Pahlevany Nejad, S. (2018). Improve health of the elderly people with M-health and technology. *Iranian Journal of Aging*, *13*(3), 288–299. doi:10.32598ija.13.3.288

Salvi, D., Ottaviano, M., Muuraiskangas, S., Martínez-Romero, A., Vera-Muñoz, C., Triantafyllidis, A., Cabrera Umpiérrez, M. F., Arredondo Waldmeyer, M. T., Skobel, E., Knackstedt, C., Liedes, H., Honka, A., Luprano, J., Cleland, J. G. F., Stut, W., & Deighan, C. (2018). An m-Health system for education and motivation in cardiac rehabilitation: The experience of HeartCycle guided exercise. *Journal of Telemedicine and Telecare*, *24*(4), 303–316. doi:10.1177/1357633X17697501 PMID:28350282

Schonfeld, D. J., & Gurwitch, R. H. (2009). Addressing disaster mental health needs of children: Practical guidance for pediatric emergency health care providers. *Clinical Pediatric Emergency Medicine*, *10*(3), 208–215. doi:10.1016/j.cpem.2009.06.002

Silva, B. M., Rodrigues, J. J., de la Torre Díez, I., López-Coronado, M., & Saleem, K. (2015). Mobile-health: A review of current state in 2015. *Journal of Biomedical Informatics*, *56*, 265–272. doi:10.1016/j.jbi.2015.06.003 PMID:26071682

Skyttner, L. (2001). *General systems theory: Ideas and applications*. World Scientific Publishing. doi:10.1142/4307

Stefaniak, J. E. (2021). *Needs assessment for learning and performance: Theory, process, and practice*. Routledge.

Stefaniak, J. E., Mi, M., & Afonso, N. (2015). Triangulating perspectives: A needs assessment to develop an outreach program for vulnerable and underserved populations. *Performance Improvement Quarterly*, *28*(1), 49–68. doi:10.1002/piq.21186

Steinhubl, S. R., Muse, E. D., & Topol, E. J. (2013). Can mobile health technologies transform health care? *Journal of the American Medical Association*, *310*(22), 2395–2396. doi:10.1001/jama.2013.281078 PMID:24158428

Tessmer, M., & Richey, R. C. (1997). The role of context in learning and instructional design. *Educational Technology Research and Development*, *45*(2), 85–115. doi:10.1007/BF02299526

Triantafyllidis, A., Kondylakis, H., Votis, K., Tzovaras, D., Maglaveras, N., & Rahimi, K. (2019). Features, outcomes, and challenges in mobile health interventions for patients living with chronic diseases: A review of systematic reviews. *International Journal of Medical Informatics*, *132*, 103984. doi:10.1016/j.ijmedinf.2019.103984 PMID:31605884

Van Wyk, T., Mahomed-Asmail, F., & Swanepoel, D. W. (2019). Supporting hearing health in vulnerable populations through community care workers using mHealth technologies. *International Journal of Audiology*, *58*(11), 790–797. doi:10.1080/14992027.2019.1649478 PMID:31419388

Watson, M. C. (2002). Normative needs assessment: Is this an appropriate way in which to meet the new public health agenda? *International Journal of Health Promotion and Education*, *40*(1), 4–8. doi:10.1080/14635240.2002.10806189

Woltmann, E., Grogan-Kaylor, A., Perron, B., Georges, H., Kilbourne, A. M., & Bauer, M. S. (2012). Comparative effectiveness of collaborative chronic care models for mental health conditions across primary, specialty, and behavioral health care settings: Systematic review and meta-analysis. *The American Journal of Psychiatry*, *169*(8), 790–804. doi:10.1176/appi.ajp.2012.11111616 PMID:22772364

World Health Organization. (2011). *mHealth: New Horizons for Health through Mobile Technologies: Based on the Findings of the Second Global Survey on eHealth (Global Observatory for eHealth Series, Volume 3)*. https://www.who.int/goe/publications/goe_mhealth_web.pdf

Yang, X., & Kovarik, C. L. (2021). A systematic review of mobile health interventions in China: Identifying gaps in care. *Journal of Telemedicine and Telecare*, *27*(1), 3–22. doi:10.1177/1357633X19856746 PMID:31319759

ADDITIONAL READING

Arthur, M. W., & Blitz, C. (2000). Bridging the gap between science and practice in drug abuse prevention through needs assessment and strategic community planning. *Journal of Community Psychology*, *28*(3), 241–255. doi:10.1002/(SICI)1520-6629(200005)28:3<241::AID-JCOP2>3.0.CO;2-X

Barry, M. M., Doherty, A., Hope, A., Sixsmith, J., & Kelleher, C. C. (2000). A community needs assessment for rural mental health promotion. *Health Education Research*, *15*(3), 293–304. doi:10.1093/her/15.3.293 PMID:10977377

Beverly, C. J., Mcatee, R., Costello, J., Chernoff, R., & Casteel, J. (2005). Needs assessment of rural communities: A focus on older adults. *Journal of Community Health*, *30*(3), 197–212. doi:10.100710900-004-1958-y PMID:15847245

Corpman, D. W. (2013). Mobile health in China: A review of research and programs in medical care, health education, and public health. *Journal of Health Communication*, *18*(11), 1345–1367. doi:10.1080/10810730.2013.778370 PMID:23915211

Ellis, K., Davis, A., & Rummery, K. (1999). Needs assessment, street-level bureaucracy and the new community care. *Social Policy and Administration*, *33*(3), 262–280. doi:10.1111/1467-9515.00150

Gagnon, M. P., Ngangue, P., Payne-Gagnon, J., & Desmartis, M. (2016). m-Health adoption by healthcare professionals: A systematic review. *Journal of the American Medical Informatics Association: JAMIA*, *23*(1), 212–220. doi:10.1093/jamia/ocv052 PMID:26078410

Garner, S. L., George, C. E., Young, P., Hitchcock, J., Koch, H., Green, G., Mahid, Z., & Norman, G. (2020). Effectiveness of an mHealth application to improve hypertension health literacy in India. *International Nursing Review*, *67*(4), 476–483. doi:10.1111/inr.12616 PMID:32767464

Goldman, K. D., & Schmalz, K. J. (2005). "Accentuate the positive!" using an asset-mapping tool as part of a community-health needs assessment. *Health Promotion Practice*, *6*(2), 125–128. doi:10.1177/1524839904273344 PMID:15912635

Hartzell, J. D., Yu, C. E., Cohee, B. M., Nelson, M. R., & Wilson, R. L. (2017). Moving beyond accidental leadership: A graduate medical education leadership curriculum needs assessment. *Military Medicine*, *182*(7), e1815–e1822. doi:10.7205/MILMED-D-16-00365 PMID:28810977

Istepanian, R., Laxminarayan, S., & Pattichis, C. S. (Eds.). (2007). *M-health: Emerging mobile health systems*. Springer Science & Business Media.

Kahn, J. G., Yang, J. S., & Kahn, J. S. (2010). 'Mobile'health needs and opportunities in developing countries. *Health Affairs*, *29*(2), 252–258. doi:10.1377/hlthaff.2009.0965 PMID:20348069

Källander, K., Tibenderana, J. K., Akpogheneta, O. J., Strachan, D. L., Hill, Z., ten Asbroek, A. H., Conteh, L., Kirkwood, B. R., & Meek, S. R. (2013). Mobile health (mHealth) approaches and lessons for increased performance and retention of community health workers in low-and middle-income countries: A review. *Journal of Medical Internet Research*, *15*(1), e17. doi:10.2196/jmir.2130 PMID:23353680

Kotz, D., Gunter, C. A., Kumar, S., & Weiner, J. P. (2016). Privacy and security in mobile health: A research agenda. *Computer*, *49*(6), 22–30. doi:10.1109/MC.2016.185 PMID:28344359

Marcolino, M. S., Oliveira, J. A. Q., D'Agostino, M., Ribeiro, A. L., Alkmim, M. B. M., & Novillo-Ortiz, D. (2018). The impact of mHealth interventions: Systematic review of systematic reviews. *JMIR mHealth and uHealth*, *6*(1), e23. doi:10.2196/mhealth.8873 PMID:29343463

Miller, K., Yost, B., Abbott, C., Thompson Buckland, S., Dlugi, E., Adams, Z., Rajagopalan, V., Schulman, M., Hilfrank, K., & Cohen, M. A. (2019). Health needs assessment of five Pennsylvania Plain populations. *International Journal of Environmental Research and Public Health*, *16*(13), 2378. doi:10.3390/ijerph16132378 PMID:31277401

Ming, L. C., Untong, N., Aliudin, N. A., Osili, N., Kifli, N., Tan, C. S., Goh, K. W., Ng, P. W., Al-Worafi, Y. M., Lee, K. S., & Goh, H. P. (2020). Mobile health apps on COVID-19 launched in the early days of the pandemic: Content analysis and review. *JMIR mHealth and uHealth*, *8*(9), e19796. doi:10.2196/19796 PMID:32609622

Mohr, D. C., Schueller, S. M., Montague, E., Burns, M. N., & Rashidi, P. (2014). The behavioral intervention technology model: An integrated conceptual and technological framework for eHealth and mHealth interventions. *Journal of Medical Internet Research*, *16*(6), e3077. doi:10.2196/jmir.3077 PMID:24905070

Naslund, J. A., Aschbrenner, K. A., Barre, L. K., & Bartels, S. J. (2015). Feasibility of popular m-health technologies for activity tracking among individuals with serious mental illness. *Telemedicine Journal and e-Health*, *21*(3), 213–216. doi:10.1089/tmj.2014.0105 PMID:25536190

Nolin, J., Wilburn, S. T., Wilburn, K. T., & Weaver, D. (2006). Health and social service needs of older adults: Implementing a community-based needs assessment. *Evaluation and Program Planning*, *29*(3), 217–226. doi:10.1016/j.evalprogplan.2006.06.003

Norman, G. R., Shannon, S. I., & Marrin, M. L. (2004). The need for needs assessment in continuing medical education. *BMJ (Clinical Research Ed.)*, *328*(7446), 999–1001. doi:10.1136/bmj.328.7446.999 PMID:15105326

Norris, A. C., Stockdale, R. S., & Sharma, S. (2009). A strategic approach to m-health. *Health Informatics Journal*, *15*(3), 244–253. doi:10.1177/1460458209337445 PMID:19713398

Ramirez, V., Johnson, E., Gonzalez, C., Ramirez, V., Rubino, B., & Rossetti, G. (2016). Assessing the use of mobile health technology by patients: An observational study in primary care clinics. *JMIR mHealth and uHealth*, *4*(2), e4928. doi:10.2196/mhealth.4928 PMID:27095507

Roess, A. (2017). The promise, growth, and reality of mobile health-another data-free zone. *The New England Journal of Medicine*, *377*(21), 2010–2011. doi:10.1056/NEJMp1713180 PMID:29116869

Shareef, M. A., Kumar, V., & Kumar, U. (2014). Predicting mobile health adoption behaviour: A demand side perspective. *Journal of Customer Behaviour*, *13*(3), 187–205. doi:10.1362/14753921 4X14103453768697

Stowell, E., Lyson, M. C., Saksono, H., Wurth, R. C., Jimison, H., Pavel, M., & Parker, A. G. (2018). Designing and evaluating mHealth interventions for vulnerable populations. *Systematic Reviews*.

Vafa, S., & Chico, D. E. (2013). A needs assessment for mobile technology use in medical education. *International Journal of Medical Education*, *4*, 230–235. doi:10.5116/ijme.5259.4a88

Vukovic, V., Favaretti, C., Ricciardi, W., & de Waure, C. (2018). Health technology assessment evidence on e-health/m-health technologies: Evaluating the transparency and thoroughness. *International Journal of Technology Assessment in Health Care*, *34*(1), 87–96. doi:10.1017/S0266462317004512 PMID:29455685

KEY TERMS AND DEFINITIONS

Environmental Affordances: Factors that pose significant implications for the patient and provider affordances and needs.

Intervention: A resource or service that is provided to address a need.

M-Health: Educational resources and health services that are supported by mobile devices.

Need: A gap between a current state of affairs and a desired state of affairs.

Needs Analysis: A process of determining causal factors that are contributing to needs and gaps in performance identified during a needs assessment.

Needs Assessment: A process of determining discrepancies or gaps in performance that may exist between a current state of affairs and a desired state of affairs.

Patient Affordances: A patient's perceivable actions that are possible in terms of how a patient will use resources and tools provided through a m-health platform.

Provider Affordances: The abilities and potential for action of those individuals responsible for providing services.

Technology Affordances: The capabilities of the technologies being used to provide services via a m-health platform.

Section 2

eHealth and mHealth Education Interventions: Exemplars in Health Behavior Change

Chapter 5
Promoting Behavioral Weight Loss and Physical Activity:
Design of Two Interventions

Courtney M. Monroe
University of South Carolina, USA

ABSTRACT

Obesity and insufficient physical activity represent ongoing pandemics. These cases describe the design process of two different electronic and mobile health interventions in the areas of behavioral weight loss and physical activity promotion. An interdisciplinary team of experts followed several guidelines of an established intervention framework to ensure the interventions were addressing significant research gaps and grounded in theory and empirical evidence. Intervention strategies were guided by the intervention mapping taxonomy of behavior change methods and integrated both custom-built and commercially available technologies. These cases detail how the chosen theories, methods, and intervention strategies were connected. Challenges and opportunities in relation to both the interventions and the fields of technology-based behavioral weight loss and physical activity more broadly are also discussed.

INTRODUCTION

The issues of obesity and insufficient physical activity represent persistent pandemics (World Health Organization, 2021a, 2021b). Electronic and mobile health (e/mhealth) interventions have increasingly been implemented and evaluated to help address these issues among adults (Beleigoli et al., 2019; Jahangiry et al., 2017; Mateo et al., 2015; McEwan et al., 2020; Monroe et al., 2015). While e/mhealth strategies hold promise for improving weight statuses and physical activity levels in the broader population, unexplored areas abound when it comes to understanding how best to leverage e/mhealth solutions for long-term maintenance of improvements in these outcomes. Growing calls have been made within the e/mhealth behavioral weight loss and physical activity fields to design and test multilevel interventions that consider the complex individual and environmental determinants of weight control and physical activity (Mezuk & Allen, 2021; Sallis, 2018; Vo et al., 2019). The two theory-based interventions de-

DOI: 10.4018/978-1-7998-9490-2.ch005

scribed as part of these two case studies – called (1) NETworks (Nutrition, Exercise, and Technology) for Weight Loss (Monroe, Geraci, Larsen, et al., 2019) and (2) Columbia Moves (Monroe, Geraci, Turner-McGrievy, et al., 2019) – were designed to help answer these calls by directly targeting both individual and interpersonal factors via novel strategies delivered through digital mediums. The focus of these two case studies in e/mhealth-based behavioral weight loss and physical activity is to describe the (1) specific need, rationale, and goals for them, (2) intervention setting and team, (3) overarching design process, (4) theoretical foundations and corresponding intervention components, design considerations, and assessment elements, and (5) corresponding challenges and recommendations for future research.

VALUE OF PROMOTING BEHAVIORAL WEIGHT LOSS AND PHYSICAL ACTIVITY

According to the Centers for Disease Control and Prevention's Behavioral Risk Factor Surveillance System 2020 data, 65% of adults in Columbia, SC – the location of the NETworks and Columbia Moves interventions – report being overweight or obese (i.e., body mass index greater than or equal to 25 kg/m^2) and 48% report being insufficiently physically active (i.e., less than 150 minutes of moderate-intensity equivalent aerobic physical activity per week). These prevalence rates for overweight/obesity and insufficient physical activity are similar to those reported by adults in South Carolina (68% and 53%) and the United States (U.S.; 67% and 50%) (Centers for Disease Control and Prevention, 2020). Likewise, the most recent World Health Organization data show that just over half of the world's adult population is overweight and obese and 28% are insufficiently physically active (World Health Organization, 2021a, 2021b).

The high prevalence of overweight and obesity, as well as insufficient physical activity leads to numerous adverse health and economic consequences in the population. Both issues negatively affect quality of life. They are also linked to premature mortality and an increased risk for cardiovascular disease, type 2 diabetes mellitus, and some cancers (U.S. Department of Health and Human Services, 2018; Williams et al., 2015). Their consequences extend beyond those related to non-communicable diseases. For example, individuals with obesity are at an elevated risk for hospitalization and mortality in relation to acquiring a COVID-19 infection (Popkin et al., 2020). While research on how physical activity might interact with the immune system to affect COVID-19 infectivity and disease progression is needed, scientific evidence from other viral infections suggests that leading a physically active lifestyle can mitigate symptom severity and shorten recovery time (Simpson & Katsanis, 2020). In the U.S., obesity accounts for $92 billion per year or 5% of total adult health expenditures (Aljunid, 2021). Inadequate physical activity is estimated to account for $117 billion per year or about 9% of total healthcare costs (Carlson et al., 2015). Both issues pose a similar, significant economic burden globally (Ding et al., 2016; Okunogbe et al., 2021).

RATIONALE FOR INTERVENTIONS

Behavioral weight loss and physical activity interventions administered in-person have produced clinically meaningful weight losses and physical activity improvements, respectively (Diabetes Prevention Program Research Group, 2002; Greaves et al., 2011; Howlett et al., 2019; West et al., 2016). However, in-person interventions are frequently time intensive, costly, and limited in their reach and availability

(Beleigoli et al., 2019; Howlett et al., 2019; Mezuk & Allen, 2021; West et al., 2016). Given that 93% of adults in the U.S. use the internet and 85% own a smartphone, e/mhealth interventions represent a promising medium for broadening the reach and availability of evidence-based interventions (Pew Research Center, 2021a, 2021b). E/mHealth technology solutions also allow for efficient communication and distribution of information and are generally cost-effective (Iribarren et al., 2017).

Theory-based e/mhealth interventions have successfully leveraged study websites, mobile phone apps, and self-monitoring tools to deliver evidence-based behavior change techniques and subsequently drive short-term improvements in weight loss and physical activity; however, their ability to facilitate long-term maintenance of these early behavior changes remains less certain (Beleigoli et al., 2019; Jahangiry et al., 2017; Mateo et al., 2015; McEwan et al., 2020; Monroe et al., 2015). Most of these interventions (Beleigoli et al., 2019; Jahangiry et al., 2017; Mateo et al., 2015; McEwan et al., 2020; Monroe et al., 2015) have largely focused on individual determinants of health behavior and either failed to directly target the larger environmental context in which persons are embedded or failed to directly target it in an effective manner, potentially limiting the ability to produce sustained improvements (Mezuk & Allen, 2021; Sallis, 2018; Vo et al., 2019). Ecological models (Richard et al., 2011) recognize that health behaviors are impacted by dynamic interactions among factors that span multiple levels of influence (e.g., individual; interpersonal; environmental). Indeed, the obesity and insufficient physical activity pandemics result from multilevel causes that require multilevel interventions guided by ecological models to address them (Sallis, 2018; Vo et al., 2019).

In conjunction with targeting well-established individual determinants of weight loss and physical activity (e.g., self-efficacy; motivation; behavioral regulation), (Anderson et al., 2006; Teixeria et al., 2012; Varkevisser et al., 2019), harnessing the influence of existing social ties represents one promising approach for enhancing social support and shaping social norms for sustainable weight loss and physical activity promotion (Feeney & Collins, 2015; Leahey et al., 2012; Samuel-Hodge et al., 2017; Scarapicchia et al., 2017; Trost et al., 2002; Wing & Jeffery, 1999). Ecological models (Richard et al., 2011) and the Community Preventive Services Task Force (Kahn et al., 2002) endorse interventions that focus on strengthening and maintaining existing social relationships that provide support for health behavior change. A small number of physical activity interventions and behavioral weight loss interventions (Burke et al., 2006; Forthofer et al., 2019; Gorin et al., 2013, 2020; Johannesson et al., 2010; Kassavou et al., 2013; Kernot et al., 2019; Maher et al., 2015; Monroe et al., 2017; Patel et al., 2017, 2019; Pedersen et al., 2018; Spring et al., 2019; Wing & Jeffrey, 1999; Zhang et al., 2016) have explicitly targeted strategies to directly engage the interpersonal environment (e.g., walking groups; competitions) among adults; this prior research included studies focused on family members, (Patel et al., 2017) support partners/friends, (Spring et al., 2019; Wing & Jeffrey, 1999) co-workers, (Johannesson et al., 2010; Patel et al., 2019; Pedersen et al., 2018) and self-selected teams (Forthofer et al., 2019; Johannesson et al., 2010; Kernot et al., 2019; Maher et al., 2015; Patel et al., 2017). These studies have demonstrated feasibility (Burke et al., 2006; Forthofer et al., 2019; Johannesson et al., 2010; Kassavou et al., 2013; Kernot et al., 2019; Maher et al., 2015; Monroe et al., 2017; Patel et al., 2017, 2019; Pedersen et al., 2018; Spring et al., 2019; Wing & Jeffrey, 1999; Zhang et al., 2016) and promise (Burke et al., 2006; Forthofer et al., 2019; Johannesson et al., 2010; Kassavou et al., 2013; Maher et al., 2015; Monroe et al., 2017; Patel et al., 2017, 2019; Pedersen et al., 2018; Zhang et al., 2016) for promoting short-term health behavior change. However, some of these interventions were not scalable, used only self-reported measures of outcomes, or employed a non-randomized controlled trial design. Thus, important questions persist about best practices for achieving sustained improvements in weight and physical activity via the direct targeting of existing social contexts.

Studies have demonstrated that providing individuals with tangible resources can improve weight losses and physical activity (Gorin et al., 2013; Jakicic et al., 2003). The NETworks pilot study built upon this evidence using a novel, e/mhealth strategy. Its purpose was to use a randomized controlled trial to evaluate the efficacy of a four-month intervention that provided health-promoting technologies to leverage the influence of existing social ties for increasing objectively measured weight losses over existing best practices (Monroe, Geraci, Larsen, et al., 2019).

Further, gamification, or the use of game-like elements in nongame contexts, offers an engaging method for harnessing the influence of existing social ties for improved physical activity outcomes by seeking to promote positive social interactions and openness to positive behavioral influences (Deterding et al., 2011; Koivisto & Hamari, 2019). The Columbia Moves pilot study (Monroe, Geraci, Turner-McGrievy, et al., 2019) was one of the few physical activity promotion studies to rigorously evaluate the efficacy of a scalable gamification approach. Its purpose was to conduct a three-month pilot randomized controlled trial among self-selected teams of insufficiently physically active adults, comparing a standard theory-based intervention delivered using e/mhealth platforms (TECH) versus an identical intervention plus gamification components (TECH+GAMIFICATION) for promoting increases in objectively measured step counts and moderate-to-vigorous physical activity (Monroe, Geraci, Turner-McGrievy, et al., 2019).

RESEARCH SETTING AND INVESTIGATIVE TEAM

The University of South Carolina (UofSC) is a Carnegie-designated Very High Research Activity and Community Engagement institute, and its Arnold School of Public Health (ASPH) is the main public health and education research entity for South Carolina citizens (The Carnegie Classification of Institutions of Higher Education, n.d.). The ASPH's mission is to "improve population health and well-being by fostering innovative education and research that promotes health and healthy environments and use that knowledge to prevent and effectively respond to disease, disability, and environmental degradation in diverse communities" (ASPH, n.d.-c, Mission, Vision and Values section). It encompasses six departments, including the Department of Health Promotion, Education, and Behavior, the Department of Exercise Science, and the Department of Epidemiology and Biostatistics. Collectively, these three interdisciplinary departments apply the social and behavioral sciences in conjunction with statistical theory and techniques to improve public health, with research and education strengths in the areas of community-based interventions, digital health, and chronic disease prevention among many others (ASPH, n.d.-b, Health Promotion, Education, & Behavior section). The ASPH also houses five centers as part of the SmartState Program, which was established in 2002 by the South Carolina General Assembly to fund Centers of Economic Excellence in research areas designed to advance the state's economy and quality of life of its citizens via the innovative work of world-class researchers. One of these five SmartState Centers is the Technology Center to Promote Healthy Lifestyles (TecHealth Center). Its mission is focused on "fostering collaborations between scholars from multiple disciplines, innovative businesses, and community partners to design and evaluate technology-assisted lifestyle behavioral interventions that will improve the health, quality of life, and economic capacity of South Carolinians and people across the globe" (ASPH, n.d.-a, About the Center section).

Columbia is the capital city of South Carolina and the community in which UofSC is embedded. It is at the center of the Columbia metropolitan statistical area, which has a population of 829,470 based on data from the 2020 census (U.S. Census Bureau, 2021a). Columbia alone has a population of 136,632 persons, with 51% self-identifying as belonging to a racial minority group, 6% self-identifying as Hispanic or Latino of any race, 49% indicating they are female, and 74% representing adults ages 18 to 64 years. The median household income in Columbia is $47,286, and 44% of persons aged 25 years and older have earned a bachelor's degree or higher (U.S. Census Bureau, 2021b).

Many TecHealth Center pilot health behavior change interventions are launched in the Greater Columbia, SC region. The NETworks (Monroe, Geraci, Larsen, et al., 2019) and Columbia Moves trials (Monroe, Geraci, Turner-McGrievy, et al., 2019) stemmed from the TecHealth Center. The principal investigator of both studies is an Assistant Professor in the TecHealth Center and has substantial experience in the design, implementation, and evaluation of community-based, e/mhealth behavioral weight loss and physical activity interventions grounded in theory. To carry out both studies, she coordinated investigative teams across three departments with combined expertise in exercise physiology, nutrition, health psychology, digital health, and biostatistics. Additionally, UofSC's Web Development and Communications Core served as technology consultants with expertise in website design and hosting, custom web app development, data capture, survey management and design, data security, audio/video production, communications, and logo/graphic design (ASPH, n.d.-d, Web Development and Communications Core section). ASPH students supported the investigate teams, assisting with various study tasks (e.g., proofreading content; informally pilot testing intervention elements).

DESCRIPTION OF CASE STUDIES

Design Process

The planning of the NETworks (Monroe, Geraci, Larsen, et al., 2019) and Columbia Moves (Monroe, Geraci, Turner-McGrievy, et al., 2019) trials involved regular meetings among members of the investigative teams and the Web Development and Communications Core. To the extent possible – given the need to balance a sound, comprehensive intervention planning process with the practical considerations of funding and time constraints – notions from an established health behavior change intervention framework called Intervention Mapping (IM) (Glanz et al., 2015) helped inform the design process for the interventions. IM provides guidelines to ensure a health behavior change intervention is grounded in theory and empirical evidence. The characteristic theme highlighted throughout the IM framework is the importance of linking theory-based behavior and environmental change methods (i.e., a technique for changing a behavioral determinant) to determinants of health behavior, and in turn, translating those methods into practical applications (i.e., specific strategy that delivers the method in a way that fits the needs of the target behavior, population, and setting).

The initial steps of IM generally focus on what needs to be changed and for whom, as well as identifying determinants that influence the health behavior or problem (Kok et al., 2016). NETworks (Monroe, Geraci, Larsen, et al., 2019) and Columbia Moves (Monroe, Geraci, Turner-McGrievy, et al., 2019) represented studies that were part of a systematic line of inquiry, reflective of the principal investigator's expertise in the areas of e/mhealth, behavioral weight loss, physical activity, and social support. Relevant empirical literature, the identification of pertinent health behavior change theories, and findings from a previous technology-delivered physical activity intervention conducted by the principal investigator collectively supported the selection of determinants of interest for the interventions. A preliminary conceptual model that specified the relationship among factors believed to be related to the outcomes of interest was then developed for the experimental intervention arm of each respective study.

The selection of theory- and evidence-based behavior change methods and subsequent delineation of their translation into practical applications is the next step in the IM process (Glanz et al., 2015). The IM taxonomy of behavior change methods (Kok et al., 2016), a review of relevant empirical literature, and ideas generated via brainstorming by the investigative team guided the selection of theory-based methods and their translation to specific intervention strategies for the NETworks (Monroe, Geraci, Larsen, et al., 2019) and Columbia Moves (Monroe, Geraci, Turner-McGrievy, et al., 2019) interventions. The IM taxonomy of behavior change methods lists and defines methods across each level of the social ecological model (Glanz et al., 2015; Kok et al., 2016) and notes the evidence base underlying their inclusion in the taxonomy. It also describes the corresponding conditions that must be met for the method to be effective when it is translated into a practical application. The NETworks and Columbia Moves interventions were characterized by practical applications focused exclusively on individual and interpersonal factors linked to behavioral weight loss and physical activity, respectively. Once behavior change methods and their practical applications were solidified, the preliminary conceptual model for the experimental intervention arm of each respective study was finalized.

Integrating the practical applications or specific intervention strategies into a single program is the next IM step (Glanz et al., 2015). At this stage, the investigative team worked especially closely with the Web Development and Communications Core to determine how best to bring together the e/mhealth intervention elements. NETworks (Monroe, Geraci, Larsen, et al., 2019) contained a combination of in-person and technology-delivered elements. Columbia Moves (Monroe, Geraci, Turner-McGrievy, et al., 2019) was characterized by elements delivered entirely through technologies. Both NETworks and Columbia Moves integrated commercially available technologies (i.e., Fitbit physical activity trackers) and custom-built technologies (i.e., study website). Approaches informed by design research and a model of user engagement in online health behavior change interventions also helped shape the custom-built technological intervention components. With the characteristics of the target population kept in mind, personalization, the use of metaphors, aesthetics, and usability were all considered when merging the intervention strategies into a single program (Ludden et al., 2015; Short et al., 2015). The investigative teams tested the technological components built by the Web Development and Communications Core and provided feedback, which informed final refinements.

The investigative teams also created an evaluation plan, which is another important step of IM (Glanz et al., 2015). This plan included measuring not only the primary behavioral and health outcomes associated with each respective intervention, but it also involved measuring key psychosocial constructs targeted by the intervention strategies, intervention fidelity, and participant engagement and satisfaction. This plan ensured that insights could be gleaned into mechanisms of the intervention effects, informing future research.

Case Study 1: NETworks for Weight Loss

Funding

The NETworks study (Monroe, Geraci, Larsen, et al., 2019) was funded by an internal grant secured via UofSC's Advanced Support for Innovative Research Excellence program (ASPIRE; Office of the Vice President for Research, n.d.). This program gives postdoctoral fellows and faculty members the opportunity to compete for funding to begin promising new research for later external funding.

Theoretical Underpinnings

Three theories informed the design of the NETworks experimental intervention arm: social cognitive theory (Glanz et al., 2015), self-determination theory (Deci & Ryan, 2008), and social network theory (Glanz et al., 2015). Considerable evidence conducted among adults has demonstrated a favorable link between several theoretical constructs and behavioral weight loss (Gorin et al., 2013; Leahey et al., 2012; Robinson, Fleming, et al., 2014; Robinson, Thomas, et al., 2014; Samuel-Hodge et al., 2017; Varkevisser et al., 2019; Verstuyf et al., 2012; Wing & Jeffery, 1999). First, four constructs from the social cognitive theory served as intervention targets (Glanz et al., 2015). The social cognitive theory purports that one's health behavior is uniquely determined by a combination of personal cognitive factors, socioenvironmental influences, and supporting behavioral factors. Specifically, social support, or the perception of encouragement and aid a person receives from their social network, was targeted via methods designed to enhance network linkages (i.e., facilitating network members to mobilize their networks) and feedback (i.e., giving information to persons about the extent to which they are performing) (Kok et al., 2016). Social support encompasses informational support (e.g., advice; factual input), tangible support (e.g., take on a responsibility to give someone free time), emotional support (e.g., encouragement), and esteem support (e.g., validation of one's feelings) (Glanz et al., 2015). Normative beliefs, inclusive of both descriptive norms (i.e., knowledge of what others are doing in terms of the behavior) and injunctive norms (i.e., knowledge of what others think about engaging in the behavior), (Glanz et al., 2015) reflected a second construct that was targeted via both feedback and the mobilization of social networks (Kok et al., 2016). Self-efficacy, or a person's confidence in their ability to perform a behavior that leads to an outcome, reflected a third construct from the social cognitive theory that was targeted through several means (Glanz et al., 2015). Enactive mastery experiences (i.e., providing progressively challenging tasks with feedback to provide an indication of capability), verbal persuasion (i.e., using messages that suggest that the person possesses specific capabilities), self-monitoring of behavior (i.e., prompting persons to keep a record of behaviors), providing contingent rewards and reinforcement (i.e., praise, encouragement, or material items that are linked to the achievement of specified behaviors to increase the rates of those behaviors), and feedback (Kok et al., 2016) were all leveraged to influence self-efficacy. This collection of methods was also employed to target behavioral regulation, which is another construct that is part of the social cognitive theory and refers to the behavioral, cognitive, and/or emotional skills needed for changing behavior (Glanz et al., 2015; Kok et al., 2016).

Second, self-determination theory – a macrotheory of human motivation – also served as a foundation for the NETworks experimental intervention arm (Deci & Ryan, 2008; Monroe, Geraci, Larsen, et al., 2019). This theory purports that autonomous and controlled forms of motivation spark and direct behavior. Autonomous motivation encompasses intrinsic motivation (i.e., behavior is driven by internal rewards) and closely related types of extrinsic motivation in which the value of the activity is integrated into one's identity. Controlled motivation includes both external regulation (i.e., behavior is a function of reward or punishment) and introjected regulation (i.e., behavior is partially internalized and driven by factors such as avoidance of shame and contingent self-esteem). According to this theory, contextual factors are used to influence motivation via their effect on the basic psychological needs of autonomy, competence, and relatedness. Both feedback and the provision of contingent rewards were leveraged to target motivation to perform desired weight control practices (Kok et al., 2016).

Third, social network theory also underpinned the NETworks experimental intervention arm (Monroe, Geraci, Larsen, et al., 2019) and refers to the mechanisms by which social relations influence behavior. Social influence was specifically targeted, which is a social network process in which one changes their behavior to be the same as those in their network (Glanz et al., 2015). Methods involving information about others' approval of one's behavior, mobilization of social support, opportunities for social comparison, and feedback were harnessed to tap into the power of social influence (Kok et al., 2016).

Intervention Strategies

The NETworks experimental intervention arm (Monroe, Geraci, Larsen, et al., 2019) implemented the previously mentioned methods via a constellation of practical strategies designed to positively influence the designated theory-based behavioral determinants. Overweight and obese adults from the Greater Columbia, SC area received the intervention. (1) Each participant was given a Fitbit Zip physical activity tracker, which tracks steps, distance, and calories burned in real-time. These data were also visible on the corresponding Fitbit app, which contains additional features such as the ability to connect with fellow Fitbit users, engage in built-in physical activity challenges, and view progress towards goals over time. (2) Participants received access to the free version of the commercially available MyFitnessPal app, which allowed them to track their overall dietary intake, caloric intake, and fat intake among other parameters. They could also connect with fellow MyFitnessPal users through the app. (3) Participants received a digital body weight scale to monitor their weight. (4) Personalized calorie, fat gram, step, and moderate-to-vigorous physical activity goals were prescribed.

Further, (5) participants were provided with two additional Fitbit Zips and digital body weight scales and asked to share them with up to two adults of their choice within their existing social network to serve as support partners. (6) All participants engaged in weekly, one-hour, in-person, group counseling sessions led by experts in behavioral weight loss. Behavioral modification strategies (e.g., self-monitoring; setting and achieving goals; problem solving; social support; planning; relapse prevention) were taught and discussed during these sessions. (7) Content from the group counseling sessions was reiterated on a custom-built study website in the form of weekly informational lessons that were accessible through a responsive web app. A weight loss progress graph based on participants' self-reported weight entries, homework assignments associated with the topics addressed in the group counseling sessions, educational resources, and group member profiles were additional components housed on the study website. (8) Participants also received supportive feedback about their progress from the study interventionists through the study website (Monroe, Geraci, Larsen, et al., 2019).

Table 1 shows the connection among the e/mhealth-related NETworks experimental intervention arm strategies and corresponding methods by which they were designed to influence the targeted, theoretical-based behavioral constructs (Kok et al., 2016; Monroe, Geraci, Larsen, et al., 2019). In short, the act of participants inviting persons in their social network to serve as support partners through the provision of a Fitbit Zip and digital body weight scale reflected a unique way to mobilize social support and enhance existing social ties for behavioral weight loss. The Fitbit and MyFitnessPal built-in app features provided a way for participants, support partners, and any of the other participants' app 'friends' to exchange social support and compare their progress. Both apps allowed participants to monitor their physical activity and diet, gave them feedback (i.e., informational, graphical, and numerical), and provided reinforcement and contingent rewards (e.g., badges for achieving milestones). Participants' personalized physical activity and dietary goals fostered mastery experiences. Interventionist online messages to participants served as a conduit for information about others' approval of their behavior, positive reinforcement, and feedback about their progress. Finally, the weekly content presented on the study website represented a supplemental way to reiterate the value of harnessing social networks and social support for behavior change, while simultaneously reinforcing concepts tied to enhancing self-efficacy and self-regulation. Notably, the in-person, group counseling sessions were a central strategy for targeting all the designated behavioral determinants.

Further, efforts to spur engagement with and adherence to the NETworks experimental intervention (Monroe, Geraci, Larsen, et al., 2019) required certain e/mhealth design considerations (Ludden et al., 2015; Short et al., 2015). The prescribed goals, interventionist feedback, and participants' autonomy to select their support partners represented the design notion of personalization. Each participant could also upload information about themselves in the profile section of the website. Further, the aesthetics of the custom-built study website were similar to those of a high-quality commercial app to the extent possible. Lastly, the study website was designed to be as user-friendly as possible. For example, tabs and dropdown menus were used to foster easy navigation. The use of a responsive web app inherently also made it easy to view and navigate website content on a screen of any size.

The investigative team measured several outcomes beyond body weight to help gain insights into the NETworks experimental intervention's (Monroe, Geraci, Larsen, et al., 2019) mechanisms of influence. Perceived social support for physical activity and diet from family and friends was gauged using validated surveys (Sallis et al., 1987). Physical activity, dietary, and body weight self-monitoring rates based on Fitbit, MyFitnessPal, and website data, respectively, were also tracked. Data regarding engagement with the website (e.g., number of log-ins) and overall intervention satisfaction (e.g., would one recommend the program to a friend; helpfulness of support partners) were also captured.

Case Study 2: Columbia Moves

Funding

The Columbia Moves study (Monroe, Geraci, Turner-McGrievy, et al., 2019) was also funded by an internal grant secured via UofSC's ASPIRE program (Office of the Vice President for Research, n.d.).

Theoretical Underpinnings

Three theories formed the basis for the TECH+GAMIFICATION intervention of Columbia Moves (Monroe, Geraci, Turner-McGrievy, et al., 2019): social cognitive theory (Glanz et al., 2015), self-determination theory (Deci & Ryan, 2008), and social network theory (Glanz et al., 2015). Specifically, the same constructs from social cognitive theory (social support; normative beliefs; self-efficacy; behavioral regulation), self-determination theory (motivation), and social network theory (social influence) that

Table 1. NETworks e/mhealth-based intervention strategies and corresponding underlying behavior change methods and determinants

Determinant	Method	Intervention Strategy
Social support	• Enhancing network linkages • Feedback	• Providing a Fitbit and digital scale to share with support partners • Interventionist electronic feedback to participants • Informational content • Fitbit app and MyFitnessPal app
Social influence	• Information about others' approval • Mobilizing social support • Providing opportunities for social comparison • Feedback	• Providing a Fitbit and digital scale to share with support partners • Interventionist electronic feedback to participants • Informational content • Fitbit app and MyFitnessPal app
Descriptive and injunctive norms	• Mobilizing social networks • Feedback	• Providing a Fitbit and digital scale to share with support partners • Informational content • Fitbit app and MyFitnessPal app
Motivation	• Feedback • Provide contingent rewards	• Interventionist electronic feedback to participants • Fitbit app and MyFitnessPal app
Self-efficacy	• Enactive mastery experiences (goal setting; set graded tasks) • Verbal persuasion • Self-monitoring of behavior • Provide contingent rewards • Feedback • Reinforcement	• Interventionist electronic feedback to participants • Informational content • Fitbit app and MyFitnessPal app • Graded, personalized step goals • Personalized dietary goals
Behavioral regulation	• Enactive mastery experiences (goal setting; set graded tasks) • Verbal persuasion • Self-monitoring of behavior • Provide contingent rewards • Feedback • Reinforcement	• Interventionist electronic feedback to participants • Informational content • Fitbit app and MyFitnessPal app • Graded, personalized step goals • Personalized dietary goals

Source: (Deci & Ryan, 2008; Glanz et al., 2015; Kok et al., 2016; Monroe, Geraci, Larsen, et al., 2019)

were targeted in NETworks were also addressed in TECH+GAMIFICATION. Substantial evidence has shown a favorable relationship between these constructs and physical activity (Anderson et al., 2006; Ball et al., 2010; Feeney & Collins, 2015; Glanz et al., 2015; McAuley & Blissmer, 2000; Scarapicchia et al, 2017; Teixeria et al., 2012; Trost et al., 2002).

An additional construct from social cognitive theory called collective efficacy (i.e., belief in the ability of a group of individuals to perform purposeful actions to achieve an outcome) also helped inform the design of the TECH+GAMIFICATION intervention (Monroe, Geraci, Turner-McGrievy, et al., 2019) through enactive team mastery experiences, self-monitoring of behavior, and the provision of contingent rewards and feedback (Beverly & Wray, 2010; Kok et al., 2016). Further, insights from behavioral economics (Glanz et al., 2015) were used to design the TECH+GAMIFICATION intervention, including precommitment (i.e., committing to a specific future action or goal achievement) (Rogers et al., 2014), loss aversion (i.e., the tendency to prefer to avoid losses over acquiring equivalent gains) (Schmidt &

Zank, 2005), and goal gradients (i.e., the notion that the next highest level or goal is attainable) (Patel et al., 2019) in conjunction with the psychological principle of the fresh start effect (i.e., the tendency for aspirational behavior around temporal markers such as the beginning of a week) (Dai et al., 2014).

Intervention Strategies

The TECH+GAMIFICATION intervention (Monroe, Geraci, Turner-McGrievy, et al., 2019) was comprised of carefully designed strategies that reflected practical manifestations of the aforementioned methods used to target the associated theoretical constructs. Insufficiently active adults from the Greater Columbia, SC area who were part of self-selected teams comprised of existing social ties (i.e., family; friends; co-workers) received the intervention. (1) Each participant received a Fitbit Alta HR physical activity tracker, which tracks steps, active minutes, heart rate, and other parameters in real-time. These data were also displayed on the corresponding Fitbit app. (2) Participants also received and committed to achieving personalized, graded, physical activity goals. They had the autonomy to choose how they achieved their goals.

Additionally, they had access to a custom-built study website, which was accessible via a responsive web app and housed the other intervention components. Gamification represented the primary, experimental intervention strategy (Deterding et al., 2011). (3) Teams chose a team name and competed against each other in a step competition delivered through the study website. The status of each team's physical activity performance was displayed on a leaderboard. Each participant could also view their team members' physical activity progress, as well as their own progress. Each participant's Fitbit data was accessible via the Fitbit application programming interface (API) and automatically pulled into the study website, allowing for near, real-time team and individual physical activity updates to be displayed. A second gamification strategy called the (4) Shoe Mascot Weekly Challenge Game was also delivered via the study website and embodied the behavioral economics principles of loss aversion and the fresh start effect. Each team had a shoe mascot avatar. The object of the game was to keep their shoe mascot on a virtual walking trail (highest level of the game) and away from sedentary objects (lower levels of the game) by fulfilling physical activity challenges. At the start of each week, all teams were presented with two weekly physical activity challenges that were associated with a point value. The challenges varied every week, meaning some were team-based (e.g., your team must collectively accumulate more steps this week compared to what your team achieved during the prior week) and others were individual-based (e.g., one team member will be randomly selected to see if they achieved their personal step goal for the week). During some weeks, teams could select which challenges they wanted to complete from a menu of options. If challenges were fulfilled, then the team would not lose points and thus stay on the highest level of the game. If the challenges were not met, then the team would lose points and eventually descend to the lower levels. Each team's status in the game was displayed on the leaderboard. Teams that won the step competition and Shoe Mascot Weekly Challenge Game received recognition in the form of a congratulatory message visible to all participants (Monroe, Geraci, Turner-McGrievy, et al., 2019).

The TECH+GAMIFICATION (Monroe, Geraci, Turner-McGrievy, et al., 2019) study website contained other standard physical activity behavior change components. (5) Information about behavior change topics (e.g., social support; setting and achieving goals; rewards for goal achievement; overcoming barriers to being active; benefits of physical activity; relapse prevention) were delivered on a weekly basis via online handouts, videos, external websites, and an expert blog. (6) Participants also received supportive feedback about their progress from the study interventionists via email and could submit questions or comments to them through an online journal.

Table 2 provides a summary of the connection among the primary TECH+GAMIFICATION intervention (Monroe, Geraci, Turner-McGrievy, et al., 2019) strategies and corresponding methods by which they were designed to influence the targeted, theoretical-based behavioral determinants. Briefly, the structure of the team step competition and Shoe Mascot Weekly Challenge Game naturally served many purposes. Both were designed to strengthen existing social network linkages and mobilize social support for physical activity. Simultaneously, these strategies provided feedback about physical activity progress (i.e., numerical and graphical), opportunities for social comparison, team mastery experiences, positive reinforcement, and a contingent reward (Kok et al., 2016).

The built-in social features on the Fitbit app gave participants an additional avenue to strengthen their social networks, exchange social support for physical activity, and compare their progress. It naturally allowed for self-monitoring of physical activity, the provision of feedback (i.e., informational, graphical, and numerical), reinforcement, and contingent rewards (e.g., fireworks for reaching step goal). Further, the personalized, graded physical activity goals facilitated individual mastery experiences. Interventionist electronic messages naturally provided feedback about participants' progress towards their goals and represented another method for delivering social support. It also provided information about others' approval of their physical activity behavior and positive reinforcement. Finally, the weekly informational content served as a supplemental way to mobilize social support, enhance social network linkages, and reiterate important concepts tied to self-efficacy and behavioral regulation (Kok et al., 2016).

Equally as important, several design considerations were reflected in the TECH+GAMIFICATION intervention (Monroe, Geraci, Turner-McGrievy, et al., 2019) to help drive engagement and adherence (Ludden et al., 2015; Short et al., 2015;). For example, personalization was reflected in the physical activity goals, interventionist feedback, and participants' autonomy to select how they wanted to achieve their goals. At a team level, both the selection of a team name and challenges to complete reflected a form of personalization. Additionally, the storyline for the Shoe Mascot Weekly Challenge Game acted as a metaphor. In doing so, it was meant to contribute to positive emotions towards physical activity and make participants' pursuit of their goals feel meaningful by connecting to their intuitive comprehension of the world. Further, the aesthetics of the custom-built study website were crafted in a way to mimic the professional look of a high-quality commercial app to the extent possible. Lastly, the study website was designed to be as user-friendly as possible. For example, the Fitbit information was seamlessly integrated with the other study website features, creating a central location to view the status of the gamified elements. Tabs and dropdown menus were used to make it easy to navigate different sections of the website, and the use of a responsive web app inherently meant that the website content would conform to fit a screen of any size without losing its usability.

To gain insights into how the TECH+GAMIFICATION intervention (Monroe, Geraci, Turner-McGrievy, et al., 2019) influenced participants' physical activity behavior change, the investigative team measured changes in two of the primary theoretical constructs using validated surveys (i.e., perceived social support from teammates and their broader social network; motivation) (Sallis et al., 1987; Wilson et al., 2006). Fitbit self-monitoring rates were also automatically tracked, reflecting one indicator of self-regulatory behavior. Data regarding engagement with the website (e.g., number of log-ins; number of hits on a website feature) and overall intervention satisfaction (e.g., would one recommend the program to a friend; likes and dislikes about the program) were also captured.

Table 2. Columbia moves e/mhealth-based TECH+GAMIFICATION intervention strategies and corresponding underlying behavior change methods and determinants

Determinant	Method	Intervention Strategy
Social support	• Enhancing network linkages • Feedback	• Step competition (leaderboard) and Shoe Mascot Game (weekly challenges) • Interventionist electronic feedback to participants • Informational content • Fitbit app
Social influence	• Information about others' approval • Mobilizing social support • Providing opportunities for social comparison • Feedback	• Step competition (leaderboard) and Shoe Mascot Game (weekly challenges) • Interventionist electronic feedback to participants • Informational content • Fitbit app
Descriptive and injunctive norms	• Mobilizing social networks • Feedback	• Step competition (leaderboard) and Shoe Mascot Game (weekly challenges) • Informational content • Fitbit app
Motivation	• Feedback • Provide contingent rewards	• Step competition (leaderboard) and Shoe Mascot Game (weekly challenges) • Interventionist electronic feedback to participants • Fitbit app
Self-efficacy	• Enactive mastery experiences (goal setting; set graded tasks) • Verbal persuasion • Self-monitoring of behavior • Provide contingent rewards • Feedback • Reinforcement	• Step competition (leaderboard) and Shoe Mascot Game (weekly challenges) • Interventionist electronic feedback to participants • Informational content • Fitbit app • Graded, personalized step goals
Collective efficacy	• Enactive team mastery experiences (goal setting; set graded tasks) • Self-monitoring of behavior • Feedback • Provide contingent rewards	• Step competition (leaderboard) and Shoe Mascot Game (weekly challenges) • Fitbit app
Behavioral regulation	• Enactive mastery experiences (goal setting; set graded tasks) • Verbal persuasion • Self-monitoring of behavior • Provide contingent rewards • Feedback • Reinforcement	• Step competition (leaderboard) and Shoe Mascot Game (weekly challenges) • Interventionist electronic feedback to participants • Informational content • Fitbit app • Graded, personalized step goals

Source: (Beverly & Wray, 2010; Deci & Ryan, 2008; Glanz et al., 2015; Kok et al., 2016; Monroe, Geraci, Turner-McGrievy, et al., 2019)

CHALLENGES AND RECOMMENDATIONS

Several challenges exist for the research fields in terms of designing e/mhealth behavioral weight loss and physical activity interventions. (1) Determining how best to integrate both research and commercial digital health solutions for behavior change interventions can be complex. Popular commercial mobile apps often have a great reach, but the extent to which they include evidence- and theory-based behavior change strategies and involve health scientists in the development process can be low (Arigo et al, 2019).

Data access is often limited or completely restricted, and the underlying design process is generally propriety. Research mobile apps are increasingly being designed with a grounding in evidence and theory, but they rarely reach the population due to various constraints (e.g., funding; app development process and evidence generation takes time; behavioral scientists generally do not have entrepreneurial skills) (Arigo et al, 2019; Sezgin, 2021). Leveraging both research and commercial apps in the same intervention can be inconvenient for users because information is not always integrated in a central location.

Some of these challenges were apparent in the NETworks (Monroe, Geraci, Larsen, et al., 2019) and Columbia Moves (Monroe, Geraci, Turner-McGrievy, et al., 2019) studies. For example, NETworks participants had to access more than one app as part of the study, and although the Columbia Moves TECH+GAMIFICIATION intervention was able to integrate the Fitbit physical activity data with the study web app, other Fitbit features (e.g., connecting with Fitbit 'friends') were still only accessible via the Fitbit app. While the Web Development and Communications Core was able to access the Fitbit API and retrieve a rich set of Fitbit data for the Columbia Moves study, it required a significant time investment upfront. Further, both the NETworks and Columbia Moves study websites were developed to look and function like some of the most well-designed commercial apps. Yet, a native app would better duplicate the look and functionality of a sophisticated commercial app and be more customizable. Unfortunately, native apps can be more costly and complicated to develop and make available for use. Calls have been made for the academic and industry sectors to find common ground and bring together their respective advantages to grow successful partnerships that can be leveraged to improve public health (Arigo et al, 2019; Sezgin, 2021).

Relatedly, the traditional randomized controlled trial has typically been used to scientifically test e/mhealth solutions. The NETworks (Monroe, Geraci, Larsen, et al., 2019) and Columbia Moves (Monroe, Geraci, Turner-McGrievy, et al., 2019) trials used this research design to isolate the effect of a single strategy as part of a multicomponent intervention on outcomes of interest. Yet, this process is quite inefficient. (2) Technology is constantly evolving, so by the time evidence is generated from a traditional randomized controlled trial, the technology that was used in it may be out-of-date. For instance, the Fitbit model used in the NETworks study has been discontinued. Beyond the frequent mismatch between the pace of research and the evolution of technological capabilities, (3) the traditional randomized controlled trial makes it difficult to efficiently test mechanisms of efficacy. Behavioral scientists are increasingly considering using other frameworks. For example, the Multiphase Optimization Strategy allows the independent effect of multiple intervention strategies on changes in mediators and outcomes of interest to efficiently be tested (Arigo et al, 2019).

(4) Another challenge concerns the theories and methods used to inform the NETworks (Monroe, Geraci, Larsen, et al., 2019) and Columbia Moves (Monroe, Geraci, Turner-McGrievy, et al., 2019) interventions. The IM taxonomy of behavior change methods stems from psychological theories that represent a codification of empirical evidence and an even larger set of behavior change techniques has been established for categorization of intervention content (Michie et al., 2013). Nevertheless, calls have been made for the conduction of additional meta-analyses of key studies to build a more robust, quantified base of support (Kok et al., 2016).

Additionally, as interventions continue to leverage e/mhealth technologies, the ability to collect longitudinal data at an intensive frequency will be enhanced, and thus, intervention timing and content can be adapted for each individual over time based on these data to optimize health behavior change. (5) Yet, traditional health behavior change theories used to inform intervention design may be inadequate to keep pace with these advancements in technological capabilities because they are based on differentiating between person, not intra-individual differences (Riley et al., 2011). (6) They also predominantly take conscious regulatory processes into consideration even though non-conscious processes may also play a role in behavior (Cleo et al., 2020; Rebar et al., 2016). While traditional theories still have a place in the intervention design process, calls have been made to adopt dynamical system models to help create theories that are a better match for informing the intra-individual dynamics of e/mhealth interventions. Calls have also been made to include non-conscious regulatory processes in theories (Rebar et al., 2016).

(7) Finally, the traditional theories that were used to inform the NETworks (Monroe, Geraci, Larsen, et al., 2019) and Columbia Moves (Monroe, Geraci, Turner-McGrievy, et al., 2019) interventions primarily focus on behavioral determinants as opposed to user engagement. While some design principles were leveraged to help foster user engagement with and adherence to the e/mhealth intervention strategies, there is a need for greater consideration of design elements and theories of engagement in the intervention development process. Gauging the target population's perspectives about design preferences via formative research or at the end of an intervention can help inform the development of future e/mhealth interventions. The science of engagement for health behavior change is in its infancy (Arigo et al., 2019), but opportunities abound to generate additional evidence in this area.

CONCLUSION

The design process for the NETworks (Monroe, Geraci, Larsen, et al., 2019) and Columbia Moves (Monroe, Geraci, Turner-McGrievy, et al., 2019) interventions involved interdisciplinary teams of experts and a sound understanding of the e/mhealth behavioral weight loss and physical activity evidence base. Intervention strategies were shaped by traditional behavior change theories, the IM taxonomy of behavior change methods (Kok et al., 2016), adaptations of other psychological principles (Glanz et al., 2015), design research (Ludden et al., 2015; Short et al., 2015), and investigator expertise. While designing these interventions required a significant upfront investment in terms of time and cost, it paid off in the form of relatively smooth and successful implementation and evaluation processes. The fields of e/mhealth-based behavioral weight loss and physical activity will always be evolving as the evidence base grows and advancements in technology push investigators to think about leveraging more dynamic theories, research designs, and design principles supported by ongoing scientific progress.

ACKNOWLEDGMENT

This research was supported by the University of South Carolina's Office of the Vice President for Research. The author would also like to thank fellow NETworks and Columbia Moves investigative team members and study participants for their support of and contributions to this research.

REFERENCES

Aljunid, S. M. (2021). Obesity, a costly epidemic. In S. Al-Sabah., A. Aminian, L. Angrisani, E. Al Haddad, & L. Kow (Eds.), Laparoscopic Sleeve Gastrectomy. Springer. https://doi.org/ doi:10. 1007/978-3-030-57373-7_2

Anderson, E. S., Wojcik, J. R., Winett, R. A., & Williams, D. M. (2006). Social-cognitive determinants of physical activity: The influence of social support, self-efficacy, outcome expectations, and self-regulation among participants in a church-based health promotion study. *Health Psychology*, *25*(4), 510–520. doi:10.1037/0278-6133.25.4.510

Arigo, D., Jake-Schoffman, D. E., Wolin, K., Beckjord, E., Hekler, E. B., & Pagoto, S. L. (2019). The history and future of digital health in the field of behavioral medicine. *Journal of Behavioral Medicine*, *42*, 67–83. doi:10.100710865-018-9966-z

Arnold School of Public Health. (n.d.a). *About the center.* https://sc.edu/study/colleges_schools/ public_health/research/research_centers/techealth/about/index.php

Arnold School of Public Health. (n.d.b). *Health promotion, education, & behavior.* https://sc.e du// study/colleges_schools/public_health/study/areas_of_study/health_promotion_education_and behavior/ index.php

Arnold School of Public Health. (n.d.c). *Mission, vision and values*. https://sc.edu/study/collegc s_schools/ public_health/about/mission_vision_values/index.php

Arnold School of Public Health. (n.d.d). *Web development and communications core.* https://sc. edu/study/ colleges_schools/public_health/internal/faculty_staff/administrative_departments/ope rations_and_accreditation/web_development_and_communciations/index.php

Ball, K., Jeffery, R. W., Abbott, G., McNaughton, S. A., & Crawford, D. (2010). Is healthy behavior contagious: Associations of social norms with physical activity and healthy eating. *The International Journal of Behavioral Nutrition and Physical Activity*, *7*, 86. doi:10.118 6/1479-5868-7-86

Beleigoli, A. M., Andrade, A. Q., Cancado, A. G., Paulo, M. N. L., Diniz, M. D. H., & Ribeiro, A. L. (2019). Web-based digital health interventions for weight loss and lifestyle habit changes in overweight and obese adults: Systematic review and meta-analysis. *Journal of Medical Internet Research*, *21*(1), e298. Advance online publication. doi:10.2196/jmir.9609

Beverly, E. A., & Wray, L. A. (2010). The role of collective efficacy in exercise adherence: A qualitative study of spousal support and type 2 diabetes management. *Health Education Research*, *25*(2), 211–223. doi:10.1093/her/cyn032

Burke, S. M., Carron, A. V., Eys, M. A., Ntoumanis, N., & Estabrooks, P. A. (2006). Group versus individual approach? A meta-analysis of the effectiveness of interventions to promote physical activity. *Sport and Exercise Psychology Review*, *2*(1), 19–35.

Carlson, S. A., Fulton, J. E., Pratt, M., Yang, Z., & Adams, E. K. (2015). Inadequate physical activity and health care expenditures in the United States. *Progress in Cardiovascular Diseases*, *57*(4), 315–323. doi:10.1016/j.pcad.2014.08.002

Centers for Disease Control and Prevention. (2020). *BRFSS prevalence & trends data.* https://www.cdc. gov/brfss/brfssprevalence/index.html

Cleo, G., Beller, E., Glasziou, P., Isenring, E., & Thomas, R. (2020). Efficacy of habit-based weight loss interventions: A systematic review and meta-analysis. *Journal of Behavioral Medicine*, *43*(4), 519–532. https://doi.or/10.1007/s10865-019-00100-w

Dai, H., Milkman, K. L., & Riis, J. (2014). The fresh start effect: Temporal landmarks motivate aspirational behavior. *Management Science*, *60*(10), 2563–2582. doi:10.1287/ mnsc.2014.1901

Deci, E. L., & Ryan, R. M. (2008). Self-determination theory: A macrotheory of human motivation, development, and health. *Canadian Psychology*, *49*(3), 182–185. doi:10.1037/ a0012801

Deterding, S., Dixon, D., Khaled, R., & Nacke, L. (Eds.). (2011). *Proceedings of the 15th international academic MindTrek conference: Envisioning future media environments*. ACM Digital Library. https://dl.acm.org/doi/10.1145/2181037.2181040

Diabetes Prevention Program Research Group. (2002). Reduction in the incidence of type 2 diabetes with lifestyle intervention or metformin. *The New England Journal of Medicine*, *346*, 393–403. doi:10.1056/ NEJMoa012512

Ding, D., Lawson, K. D., Kolbe-Alexander, T. L., Finkelstein, E. A., Katzmarzyk, P. T., van Mechelen, W., & Pratt, M. (2016). The economic burden of physical inactivity: A global analysis of major non-communicable diseases. *Lancet*, *388*(10051), 1311–1324. doi:10.10 16/S0140-6736(16)30383-X

Feeney, B. C., & Collins, N. L. (2015). A new look at social support: A theoretical perspective on thriving through relationships. *Personality and Social Psychology Review*, *19*(2), 113–147. doi:10.1177/1088868314544222

Forthofer, M., Wilcox, S., Kinnard, D., Hutto, B., & Sharpe, P. A. (2019). Sumter county on the move! Evaluation of a walking group intervention to promote physical activity within existing social networks. *Journal of Physical Activity & Health*, *16*(1), 22–28. doi:10.1123/jpah.2017-0603

Glanz, K., Rimer, B. K., & Viswanath, K. (Eds.). (2015). *Health behavior: Theory, research, and practice*. Jossey-Bass.

Gorin, A. A., Powers, T. A., Gettens, K., Cornelius, T., Koestner, R., Mobley, A. R., Pescatello, L. S., & Huedo-Medina, T. B. (2020). A randomized controlled trial of a theory-based weight loss program for couples. *Health Psychology*, *39*(2), 137–146. doi:10.1037/hea000080 8

Gorin, A. A., Raynor, H. A., Fava, J., Maguire, K., Robichaud, E., Trautvetter, J., Crane, M., & Wing, R. R. (2013). Randomized controlled trial of a comprehensive home environment-focused weight-loss program for adults. *Health Psychology*, *32*, 128–137. doi:10.1037/a0026959

Greaves, C. J., Sheppard, K. E., Abraham, C., Hardeman, W., Roden, M., Evans, P. H., & Schwarz, P.The IMAGE Study Group. (2011). Systematic review of reviews of intervention components associated with increased effectiveness in dietary and physical activity interventions. *BMC Public Health*, *11*, 119. Advance online publication. doi:10.1186/1471-2458-11-119

Howlett, N., Trivedi, D., Troop, N. A., & Chater, A. M. (2019). Are physical activity interventions for healthy inactive adults effective in promoting behavior change and maintenance, and which behavior change techniques are effective? A systematic review and meta-analysis. *Translational Behavioral Medicine*, *9*(1), 147–157. doi:10.1093/tbm/ iby010

Iribarren, S. J., Cato, K., Falzon, L., & Stone, P. W. (2017). What is the economic evidence for mHealth? A systematic review of economic evaluations of mHealth solutions. *PLoS One*, *12*(2), e0170581. Advance online publication. doi:10.1371/journal.pone.0170581

Jahangiry, L., Farhangi, M. A., Shab-Bidar, S., Rezaei, F., & Pashaei, T. (2017). Web-based physical activity interventions: A systematic review and meta-analysis of randomized controlled trials. *Public Health*, *152*, 36–46. doi:10.1016/j.puhe.2017.06.005

Jakicic, J. M., Winters, C., Lang, W., & Wing, R. R. (1999). *Effects of intermittent exercise and use of home exercise equipment on adherence, weight loss, and fitness in overweight women: A randomized trial.* https://doi.org/ doi:10.1001/jama.282.16.1554

Johannesson, M., Ostling, R., & Ranehill, E. (2010). The effect of competition on physical activity: A randomized trial. *B.E. The B.E. Journal of Economic Analysis & Policy Pol*, *10*(1). Advance online publication. doi:10.2202/1935-1682.2555

Kahn, E. B., Ramsey, L. T., Brownson, R. C., Heath, G. W., Howze, E. H., Powell, K. E., Stone, E. J., Rajab, M. W., & Corso, P. (2002). The effectiveness of interventions to increase physical activity: Review and update. *American Journal of Preventive Medicine*, *34*(12), 1996–2001. doi:10.10160749-3797(02)00434-8

Kassavou, A., Turner, A., & French, D. P. (2013). Do interventions to promote walking in groups increase physical activity? A meta-analysis. *The International Journal of Behavioral Nutrition and Physical Activity*, *10*, 18. doi:10.1186/1479-5868-10-18

Kernot, J., Lewis, L. K., Olds, T., & Maher, C. (2019). Effectiveness of a Facebook-delivered physical activity intervention for postpartum women: A randomized controlled trial. *Journal of Physical Activity & Health*, *16*(2), 125–133. doi:10.1123/jpah.2017-0573

Koivisto, J., & Hamari, J. (Eds.). (2019). *GamiFIN conference.* https://trepo.tuni.fi/bitstream/handle/10024/117608/Gamification_of_physical_activity_2019.pdf?sequence=2

Kok, G., Gottlieb, N. H., Peters, G. Y., Mullen, P. D., Parcel, G. S., Ruiter, R. A. C., Fernandez, M. E., Markham, C., & Bartholomew, L. K. (2016). A taxonomy of beahaviour change methods: An intervention mapping approach. *Health Psychology Review*, *10*(3), 297–312. doi:10.1080/17437199.2015.1077155

Leahey, T. M., Kumar, R., Weinberg, B. M., & Wing, R. R. (2012). Teammates and social influence affect weight loss outcomes in a team-based weight loss competition. *Obesity (Silver Spring, Md.)*, *20*, 1413–1418. doi:10.1038/oby.2012.18

Ludden, G. D. S., van Rompay, T. J. L., Kelders, S. M., & van Gemert-Pijnen, J. E. W. C. (2015). How to increase reach and adherence of web-based interventions: A design research viewpoint. *Journal of Medical Internet Research*, *17*(7), e172. Advance online publication. doi:10.2196 /jmir.4201

Maher, C. F., Ferguson, M., Vandelanotte, C., Plotnikoff, R., De Bourdeaudhuij, I., Thomas, S., Nelson-Field, K., & Olds, T. (2015). A web-based, social networking physical activity intervention for insufficiently active adults delivered via Facebook app: Randomized controlled trial. *Journal of Medical Internet Research, 17*(7), e174. Advance online publication. doi:10.2196/jmir.4086

Mateo, G. F., Granado-Font, E., Ferre-Grau, C., & Montana-Carreras, X. (2015). Mobile phone apps to promote weight loss and increase physical activity: A systematic review and meta-analysis. *Journal of Medical Internet Research, 17*(11), e253. Advance online publication. doi:10.2196/jmir.4836

McAuley, E., & Blissmer, B. (2000). Self-efficacy determinants and consequences of physical activity. *Exercise and Sport Sciences Reviews*, *28*(2), 85–88.

McEwan, D., Rhodes, R. E., & Beauchamp, M. R. (2020). What happens when the party is over? Sustaining physical activity behaviors after intervention cessation. *Behavioral Medicine (Washington, D.C.)*, *48*(1), 1–9. doi:10.1080/08964289.2020.1750335

Mezuk, B., & Allen, J. (2021). Rethinking the goals of diabetes prevention programs. *Diabetes Care*, *44*(11), 2457–2459. doi:10.2337/dci21-0038

Michie, S., Richardson, M., Johnston, M., Abraham, C., Francis, J., Hardeman, W., Eccles, M. P., Cane, J., & Wood, C. E. (2013). The behavior change technique taxonomy (v1) of 93 hierarchically clustered techniques: Building an international consensus for the reporting of behavior change interventions. *Annals of Behavioral Medicine*, *46*(1), 81–95. doi:10.1 00712160-013-9486-6

Monroe, C. M., Bassett, D. R. Jr, Fitzhugh, E. C., Raynor, H. A., & Thompson, D. L. (2017). Effect of adding online social support tools to an adult walking program: A pilot randomized controlled trial. *Health Promotion Practice*, *18*(1), 84–92. doi:10.1177/1524839915626 674

Monroe, C. M., Geraci, M., Larsen, C. A., & West, D. S. (2019). Feasibility and efficacy of a novel technology-based approach to harness social networks for weight loss: The NETworks pilot randomized controlled trial. *Obesity Science & Practice*, *5*(4), 354–365. doi:10. 1002/osp4.352

Monroe, C. M., Geraci, M., Turner-McGrievy, G., Wallace, K., Jake-Schoffman, D. E., Bucko, A., & Brazendale, K. (2019, June). *Leveraging a social network approach via gamification and mobile technology to increase physical activity among adults: a cluster randomized controlled trial* [Conference presentation]. International Society of Behavioral Nutrition and Physical Activity Annual Meeting, Prague, Czech Republic.

Monroe, C. M., Thompson, D. L., Bassett, D. R. Jr, Fitzhugh, E. C., & Raynor, H. A. (2015). Usability of mobile phones in physical activity-related research: A systematic review. *American Journal of Health Education*, *46*, 196–206. doi:10.1080/19325037.2015.1044141

Office of the Vice President for Research. (n.d.). *ASPIRE*. https://sc.edu/about/offices_and_divi sions/research/internal_funding_awards/faculty/aspire/

Okunogbe, A., Nugent, R., Spencer, G., Ralston, J., & Wilding, J. (2021). Economic impacts of overweight and obesity: Current and future estimates for eight countries. *BMJ Global Health*, *6*(10), e006351. Advance online publication. doi:10.1136/bmjgh-2021-006351

Patel, M. S., Benjamin, E. J., Volpp, K. G., Fox, C. S., Small, D. S., Massaro, J. M., Lee, J. J., Hilbert, V., Valentino, M., Taylor, D. H., Manders, E. S., Mutalik, K., Zhu, J., Wang, W., & Murabito, J. M. (2017). Effect of a game-based intervention designed to enhance social incentives to increase physical activity among families: The BE FIT randomized clinical trial. *JAMA Internal Medicine*, *177*(11), 1586–1593. doi:10.1001/jamainternmed.2017.3458

Patel, M. S., Small, D. S., Harrison, J. D., Fortunato, M. P., Oon, A. L., Rareshide, C. A. L., Reh, G., Szwartz, G., Guszcza, J., Steier, D., Kalra, P., & Hilbert, V. (2019). Effectiveness of behaviorally designed gamification interventions with social incentives for increasing physical activity among overweight and obese adults across the United States: The STEP UP randomized clinical trial. JAMA Internal Medicine, 179(12), 1624-1632. https://doi.org/ed.2019.3505 doi:10.1001/jamainternm

Pedersen, C., Halvari, H., & Williams, G. C. (2018). Worksite intervention effects on motivation, physical activity, and health: A cluster randomized controlled trial. *Psychology of Sport and Exercise*, *35*, 171–180. doi:10.1016/j.psychsport.2017.11.004

Pew Research Center. (2021a, April 7). *Internet/broadband fact sheet.* https://www.pewresearch. org/internet/fact-sheet/internet-broadband/

Pew Research Center. (2021b, April 7). *Internet/broadband fact sheet.* https://www.pewresearch. org/internet/fact-sheet/mobile/

Popkin, B. M., Du, S., Green, W. D., Beck, M. A., Algaith, T., Herbst, C. H., Alsukait, R. F., Alluhidan, M., Alazemi, N., & Shekar, M. (2020). Individuals with obesity and COVID-19: A global perspective on the epidemiology and biological relationships. *Obesity Reviews*, *21*, e13128. Advance online publication. doi:10.1111/obr.13128

Rebar, A. L., Dimmock, J. A., Jackson, B., Rhodes, R. E., Kates, A., Starling, J., & Vandelanotte, C. (2016). A systematic review of the effects of non-conscious regulatory processes in physical activity. *Health Psychology*, *10*(4), 395–407. doi:10.1080/ 17437199.2016.1183505

Richard, L., Gauvin, L., & Raine, K. (2011). Ecological models revisited: Their uses and evolution in health promotion over two decades. *Annual Review of Public Health*, *32*, 307–326. doi:10.1146/annurev-publhealth-031210-101141

Riley, W. T., Rivera, D. E., Atienza, A. A., Nilsen, W., Allison, S. M., & Memelstein, R. (2011). Health behavior models in the age of mobile interventions: Are our theories up to task? *Translational Behavioral Medicine*, *1*, 53–71. doi:10.100713142-011-0021-7

Robinson, E., Fleming, A., & Higgs, S. (2014). Social norms and weight loss prompting healthier eating: Testing the use of health and social norm based messages. *Health Psychology*, *33*(9), 1057–1064. doi:10.1037/a0034213

Robinson, E., Thomas, J., Aveyard, P., & Higgs, S. (2014). What everyone else is eating: A systematic review and meta-analysis of the effect of informational eating norms on eating behavior. *Journal of the Academy of Nutrition and Dietetics*, *114*(3), 414–429. doi:10.1016/j.jand.2013.11.009

Rogers, T., Milkman, K. L., & Volpp, K. G. Commitment devices: Using initiatives to change behavior. (2014). *JAMA*, *311*(20), 2065-2066. https://doi.org/ doi:10.1001/jama.2014.3485

Sallis, J. F. (2018). Needs and challenges related to multilevel interventions: Physical activity examples. *Health Education & Behavior*, *45*(5), 661–667. doi:10.1177/109019811879 6458

Sallis, J. F., Grossman, R. M., Pinski, R. B., Patterson, T. L., & Nader, P. R. (1987). The development of scales to measure social support for diet and exercise behaviors. *Preventive Medicine*, *16*, 825–836. doi:10.1016/0091-7435(87)90022-3

Samuel-Hodge, C. D., Holder-Cooper, J. C., Gizlice, Z., Davis, G., Steele, S. P., Keyserling, T. C., Kumanyika, S. K., Brantely, P. J., & Svetkey, L. P. (2017). Family partners in lifestyle support (PALS): Family-based weight loss for African American adults with type 2 diabetes. *Obesity (Silver Spring, Md.)*, *25*, 45–55. doi:10.1002/oby.21700

Scarapicchia, T. M. F., Amireault, S., Faulkner, G., & Sabiston, C. M. (2017). Social support and physical activity participation among healthy adults: A systematic review of prospective studies. *International Review of Sport and Exercise Psychology*, *10*(1), 50–83. doi:10.1080/17 50984X.2016.1183222

Schmidt, U., & Zank, H. (2005). What is loss aversion? *Journal of Risk and Uncertainty*, *30*(20), 157–167. doi:10.100711166-005-6564-6

Sezgin, E. (2021). Can we use commercial mobile apps instead of research mobile apps in healthcare research? *Frontiers in Public Health*, *9*, 685439. doi:10.3389/fpubh.202 1.685439

Short, C. E., Rebar, A. L., Plotnikoff, R. C., & Vandelanotte, C. (2015). Designing engaging online behaviour change interventions: A proposed model of user engagement. *The European Health Psychologist*, *17*(1), 32–38.

Simpson, R., & Katsanis, E. (2020). The immunological case for staying active during the COVID-19 pandemic. *Brain, Behavior, and Immunity*, *87*, 6–7. doi:10.1016/j.bbi.2020. 04.041

Spring, B., Pfammatter, A. F., Hoffman, S. A., Pellegrini, C., McFadden, H. G., Siddique, J., Hedeker, D., & Collins, L. (2019). Determining the optimal 6-month weight loss treatment package: Results of the opt-in study. *Annals of Behavioral Medicine*, *53*, S443–S443.

Teixeria, P. J., Carraca, E. V., Markland, D., Silva, M. N., & Ryan, R. M. (2012). Exercise, physical activity, and self-determination theory: A systematic review. *The International Journal of Behavioral Nutrition and Physical Activity*, *9*, 78. doi:0.1186/1479-5868-9-78

The Carnegie Classification of Institutions of Higher Education. (n.d.). *About Carnegie classification*. https://carnegieclassifications.iu.edu/

Trost, S. G., Owen, N., Bauman, A. E., Sallis, J. F., & Brown, W. (2002). Correlates of adults' participation in physical activity: Review and update. *Medicine and Science in Sports and Exercise*, *4*(1), 1996–2001. doi:10.1249/01.MSS.0000038974.76900.92

U.S. Census Bureau. (2021a). *2020 Population and Housing State Data*. https://www.ce nsus.gov/library/visualizations/interactive/2020-population-and-housing-state-data.html

U.S. Census Bureau. (2021b). *QuickFacts*. https://www.census.gov/quickfacts/fact/table / columbiacitysouthcarolina,US/RHI125219

U.S. Department of Health & Human Services. (2018). *2018 Physical activity guidelines advisory committee scientific report.* https://health.gov/sites/default/files/2019-09/PAG_Advisory_Committee_Report.pdf

Varkevisser, R. D. M., van Stralen, M. M., Kroeze, W., Ket, J. C. F., & Steenhuis, I. H. M. (2019). Determinants of weight loss maintenance: A systematic review. *Obesity (Silver Spring, Md.)*, *20*, 171–211. doi:10.1111/obr.12772

Verstuyf, J., Patrick, H., Vansteenkiste, M., & Teixeira, P. (2012). Motivational dynamics of eating regulation: A self-determination theory perspective. *The International Journal of Behavioral Nutrition and Physical Activity*, *9*(1), 21. doi:10.1186/1479-5868-9-21

Vo, L., Albrecth, S. S., & Kershaw, K. N. (2019). Multilevel interventions to prevent and reduce obesity. *Current Opinion in Endocrine and Metabolic Research*, *4*, 62–69. doi:10.101 6/j.coemr.2018.11.002

West, D. S., Coulon, S. M., Monroe, C. M., & Wilson, D. K. (2016). Evidence-based lifestyle interventions for obesity and type 2 diabetes: The Look AHEAD intensive lifestyle intervention as exemplar. *The American Psychologist*, *71*(7), 614–627. doi:10.1037/a0040394

Williams, E. P., Mesidor, M., Winters, K., Dubbert, P. M., & Wyatt, S. B. (2015). Overweight and obesity: Prevalence, consequences, and causes of a growing public health problem. *Current Obesity Reports*, *4*, 363–370. doi:10.100713679-015-0169-4

Wilson, P. M., Rodgers, W. M., Loitz, C. C., & Scime, G. (2006). "It's who I am…Really!" The importance of integrated regulation in exercise contexts. *Journal of Applied Biobehavioral Research*, *11*(2), 79–104. doi:10.1111/j.1751-9861.2006.tb00021.x

Wing, R. R., & Jeffery, R. W. (1999). Benefits of recruiting participants with friends and increasing social support for weight loss and maintenance. *Journal of Consulting and Clinical Psychology*, *67*(1), 132–138. doi:10.1037/0022-006X.67.1.132

World Health Organization. (2021a). *Obesity and overweight.* https://www.who.int/news-room/f act-sheets/detail/obesity-and-overweight

World Health Organization. (2021b). *Physical activity.* https://www.who.int/news-room/fact-she ets/detail/physical-activity

Zhang, J., Brackbill, D., Yang, S., Becker, J., Herbert, N., & Centola, D. (2016). Support or competition? How online social networks increase physical activity: A randomized controlled trial. *Preventive Medicine Reports*, *4*, 453–458. doi:10.1016/j.pmedr.2016.08.008

ADDITIONAL READING

Alzahrani, A. S., Gay, V., Alturki, R., & AlGhamdi, J. M. (2021). Towards understanding the usability attributes of AI-enabled eHealth mobile applications. *Journal of Healthcare Engineering*, *2021*, 5313027. Advance online publication. doi:10.1155/2021/5313027

Connell, L. E., Carey, R. N., de Bruin, M., Rothman, A. J., Johnston, M., Kelly, M. P., & Michie, S. (2019). Links between behavior change techniques and mechanisms of action: An expert consensus study. *Annals of Behavioral Medicine, 53*(8), 708-720. https://doi.org/ 082 doi:10.1093/abm/ka

Fernandez, M. E., Ruiter, R. A. C., Markham, C. M., & Kok, G. (2019). Intervention mapping: Theory- and evidence-based health promotion program planning: Perspective and examples. *Frontiers in Public Health, 7*, 209. doi:10.3389/fpubh.2019.00209

Hekler, E. B., Michie, S. M., Pavel, M., Rivera, D. E., Collins, L. M., Jimison, H. B., Garnett, C., Parral, S., & Spruijt-Metz, D. (2016). Advancing models and theories for digital behavior change interventions. *American Journal of Preventive Medicine, 51*(5), 825–832. doi:10.1016/j.amepre.2016.06.013

Joseph, R. P., Royse, K. E., & Benitez, T. J. (2019). A systematic review of electronic and mobile health (e- and mHealth) physical activity interventions for African American and Hispanic women. *Journal of Physical Activity & Health, 16*(3), 230–239. doi:10.1123/jpah.20 18-0103

Lopes, Pereira, A., Magalhães, P., Oliveira, A., & Rosário, P. (2019). Gamification: focus on the strategies being implemented in interventions: A systematic review protocol. *BMC Research Notes, 12*(1), 100–100. doi:10.118613104-019-4139-x

Perski, O., Blandford, A., West, R., & Michie, S. (2017). Conceptualising engagement with digital behaviour change interventions: A systematic review using principles from critical interpretive synthesis. *Translational Behavioral Medicine, 7*, 254–267. doi:10.1007 13142-016-045 3-1

Schembre, S. M., Liao, Y., Robertson, M. C., Dunton, G. F., Kerr, J., Haffey, M. E., Burnett, T., Basen-Engquist, K., & Hicklen, R. S. (2018). Just-in-time feedback in diet and physical activity interventions: Systematic review and practical design framework. *Journal of Medical Internet Research, 20*(3), e106. Advance online publication. doi:10.2196/jmir.8701

KEY TERMS AND DEFINITIONS

API (Application Programming Interface): Collection of functions allowing two pieces of software to communicate with each other.

Behavioral Economics: Application of psychological principles to economic decision-making processes (can be adapted for application to health behavior decisions).

Engagement: Level of interaction with intervention features.

Gamification: The influence affordances (i.e., components and mechanics that structure games) have on psychological outcomes and experiences, and in turn, motivation and behavioral outcomes.

Self-Determination Theory: Comprehensive framework for the study of human motivation.

Social Cognitive Theory: An interpersonal-oriented theory that describes the collective influence of cognitive, socioenvironmental, and behavioral factors on health behavior.

Social Network Theory: The role of social relationships in spreading information, channeling influence, and enabling health behavior change.

Social Support: Perception of the provision of aid or comfort one receives from their social network to help them cope with stressors.

Chapter 6
Exemplars in eHealth Education Interventions:
The Case Study of Cardiovascular Health

Patrick J. Dunn
https://orcid.org/0000-0002-3997-8335
Walden University, USA & American Heart Association, USA

Hadi Danawi
Walden University, USA

ABSTRACT

Digital health tools have been used in a wide variety of healthcare services including promoting healthy behaviors and improving health outcomes in people with chronic conditions including cardiovascular disease. However, there is no "one size fits all" approach for these digital health tools. The need for individualized designs in order to maximize usability, effectiveness, and sustainability of use among patients has been highlighted. Intelligent health solutions are used to guide the design of effective and personalized tools for patients with cardiovascular diseases. The integration of health behavior theories and well-defined care plans in the intervention/tool are key to ensure maximum effectiveness and benefits to the patients. To this end, this chapter aims to provide a background on digital health tools in cardiovascular health and a detailed overview of the various components of intelligent health solutions that guide the tool design process.

INTRODUCTION TO DIGITAL HEALTH TOOLS

The concept of digital health tools has been rapidly evolving since its first introduction in the year 2000 (Guo et al., 2020). Digital health tools encompass a wide range of technologies including mobile applications, health information technology, smart wearable devices, remote monitoring, health platforms, telehealth, and telemedicine (Guo et al., 2020).

DOI: 10.4018/978-1-7998-9490-2.ch006

Recent data showed that the number of these tools are continuously increasing. The number of health applications available in the App Store currently exceed 318,000 applications and more than 200 new applications are added on a daily basis (IQVIA, 2017). This booming trend resulted from the World Health Organization (WHO) resolution issued in 2005 that urged countries to prioritize the development of an action plan for implementing and expanding eHealth services to promote equitable, affordable, and universal access to healthcare services (WHO, 2021). This resolution recognized the potential of health technologies to improve population health outcomes by advancing medical services and allowing the exchange and sharing of health information (WHO, 2021). The United Nations 2030 Sustainable Development Goal (SDG) Agenda has also highlighted the potential of health technologies to accelerate progress towards achieving health-related SDGs (WHO, 2021). With this recognition, there has been a growing global consensus in the health community that the use of digital health tools will contribute to ensuring that 1 billion more people will benefit from universal health coverage, will be better protected from health emergencies, and will have enhanced health and well-being (WHO, 2021).

Digital health tools have been used in a wide variety of healthcare services including promoting healthy behaviors (for example: smoking cessation, healthy eating, and physical activity), improving health outcomes in people with chronic conditions such as cardiovascular disease, diabetes, and mental health conditions, and providing remote access to treatments (for example: computerized cognitive behavioral therapy for mental health and somatic problems) (Ghose et al., 2021; Murray et al., 2016). Despite its application in various healthcare services, digital health tools have many drawbacks and challenges. The main aspects challenging the application of most digital health tools is its cost, the availability of information technology, and the literacy level of the consumer, in addition to privacy issues (such as data privacy and algorithm bias) (Rudolph et al., 2008; Paul and Das, 2017a; 2017b). However, digital health tools also create new opportunities in the field of health and offer various benefits for traditional healthcare services. These technologies can aid in disease prevention, early diagnosis, and management of chronic conditions (FDA, 2020). In addition to giving healthcare providers a more holistic view of patient health through access to relevant data, digital health tools also provide an opportunity for patients to have more control over their health enabling them to make better informed decisions (FDA, 2020). The use of digital health technologies aims to enhance efficiency, improve access and quality of health services while reducing associated cost, and ensure healthcare services that are more personalized for patients (FDA, 2020). The recent COVID-19 pandemic has accentuated the necessity of digital health tools, where lockdowns and public health measures have prompted health care professionals to adopt different remote strategies and ehealth tools to provide healthcare services to their patients (Monaco et al., 2021).

To this end, this chapter aims to provide a background on digital health tools in cardiovascular health - a major public health concern globally. The chapter also provides a detailed overview of the various components of intelligent health solutions that is developed by the American Heart Association (AHA) to guide the tool design process.

AN OVERVIEW OF DIGITAL HEALTH TOOLS IN CARDIOVASCULAR HEALTH: A NEED FOR AN INTERVENTION

Similar to other healthcare services, the use of digital health solutions is promising for improving cardiovascular health outcomes in patients (Eapen et al., 2016). Cardiovascular diseases (CVD) is a term used to describe health conditions affecting the heart or blood vessels. CVD, covering a wide range of health conditions, including ischemic heart disease, cerebrovascular disease, hypertensive heart disease, peripheral vascular disease, rheumatic heart disease, cardiomyopathies and arrhythmias, are the leading cause of death globally (Eckel et al., 2014; Santo et al., 2016; Vos et al., 2017). According to the Global Burden of Disease Report (2017), the burden of CVD continues to increase globally. In 2019, it was estimated that there are over 523 million CVD cases and 18.6 million deaths recorded globally due to CVD (Roth et al., 2020). As such, CVD is recognized as a major public health concern worldwide and various risk factors associated with CVD (for example obesity) are on the rise globally. Preventing CVD from occurring and addressing associated risk factors are important to improve public and community health, prevent disability and pre-mature deaths, and reduce associated healthcare costs.

Besides addressing the biological risk factors, proper CVD management and prevention is based on addressing modifiable behavioral risk factors by promoting healthy lifestyle (such as regular physical activity and healthy diet) (Artinian et al., 2010; Spring et al., 2013) and adhering to prescribed medications (Roth et al., 2020). However, delivering comprehensive risk factor management to diverse populations have proven to be challenging due to practical, logistical, financial, and geographical obstacles (Santo et al., 2016). Moreover, communication between patients and cardiologists and other healthcare providers regarding behavioral changes and health education is often limited, as the doctor's visits are usually short and focuses mainly on the patients' response to treatment (Dunn & Walker, 2019). The Center for Disease and Prevention's (CDC) 2016 National Health Survey reported that only 23.5% of adults meet the recommended physical activity level for aerobic and muscle-strengthening activity and 75% have a diet low in vegetables, fruits, dairy, and oils (Roger et al., 2020). In addition, 15.5% of adults are smokers and 67% are overweight or obese (Angell et al., 2020). Therefore, the American Heart Association have emphasized the need to reach patients in ways that will lead to successful and sustainable behavioral changes (Dunn & Walker, 2019).

Behavioral change is key in preventing CVD outcomes; it is defined by the Encyclopedia of Human Behavior (2012) as a process of behavior change by which a change in a stimulus event or condition that immediately follows a response decreases the future frequency of that response. Health behavioral change is required when patients perform what is considered as a risk behavior (e.g., smoking, excessive drinking) or do not meet healthy behavior recommendations (e.g., performing physical activity) (Ratz and Lippke, 2021). Several behavior change techniques (BCTs) are applied in digital health tools and interventions, including behavioral practice and rehearsal (such as hands-on training and interactive discussion), demonstration of behavior (through giving presentations, video clips, and distributing educational material), instruction on how to perform behavior, and practical social support to induce change in patients (Virtanen et al., 2021).

With the rising burden of CVD, the state of cardiovascular health in the United States and around the world is far from ideal (Roger et al., 2020). The American Heart Association has made a transformative shift from reducing the impact of cardiovascular disease to improving healthy life expectancy (Angell et al., 2020). To achieve the goal of improving the quality and quantity of life (healthy life expectancy), the reach of services to prevent and manage CVD must increase to under-resourced communities and hard to reach places (Harrington et al., 2020).

Applications of digital health tools in CVD health can help healthcare professionals reach a wider group of people in more efficient and effective ways to induce behavioral change (Santo et al., 2016). These tools have many potential applications in CVD health. Digital health applications that target behavioral changes such as smoking cessation, increasing physical activity, promoting health diets, and enhancing adherence to medications are used to improve CVD health outcomes (Eapen et al., 2016; Santo et al., 2016). Moreover, mobile applications can also improve the health literacy[1] of CVD patients and can monitor and manage their health conditions through record keeping and automatic reminders. Smartwatches can provide continuous rhythm monitoring and help in the diagnosis of arrhythmias. Inflatable blood pressure cuffs that are connected to phone applications are another example of monitoring applications in CVD health. In addition, recent innovations in artificial intelligence (AI) and machine learning (ML) can allow the development of new medicines and more accurate prediction of CVD outcomes (Fogel & Kvedar, 2018; Santo et al., 2016; Topol, 2019).

TARGET POPULATION AND SETTINGS

The most common target populations for digital health interventions are individuals with heart failure, diabetes, and high blood pressure. These innovative tools provide solutions focused on healthy behaviors such as physical activity, nutrition, weight management, tobacco cessation and stress management. Emerging solutions include atrial fibrillation detection, home-based cardiac rehabilitation supported by a digital platform, and stroke rehabilitation. At the core of all these solutions is an increasing emphasis on mental health to address the stress and emotions related to CVD, behavior change, motivation and engagement.

NATURE OF EDUCATIONAL INTERVENTIONS

Digital solutions have promise in the prevention and management of CVD because they are complex conditions that require a high level of patient engagement and rely on biometrics and behaviors. Educational interventions provide people with the required knowledge about key concepts in order to evaluate information about health interventions and may help them evaluate the trustworthiness of health interventions and make informed decisions (Cusack, 2018). There are different forms of digital educational interventions, including digital therapeutics, remote patient monitoring (RPM), telemedicine, guideline directed medical therapy (GDMT) and cognitive based solutions designed for learning and behavior change. The technologies associated with these solutions include artificial intelligence (AI), machine learning (ML), natural language processing (NPL), gaming, chat bots, computer vision, virtual and augmented reality, biosensors, social navigators, and connected devices. Advanced solutions, such as digital therapeutics will typically combine technologies, such as advanced biometrics with AI/ML. Some solutions use gaming to increase engagement. These advanced solutions also will combine human and artificial intelligence to leverage the time and skill of the healthcare professional, while creating a more personalized experience.

EFFECTIVENESS OF DIGITAL HEALTH TOOLS IN IMPROVING HEALTH OUTCOMES

Despite the fast proliferation of digital health tools and the increased interest in health applications among patients, there has been limited evidence on their effectiveness in improving targeted health outcomes in general (Krebs & Duncan, 2015). This is due to difficulties encountered in developing a knowledgebase for guiding decisions about digital health tools (Murray et al., 2016). In general, evaluating the effectiveness of digital health tools has been hindered by the rapid change in digital product development, which mandates these tools to be constantly evolving to keep up with the changing trends (Patrick et al., 2016). As such, efficacy trials that extend for a prolonged period of time may become obsolete in supporting current decisions about these tools (Murray et al., 2016). The absence of data on the effectiveness of health applications in improving health outcome are also a result of lack of standards for collecting data across health applications and the absence of healthcare regulation for these applications (Wisniewski et al., 2019). In its 2020–2025 global strategy on digital health, the WHO highlighted the importance of developing metrics for the monitoring and evaluation of the effectiveness of digital health strategies and tools (WHO, 2021). Recently, governments and donors have added more stringent guidelines on digital health innovations, calling for better evaluation of quality and effectiveness of these interventions (WHO, 2019).

Although there have been some studies evaluating the effectiveness of digital health technologies targeting cardiovascular health outcomes (Agarwal et al., 2011; Magid et al., 2013; Thomas et al., 2014), the evidence of effect is still at an early stage (Solberg Nes, 2020). There is a lack of robust scientific evidence to date to support the use of these digital health tools in cardiovascular health. In fact, few of these tools have been designed or evaluated in a clinical setting (Green et al., 2008; Solberg Nes, 2020). In addition, many of the health applications available to the public have not been designed with input from professionals and are often developed without guidance from evidence-based standards (Santo et al., 2016). A review showed that only 15% of these applications are associated with medical organizations or societies (Margolis et al., 2013). Even those applications designed with support from health organizations, evidence on their effectiveness is still limited. Recent reviews found that studies evaluating the effectiveness of digital health tools on improving cardiovascular health outcomes had low-quality evidence due to the limited number of RCTs, small sample sizes, and/or the short duration of the studies (Coorey et al., 2018). In addition, the literature showed conflicting evidence regarding the effectiveness and benefits of digital tools in improving CVD health outcomes. Even those tools whose effectiveness have been established, the literature reports low effect size and lack of sustained use of them (Morrison, 2015). Reviews also found that many mobile health applications are developed with limited consideration to theoretical frameworks to guide behavioral changes (Flores-Mateo et al., 2015).

Underutilization of eHealth/mHealth Intervention

CVD are high volume, high-cost conditions that can be prevented with the right targeted intervention, but these interventions are highly under-utilized. For example, only one in four patients that are eligible for cardiac rehabilitation following a cardiovascular event participate in a program (Beatty et al., 2018; Ritchey et al., 2020). Health technology has the potential to increase access to healthcare services and democratize access to health information (Topol, 2015). While much of the promise of digital intervention are yet to be realized, newer technology such as AI, virtual reality/augmented reality (VR/AR) and advanced biosensing continue to emerge. COVID-19 has been a catalyst in transforming the role of technology allowing many patients access to healthcare services and information without the risk of exposure.

Digital interventions, however, cannot result in positive health outcomes if they are not utilized. Digital interventions, therefore, are placing even greater emphasis on using a human centered design,

Figure 1. A layered, AI-ML approach to digital health
SDOH: Social determinants of health (demographic, social, cultural); Medical (diagnosis, treatment, genetics); Behavioral (lifestyle, mental health, biometric); Personality (learning style, motivation, digital preferences).

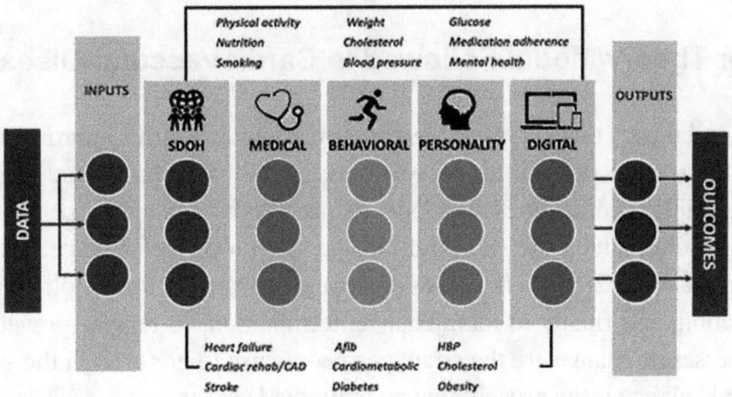

being more patient and person centered, addressing social navigation, and following a science-based approach rooted in behavior change (Bhavnani et al., 2017). Beyond simply providing access to information, and the ability to track and share information between the patient and their healthcare team, many digital interventions are following best practices in health coaching and self-care (Artinian et al., 2010; Riegel et al., 2017), facilitating the improvement in digital health literacy (Magnani et al., 2018; Smith & Magnani, 2019), using creative methods of delivering motivational interviewing, and making the solution highly personalized by identifying and addressing the social, medical, lifestyle and behavior, learning and digital preferences, and even personality traits of the individual. This layered approach is more aligned with an AI/ML solution which focuses on only one issue, such as the condition, the behavior, or the social determinant (Figure 1).

Intelligent Health Solutions to Guide the Design of Effective and Personalized Digital Health Tools

For effective applications of digital health tools, information on the adoption and effectiveness of using these tools among different population groups is needed. In addition, the literature has demonstrated that users' characteristics (attitudes, beliefs, perceptions) and the contextual and cultural factors that influence the patients' health can impact the effectiveness of these tools (Murray et al., 2016). The latter is particularly important in cardiovascular health because associated behavioral risk factors may be influenced by a wide range of social and cultural factors, such as perception of disease risks, interaction with and trust in the healthcare system, social support, etc. (Borzecki et al., 2005; Bosworth & Oddone, 2002). To overcome these challenges, the need for a more in-depth understanding about patients' engagement with digital health tools is required (Morrison, 2015). For example, in digital tools that promote behavioral change through enhancing health literacy, the content of the health education needs to be delivered to patients in a manner that is acceptable and understandable, motivating patients to adopt the targeted behavioral change (Magnani et al., 2019). Although healthcare providers know who their patients are, their health status and what they are doing to address their health problems, their motivation to act in a certain way is not well understood (Smith and Magnani, 2019). And without this information, healthcare providers face challenges in communicating health information and engaging patients in a way that enable behavioral changes. Thus, the need for understanding the different communication preferences among patients is necessary to develop effective digital tools and interventions.

Health Behavior Theory/Model Followed in Cardiovascular Diseases eTools

The primary behavioral theory that serves as the conceptual model for this approach is the transtheoretical model (TTM). The transtheoretical model was developed by Prochaska and DiClemente (1983) as a way to integrate multiple theories into one model focused on behavior change. The core constructs of the transtheoretical model include the stages of change, the process of change, decision balance, and self-efficacy (Prochaska et al., 2008). The stages of change go from precontemplation, to contemplation, to preparation, to action, and finally to maintenance, termination, or relapse prevention (Prochaska et al., 2008). The processes of change are the strategies people use to go through the stages (Prochaska et al., 2008). Decisional balance is the process that an individual uses to make their decision, including the risks and benefits of the change compared to the risks and benefits of the status quo (Prochaska et al., 2008). Self-efficacy and temptation are factors that either build or erode the person's confidence that they could make the change if they decide to do so (Prochaska et al., 2008).

Additionally, three educational theories are used to support the behavior change. Bloom's taxonomy is a hierarchical educational framework beginning with foundational skills that build to the point of mastery (Krathwohl, 2002). A revised taxonomy takes into account the cognitive process dimension that is a broader range of factors that impact teaching and learning. This taxonomy includes remembering, understanding, applying, analyzing, evaluating, and creating (Krathwohl, 2002). This educational approach can be applied to the progression of health literacy (Table 3).

This applies not only to teaching reading, vocabulary, and math to children, but also to teaching terms, concepts, and decision making to adults that can be applied to health literacy. The theory of multiple intelligences is used to emphasize the individualization and pluralization of instruction (Gardner, 2002). In his theory, Gardner warns of the use of "learning style" – which is not to be confused with "multiple intelligence", as it may lead to confusion since its notion is not coherent and there is no evidence that learning styles analysis yields more successful outcomes than a "one size fits all approach" (Strauss, 2013). The zone of proximal development and problem-based learning are theories of cognitive development that use the metaphor of a scaffold to support individuals' learning needs through their learning zone (Richard-Amato, 2003). The use of plain language is an example of establishing understanding at the base of the learning zone. Bloom's taxonomy, the theory of multiple intelligences, and the zone of proximal development can be applied to the development of health literacy skills for patients with cardiovascular disease and diabetes.

Remote Patient Monitoring

Remote patients monitoring (RPM) has been studied extensively in blood pressure control and heart failure. Traditional forms of remote patient monitoring include biometric measures, such as weight, blood pressure, and glucose monitoring. Remote monitoring also includes subjective measures of symptoms, mood, medication adherence, tobacco use, and lifestyle factors, such as activity and nutrition. With the advent of and continued innovation in wearable technology breakthroughs have occurred in detection of

Table 1. Comparison of the revised Bloom's taxonomy to the progression of health literacy

Bloom's Taxonomy	Health Literacy Skills
Remembering	Navigation
Understanding	Communication
Applying	Decision making
Analyzing	Numeracy
Learning	Reading comprehension

irregular heartbeats, such atrial fibrillation. The Apple Heart Study results were reported at ACC (2019) demonstrating the value of early detection of chronic conditions.

Blood Pressure

Improving the diagnosis, treatment, and control of hypertension is critical for achieving cardiovascular health of all Americans. Of the 116.4 million American adults estimated to have hypertension, nearly half do not have their condition under control, with many cases going undiagnosed (Welton et al., 2017).

Ensuring accurate blood pressure (BP) measurement is an essential component to both identifying and managing hypertension. The diagnosis and management of hypertension has been primarily based on the measurement of BP in the healthcare setting. But BP may differ considerably when measured in the office versus outside the office. Many patients who have elevated BP when measured in the office have normal BP when measured outside the office, a phenomenon dubbed white-coat hypertension. Other patients have normal in-office BP readings and elevated readings when measured outside the office, known as masked hypertension.

Regular out-of-office BP measurements provided through self-monitored blood pressure (SMBP) readings help exclude these misclassifications to ensure patients are diagnosed and managed more accurately. SMBP is associated with a reduction in BP and improved BP control. Additional evidence indicates that the benefits of SMBP are greatest when given with co-interventions (e.g., educational materials or classes, behavioral change management, medication management, telemonitoring, etc.). In response, the AHA and the U.S. Department of Health and Human Services (DHHS) launched the National Hypertension Control Initiative (NHCI) to improve BP and hypertension risk factor control in these more vulnerable communities. The ultimate goal was to create a healthier, more equitable country.

In a meta-analysis conducted in 2015, there was evidence that self-measurement of BP was superior to usual care (24 trials) in reducing systolic (3.1 mmHg) and diastolic (2.0 mm Hg) BP at 6 months. The researchers also provided evidence that self-measurement of BP interventions compared with usual care (13 trials) improved antihypertensive medication adherence (standardized mean difference, 0.21; 95% CI, 0.08–0.34) (Burke et al., 2015).

RPM may serve as a vital conduit for improving hypertension control and reducing the economic burden that stems from the costly hospital stays that result from acute events related to hypertension. There is an opportunity to get serial measurements outside of the healthcare setting and provide greater awareness of blood pressure numbers and trends.

The challenge is the validity and reliability of the measures. While all blood pressure devices go through a clearance process with the Food and Drug Administration (FDA), that does not mean that these devices are valid measures of blood pressure. The Validated Device List, developed by the American Medical Association and administered by NORC is a process to ensure the validity of the measurement.

Heart Failure

Patients with heart failure (HF) should receive specific education to facilitate HF self-care. After discharge many patients may need disease management programs. Lack of social support for patient with HR is associated with higher hospitalization rates. Effective systems of care coordination should pay special attention to care transitions. Every patient should have a clear, detailed, and evidence-based plan of care. Systems of care should be designed to improve communications, be patient centered, and multidisciplinary. Weight, symptoms and medication adherence outside of the healthcare setting, which can lead to early identification of signs of decompensation, is essential in disease management.

Although recent systematic reviews and meta-analyses have shown a positive effect of RPM on HF-related admissions, and mortality, the bulk of the literature consists of low-quality and inconsistent evidence. More importantly, evidence from randomized trials has been unfavorable, with inconsistent, and some showing no or negative effect (Burke et al., 2015). In addition, heart failure RPM programs are challenged by reporting bias, where only positive information is reported.

In summary, there are various aspects that need to be considered in the development of digital health interventions/tools to ensure effectiveness during application. These include designing a human centered approach in the intervention to increase uptake and utilization, the integration of evidence-based health behavior theories to effectively induce change, and methods for evaluating the effectiveness of these digital health tools.

EXEMPLAR: INTELLIGENT HEALTH SOLUTIONS

One example of a tool developed by the American Heart Association (2021) Center for Health Technology and Innovation used to guide the digital health design process is the Intelligent Health Solutions (IHS), which gives CVD patients access to the American Heart Association's digital Care Plans. The Care Plan, which will be discussed in detail below, is a digital health tool designed to help users better understand and manage their CVD conditions. The IHS digital Care Plan is tailored for each user based on their heart health needs and priorities. It is over 10 years in the making, working with scientific advisors with expertise in cardiology, technology, and behavior change and multiple technology platforms focused on cardiovascular disease, including high blood pressure, heart failure, cardiac rehabilitation, atrial fibrillation, and stroke (Eapen et al., 2016). While definitive health impact is still being evaluated, early adopters of this model have demonstrated improved blood pressure control, better adherence to guideline based medical therapy (GDMT), improved detection of atrial fibrillation, and improved participation in digital and hybrid forms of cardiac rehabilitation (Thomas et al., 2014, Burke et al., 2015; McConnell et al., 2018).

The IHS has evolved over time based on use and prior experiences, including:

- **Science-based**: With well over 400,000 health related apps in the app stores (Datta, 2020) there is a lot of 'digital snake oil' available to patients and consumers. The first step in any digital solution is to be innovative, but science and evidence based trusted sources should be prioritized, and the user should be able to review the science themselves.

- **Modular approach**: Patients with heart disease, heart failure, stroke and diabetes have multiple conditions. Ignoring the other conditions or having multiple care plans is not optimal, so the plan needs to build on the needs of the user.
- **Adaptive:** There is no single solution that will meet the needs of all of the users. Some people are hard to motivate and engage in their health, while other people are highly motivated. Some users need a motivational approach and others need direction. The solution must adapt so that it can engage a larger segment of the population.
- **Person centered:** While the focus of many digital solutions has been on the health professional and the health system, the patient is the primary user, and the solutions must focus on their needs. Patients are less focused on the achievement of clinical guidelines and more interested in solutions that will make them feel better and improve their quality of life.
- **Multi-lingual and culturally appropriate:** Digital health solutions are used around the globe and therefore need to be delivered in multiple languages. Language translations, however, is only the first step. Colloquialisms within a language needs to be addressed. Also, the program must be culturally appropriate, especially concerning dietary patterns and medical practice patterns.
- **Mobile friendly:** The world is going mobile so solutions should be optimized for a mobile experience. While early versions of digital solutions were primarily desktop and web browser based, many users, especially in developing countries and under resourced communities have bypassed the desktop computer and do many activities, such as online banking from their mobile device. Health technologies should evaluate the type of media being used to ensure that it is a good experience for their users.

The IHS digital Care Plan is a collection of evidence-based content, data collection, communication, and decision rules designed to assist a patient in their self-management care and the core is the Care Plan engine. The purpose of the care plan engine is to prioritize and personalize the delivery of Care Plan services and resources. The Care Plan engine will feed data analytics, supporting a robust research agenda. Insights derived from analysis and research will continually update the operation and effectiveness of the Care Plan Engine.

These plans are designed to help patients:

- Understand and control risk factors for these conditions.
- Develop health literacy and numeracy (understanding what numbers and measures mean).
- Navigate the health care system.
- Improve communication with health care providers.
- Improve decision-making skills.

Accessible and Actionable Education

While extensive data and scientific text are standard in academia, they are not optimal to provide information to patients and other health care consumers. Most people seek smaller bits of information, such as tips, lists and other easily digestible packages. They seek this information from a variety of channels,

Figure 2. Care plan development

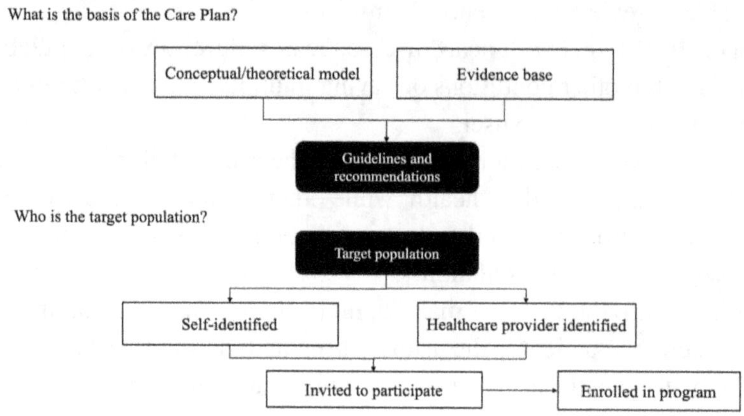

including mobile, digital, and print. This is a central idea of providing clear, simple, small chunks of information that are accessible and enable actionable plans for heart-healthy living.

Making health education accessible is critical, but when it comes to health behaviors, education must be converted into action. For some women and men with cardiovascular health problems, reading information may be enough to motivate them to make behavior changes that will improve their heart health. However, there are many health care consumers who are not motivated simply by education. These people have different motivations and priorities, so it is important for health care providers to understand these differences to activate desired behaviors.

Knowledge (Education)

Building knowledge and skill includes access to AHA educational resources, such as videos, quizzes, blogs, and weblinks. All three of these functional areas are curated by the Care Plan Engine, providing the most relevant and personal Care Plan possible. While strategies for patient education focus on the use of plain language with clear and concise messaging, it is unclear how these strategies are used to build knowledge and health literacy in patients with cardiovascular disease. Care plans are designed to build knowledge and skills by using teaching and learning strategies and adult learning theory. The educational resources associated with the care plans go through the same Science and Medicine review process to ensure accuracy and alignment with the evidence-based guidelines. These resources are specifically designed to build health literacy and self-management skills by empowering the patient and supporting self-efficacy. While low health literacy is associated with poor health outcomes it is linked to behaviors that impact the prevention, treatment, and self-management of the health condition (Table 2; See also Magnani et al., 2018)). These resources are multi-media, including web links, videos, and other interactive, web-enabled tools. All content is tagged by condition, by level, and and cardiovascular health domain (physical activity, nutrition, weight, tobacco, cholesterol, blood pressure, glucose, medication, and mental health) so that the most relevant content can be served up to the patient. Key health literacy concepts include conditions, diagnostic procedures, interventions, medications, physical activity, and nutrition. While, key numeracy concepts include target metrics, medication instructions and nutrition labels.

Table 2. Components of health literacy (Magnani et al., 2018)

Health Literacy	Covered in Care Plan	Comments
Literacy	✓	Education plan
Interaction	✓	Communication plan
Comprehension	✓	Scaffolding
Numeracy	✓	Assessment plan – biometrics
Information seeking	✓	Content management system
Application/function	✓	Action plans
Decision making/critical thinking	✓	Decision making and shared decision making
Evaluation	✓	Evaluation plan
Responsibility	✓	Smart goals
Confidence	✓	Self-efficacy
Navigation	✓	Literacy – navigation

The development of health literacy skills is a process that moves from knowledge to skills, to decision making. Patients with higher levels of education, knowledge, and skill are more likely to advance into critical health literacy, including communication and decision making (Smith & Magnani, 2019). Socioeconomic factors can play a large role in the progression to critical health literacy (Heijmans et al., 2015) and those in most need of health information have the least access to it (Rowlands et al., 2015).

Applying these models and educational approaches to broader definition of critical and functional health literacy as described by Nutbeam (2008) and D'Eath et al. (2012) is depicted in Figure 3. This results in a progression of health literacy skills from reading and comprehension to numeracy, to navigation, to communication, and finally to decision making. In practical terms, using blood pressure as an example, the patient can understand blood pressure and why it is important, then can distinguish between good and bad blood pressure readings, then know what to do with a blood pressure reading, such as rechecking, or calling 911; then know what information to share with their physicians, such as side effects from the medication, and finally to make good, well-informed decisions, such as lowering sodium intake.

It is apparent from both patients and healthcare professionals that the process of gaining knowledge and learning skills is compromised by the stress and anxiety associated with dealing with this new, life changing condition. It is critical, therefore, to address the emotional state of the patients prior to beginning an instructional intervention. This can range from formal methods, such as counseling and therapy, to informal methods, such as support groups, and if necessary, may include medications.

The behavioral strategy is designed to engage and motivate the patients to make lifestyle changes, ranging from weight loss, dietary modifications, increasing physical activity, cessation from tobacco, and taking medications as prescribed. The support structure of the patient, including friends and family, connections with other patients, access to trusted information, and access to healthcare providers was a key driver in building a behavioral strategy. Patients that were more isolated and lacked a support system had a very difficult time acquiring the knowledge and skills necessary to manage their health.

Finally, once the emotional state of the patient is addressed and a behavioral strategy is in place an instructional approach can be implemented. If the first two steps are ignored, however, the perception among patients and healthcare professionals is that an instructional approach has very little chance of suc-

Figure 3. Model for building health literacy skills

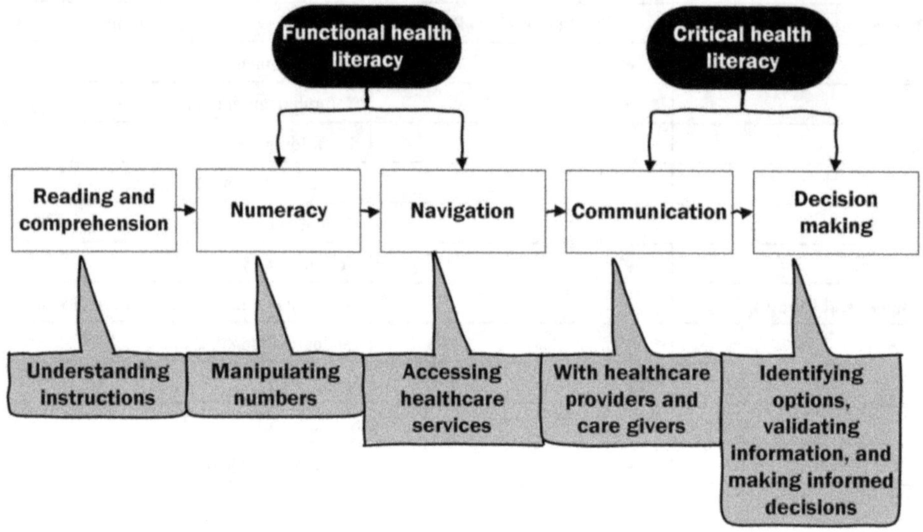

cess. Instructional strategies include the use of technology, including apps and devices, videos and print materials, and direct patient educational approaches. Patient education included informal methods, such as conversations between patients and healthcare professionals, patients interacting with other patients, and the patient's own experiences. These informal methods resulted in incidental learning opportunities where patients could build their own experiential knowledge base. Formal educational methods included discharge instructions, group education and health coaching. In the case of cardiovascular disease and diabetes, programs, such as cardiac rehabilitation, diabetes self-management, therapeutic lifestyle change programs, and online support networks were perceived by patients to provide the best learning opportunities. The key theme that runs through all three of the steps in the health literacy instructional model is the social and emotional support system (Figure 4). Patients that do not have a support system, and are managing their health by themselves, do not develop the knowledge and skills as easily as those patients that have good support systems (Dunn et al., 2017).

Educational models, designed for the classroom, have been used in adult education programs, such as English as a second language (ESL), but not specifically in adult health education. These educational models include Bloom's Taxonomy (Krathwohl, 2002), Vygotsky's Zone of Proximal Development (Shabani et al., 2010), and Gardner's Theory of Multiple Intelligences (Gardner, 2002).

This opens the door to the use of digital tools, offering multimedia formats for the delivery of information, as well as the ability to segment groups and curate content based on the motivations and world view of the individuals. Rather than applying a one-size-fits-all approach, providing multiple educational formats, such as one-on-one, group, informal, digital, and social, may reach and engage a larger number of patients. Additionally, while some patients prefer to follow the directions of their healthcare provider, other patients want to be provided with choices, or alternatives, and others would prefer to do their own research.

Vygotsky's zone of proximal development and problem-based learning theories use the metaphor of a scaffold, to support the individual's learning needs (Richard-Amato, 2003). Just like a scaffold is built around a building as it is being constructed, a support system is built around the learner. The key is

Figure 4. Integrated approach to building health literacy skills – health literacy instructional model

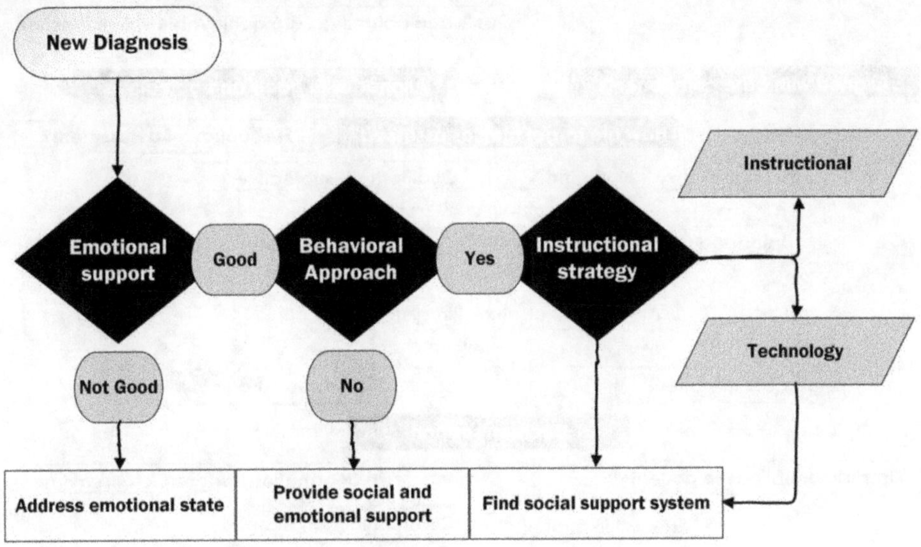

finding the learning zone and building through the zone. Simplifying the message too much runs the risk of being below the zone, and not engaging to the patient, while using jargon and complicated concepts runs the risk of being above the zone and overwhelming the patient. All three educational theories are combined into a model for building health literacy skills (Figure 5).

Figure 5. Education plan – Capturing the learning zone

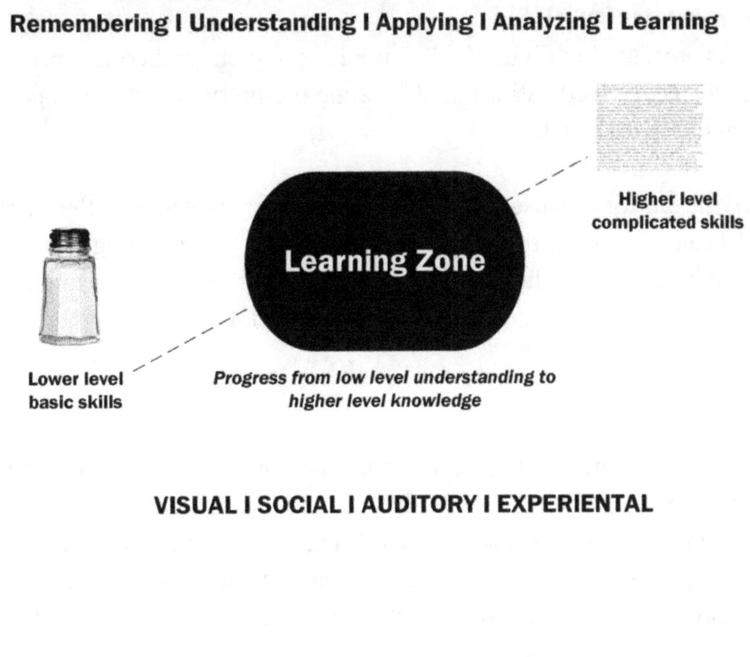

Figure 6. Assessment plan

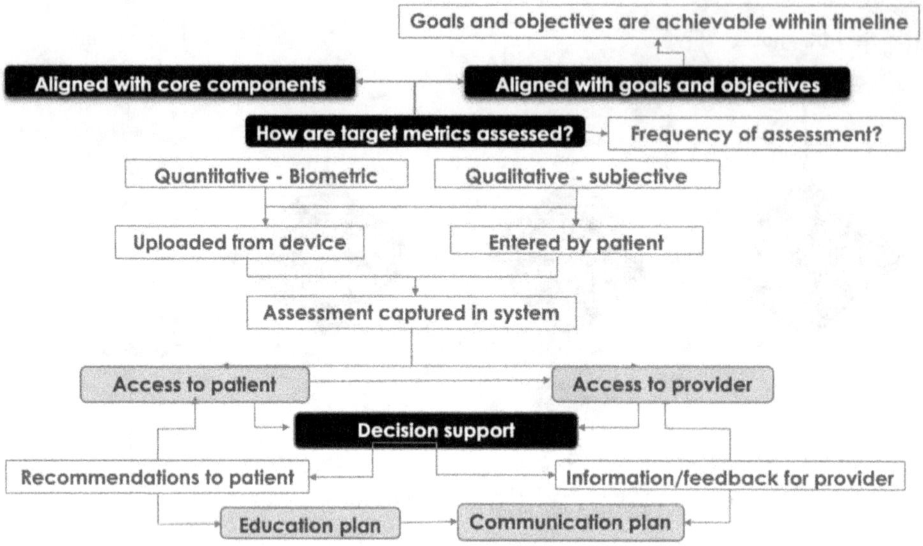

Coaching (Goal/Action Planning and Assessment)

- **Priority Areas:** The first step in the Care Planning process is to set the priorities. Priority areas are categorized on 3 levels, conditions, behaviors, and biometrics. The patient may select as many priority areas as necessary to achieve their objective. It is recommended that at least 1 condition, 1 behavior, and 1 metric be chosen.
- **Goal Examples:** The patient must select at least 1 and no more than 3 goals. There does not have to be a goal for each priority area. For example, the patient may select heart failure, diabetes, and obesity, and select a goal of losing 10 pounds. Goals should be specific, measurable, achievable, realistic, and timebound (SMART).
- **Assessments:** As presented in Figure 6, the initial assessment will collect participant information including their diagnosis, medications, and baseline biometrics. It includes participants that have not had an event or any risk factors.

On the provider end, the platform is used for surveillance of key metrics. In the Care Plan Engine, the LS7+Meds+mental health becomes the surveillance system. Dashboarding can be used to add data from the medical status survey and filter by condition, age, gender, ethnicity, and location. Healthcare providers use this surveillance system as a population health tool.

Communication Plan

The communication plan, presented in Figure 7, includes communication between the patient, caregivers, and healthcare providers. Communication also includes connection to other AHA digital assets, including the Patient Support Network, and to other 3rd party best in class apps.

The communication plan is designed to connect the patient and their healthcare team outside of the healthcare system. This communication is done through secure messaging and feedback to both the

Figure 7. Communication plan

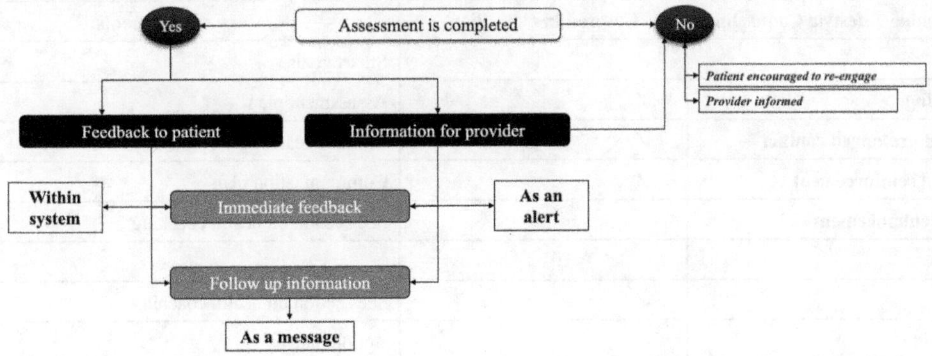

patient and the healthcare team on the progress of the patient. This feedback may come in the form of alerts or follow up messages. Specific components of the communication plan include communication with and among healthcare professionals and care givers. This includes alerts and follow up messages to patient and healthcare professionals, two-way communication between the patient and the healthcare provider, and updates/dashboards for the patient and the healthcare provider.

Alerts are designed to inform the healthcare provider without creating noise. Alerts are used only in cases where timely intervention is necessary

The communication plan is a method for implementing best practices in health coaching as described in Table 3. The Care Plan is intended to be monitored and implemented by a human coach, working in conjunction with the technology platform. Rather than technology replacing the role of the human/health coach, the purpose is to leverage the skills and time of the healthcare professional. From a technology perspective this is a human-enabled AI approach (Fogel & Kvedar, 2018). The communication plan is also intended to get the patient on the right side of the argument by using challenges, reflections, and journaling. These approaches mirror many of the strategies used in motivational interviewing (Miller & Rollnick, 2002). Televisits, with the camera on, can provide even greater insights into the patient's readiness for change, self-efficacy, and emotional state.

Engagement Plan

An often-overlooked element of a plan of care is the level of patient interaction, or engagement. Key elements of the engagement plan include making it as user/patient friendly as possible and making the content interesting so that the patient continues to use the system. To make the Care Plan more interesting it needs to be highly personalized, relevant, interactive, and social. The Care Plans are personalized using a modular approach, so that content can be expanded or filtered based on the patient's condition. For example, if the patient has heart failure and diabetes, both conditions can be addressed simultaneously through the Care Plan. The patient sets their own goals and action plan, including the core component, targeted metric, timeline, and accountability. Likewise, the plans can be more relevant by giving the patient the ability to prioritize their goals and action plans. For example, the patient might wish to prioritize blood pressure control and physical activity. Patient centeredness and evidence/science based are reconciled using a shared decision-making model by providing the patient with evidence-based choices when selecting their goals and action plans. Care Plans are made interactive by providing

Table 3. Components of health coaching/lifestyle counseling (Artinian et al., 2010)

Health Coaching/Lifestyle Counseling	Covered in Care Plan	Comments
Goal setting	✓	Smart goals
Self-monitoring	✓	Assessment plan
Frequent and prolonged contact	✓	Communication plan
Feedback and reinforcement	✓	Communication plan
Self-efficacy enhancement	✓	See section on health coaching
Incentives		
Modeling	✓	See section on health coaching
Problem solving	✓	Action plans
Relapse prevention	✓	Part of readiness for change
Motivational interviewing	✓	See section on health coaching

two-way communication between the patient, care givers, healthcare professionals, and other patients. Also, educational content includes quizzes on knowledge, and surveys. Patients are given a voice to share their preferences and experiences and can even share their own data by becoming part of research studies. These preferences can provide even deeper insights into key issues, and from the perspective of the patient. Finally, the Care Plans can connect to social networks so that patients can interact with other patients. The social and emotional support provided through the care plans can reduce the level of anxiety of the patient, provide an opportunity for the patient to share experiences and learn from other patients, and can be an instructional platform.

While the emphasis is on empowering the patient to be a more active participant in their health, the system is also designed to give the healthcare professional more tools in their role as a health coach. A more detailed and personalized approach can be developed by digging deeper into multiple dimensions of health and developing a more personalized coaching strategy. Table 5 shows how the social, medical, lifestyle, and learning signatures can be used to help the patient and the healthcare professional create a highly personalized strategy using shared decision making.

An even more personalized coaching strategy can be created by assessing the preferences of the patient. This includes both dynamic factors, such as readiness for change, self-efficacy, and health literacy, with static factors such as:

- Is the person proactive or reactive?
- What is their goal orientation? Individual, group, or neither
- Are they self-directed?
- Are they independent or interdependent?
- Do they prefer direction or choices?

- **Listener:** The listener is for the patient that is not proactive and engaged in their health. This person is not sure if they want to participate in the program. The goal here is to listen to the person

Table 4. Social, medical, lifestyle, and learning Signatures

<table>
<tr><th>Signatures</th><th>Elements</th><th>Examples</th><th>Strategy</th></tr>
<tr><td>Social</td><td>Demographic
Social
Cultural</td><td>African American
Female
Low income</td><td rowspan="4">Focus on family health;
Begin preparing low sodium meals;
Wants a list of low sodium recipes and articles on low sodium cooking;
Will begin participating in a social group at her church.</td></tr>
<tr><td>Medical</td><td>Diagnosis
Treatment
Genetics</td><td>High blood pressure
Taking BP meds
Family history of stroke</td></tr>
<tr><td>Lifestyle</td><td>Behavioral
Mental health
Biometric</td><td>High sodium diet
Feels stressed out
Obese</td></tr>
<tr><td>Learning</td><td>Learning preference
Motivation
Digital</td><td>Prefers choices
Wants to feel better
Uses email and internet</td></tr>
</table>

Based on the personality and preferences of the patient the IHS has created four coaching strategies.

and help them get on the right side of the argument. Go light on instruction and heavy on reflection. Get the person to reflect on their goals and plans and look for motivational statements.

- **Motivator:** This person knows they need to make some changes to improve their health but has not decided to make a commitment. Some instruction is good here, but the focus should be on challenges, forming habits, and seeing some early success. The goal here is to get the person on the right track. Once they start to see some success, they will begin to make more progress.
- **Director:** This is for the proactive patient that wants to grow in their knowledge and achieve their goals. The coach is in charge and provides direction to the person. The pace and level of information can increase at this stage. The goal here is to keep the person accountable to their plan. Once they achieve their goal, a new, revised SMART goal should be developed.
- **Expert:** This approach is for the most proactive patient. Instruction is not necessary because the person had already done this. The goal here is to keep the person on track. The coach can provide expertise but should not get in the way of the pace and achievement of the person. The goal of the coach is to be supportive and collaborative with the person.

CHALLENGES AND RECOMMENDATIONS

While COVID-19 has accelerated the use of digital interventions, there are still challenges to overcome. One challenge is the ability to study these interventions. Not all digital interventions will achieve the same outcome and there is still a lot of 'digital snake-oil' out there. Digital interventions, by their very nature are highly innovative. Traditional research models, such as the randomized clinical trial are expensive and take a long time to conduct. It is difficult to ask an innovator to stop innovating during the duration of the trial and run the risk of reporting on obsolete technology or running the risk of falling behind competitors. Outcomes must be demanded, but innovation must also occur in evaluation methods. Another challenge is lack of adoption of digital health technology. Technology has become a focal point in many people's lives from Facebook to Google, to Amazon, but adoption of health technologies has been much slower. Finally, effective digital interventions much address the digital divide and design their solutions so that people of all age, gender, race and region can benefit.

To address these challenges and to fulfill the promise that digital interventions can result in better health outcome, the following recommendations are proposed:

- Build digital interventions that are science based and can be studied to demonstrate positive outcome.
- Use human centered design to build solutions that are intuitive, easy to use and will meet the needs of the users.
- Design digital interventions to leverage emerging technologies and that emphasize increasing or improving human interaction between patients and their healthcare team.
- Build digital interventions with equity in mind.

CONCLUSION

There is no "one size fits all" approach for these digital health tools; research have emphasized the need for individualized designs in order to maximize usability, effectiveness, and sustainability of use among patients (Chew et al., 2020). Research-based models and frameworks ought to be integrated in the design of the digital health tools, where they help identify the characteristics of the users and automatically tailor and personalize the content of the intervention/tool in order to ensure maximum effectiveness and benefits to the patients. This applies to all types of digital health tools and interventions targeting various clinical settings, including those targeting cardiovascular health. Taking into consideration the wide range of patients, their characteristics, and their cultural and social context is key to developing effective tool designs.

REFERENCES

Agarwal, R., Bills, J. E., Hecht, T. J., & Light, R. P. (2011). Role of home blood pressure monitoring in overcoming therapeutic inertia and improving hypertension control: A systematic review and meta-analysis. *Hypertension*, *57*(1), 29–38. doi:10.1161/HYPERTENSIONAHA.110.160911 PMID:21115879

American Heart Association. (2021). *Center for Health Technology and Innovation.* Retrieved from: https://www.ahahealthtech.org

Angell, S. Y., McConnell, M. V., Anderson, C. A., Bibbins-Domingo, K., Boyle, D. S., Capewell, S., Ezzati, M., De Ferranti, S., Gaskin, D. J., Goetzel, R. Z., Huffman, M. D., Jones, M., Khan, Y. M., Kim, S., Kumanyika, S. K., McCray, A. T., Merritt, R. K., Milstein, B., Mozaffarian, D., ... Warner, J. J. (2020). The American Heart Association 2030 impact goal: A presidential advisory from the American Heart Association. *Circulation*, *141*(9), e120–e138. doi:10.1161/CIR.0000000000000758 PMID:31992057

Artinian, N. T., Fletcher, G. F., Mozaffarian, D., Kris-Etherton, P., Van Horn, L., Lichtenstein, A. H., Kumanyika, S., Kraus, W. E., Fleg, J. L., Redeker, N. S., Meininger, J. C., Banks, J. A., Stuart-Shor, E. M., Fletcher, B. J., Miller, T. D., Hughes, S., Braun, L. T., Kopin, L. A., Berra, K., ... Burke, L. E. (2010). Interventions to promote physical activity and dietary lifestyle changes for cardiovascular risk factor reduction in adults: A scientific statement from the American Heart Association. *Circulation, 122*(4), 406–441. doi:10.1161/CIR.0b013e3181e8edf1 PMID:20625115

Batterham, R. W., Hawkins, M., Collins, P. A., Buchbinder, R., & Osborne, R. H. (2016). 2016/03/01/). Health literacy: Applying current concepts to improve health services and reduce health inequalities. *Public Health, 132*, 3–12. doi:10.1016/j.puhe.2016.01.001 PMID:26872738

Beatty, A. L., Doll, J. A., Schopfer, D. W., Maynard, C., Plomondon, M. E., Shen, H., & Whooley, M. A. (2018). Cardiac rehabilitation participation and mortality after percutaneous coronary intervention: Insights from the veterans affairs clinical assessment, reporting, and tracking program. *Journal of the American Heart Association, 7*(19), e010010. doi:10.1161/JAHA.118.010010 PMID:30371315

Bhavnani, S. P., Parakh, K., Atreja, A., Druz, R., Graham, G. N., Hayek, S. S., Krumholz, H. M., Maddox, T. M., Majmudar, M. D., Rumsfeld, J. S., & Shah, B. R. (2017). 2017 Roadmap for innovation—ACC health policy statement on healthcare transformation in the era of digital health, big data, and precision health: A report of the American College of Cardiology Task Force on Health Policy Statements and Systems of Care. *Journal of the American College of Cardiology, 70*(21), 2696–2718. doi:10.1016/j.jacc.2017.10.018 PMID:29169478

Borzecki, A. M., Oliveria, S. A., & Berlowitz, D. R. (2005). Barriers to hypertension control. *American Heart Journal, 149*(5), 785–794. doi:10.1016/j.ahj.2005.01.047 PMID:15894958

Bosworth, H. B., & Oddone, E. Z. (2002). A model of psychosocial and cultural antecedents of blood pressure control. *Journal of the National Medical Association, 94*(4), 236. PMID:11991336

Burke, L. E., Ma, J., Azar, K. M., Bennett, G. G., Peterson, E. D., Zheng, Y., Riley, W., Stephens, J., Shah, S. H., Suffoletto, B., Turan, T. N., Spring, B., Steinberger, J., & Quinn, C. C. (2015). Current science on consumer use of mobile health for cardiovascular disease prevention: A scientific statement from the American Heart Association. *Circulation, 132*(12), 1157–1213. doi:10.1161/CIR.0000000000000232 PMID:26271892

Center for Disease Control and Prevention (CDC). (2021). *What Is Health Literacy?* https://www.cdc.gov/healthliteracy/learn/index.html

Chew, A. M. K., Ong, R., Lei, H.-H., Rajendram, M., K v, G., Verma, S. K., Fung, D. S. S., Leong, J. J., & Gunasekeran, D. V. (2020). Digital health solutions for mental health disorders during COVID-19. *Frontiers in Psychiatry, 11*, 898. doi:10.3389/fpsyt.2020.582007 PMID:33033487

Conard, S. (2019). Best practices in digital health literacy. *International Journal of Cardiology, 292*, 277–279. doi:10.1016/j.ijcard.2019.05.070 PMID:31230937

Coorey, G. M., Neubeck, L., Mulley, J., & Redfern, J. (2018). Effectiveness, acceptability and usefulness of mobile applications for cardiovascular disease self-management: Systematic review with meta-synthesis of quantitative and qualitative data. *European Journal of Preventive Cardiology, 25*(5), 505–521. doi:10.1177/2047487317750913 PMID:29313363

Cusack, L., Del Mar, C. B., Chalmers, I., Gibson, E., & Hoffmann, T. C. (2018). Educational interventions to improve people's understanding of key concepts in assessing the effects of health interventions: A systematic review. *Systematic Reviews, 7*(1), 68. doi:10.118613643-018-0719-4 PMID:29716639

D'Eath, M., Barry, M. M., & Sixsmith, J. (2012). *A Rapid Evidence Review of Interventions for Improving Health Literacy*. Academic Press.

Datta, G. (2020). *Mobile Health Apps Conformity Assessment & Certification Guidance Concept Note*. https://www.healthit.gov/isa/sites/isa/files/webform/uscid_webform/2126/Mobile%20Health%20App%20CA%20%26%20Certification%20Guidance%20Concept%20Note%20%20-%20Gora%20Datta.pdf

Dunn, P., & Cianflone, D. (2020). Special Issue on Digital Health Literacy. *International Journal of Cardiology, 299*, 301–302. doi:10.1016/j.ijcard.2019.08.055 PMID:31493913

Dunn, P., & Conard, S. (2018). Improving health literacy in patients with chronic conditions: A call to action. *International Journal of Cardiology, 273*, 249–251. doi:10.1016/j.ijcard.2018.08.090 PMID:30193793

Dunn, P., Margaritis, V., & Anderson, C. L. (2017). Understanding Health Literacy Skills in Patients with Cardiovascular Disease and Diabetes. *Qualitative Report, 22*(1), 33–46. doi:10.46743/2160-3715/2017.2548

Eapen, Z. J., Turakhia, M. P., McConnell, M. V., Graham, G., Dunn, P., Tiner, C., Rich, C., Harrington, R. A., Peterson, E. D., & Wayte, P. (2016). Defining a mobile health roadmap for cardiovascular health and disease. *Journal of the American Heart Association, 5*(7), e003119. doi:10.1161/JAHA.115.003119 PMID:27405809

Eckel, R. H., Jakicic, J. M., Ard, J. D., de Jesus, J. M., Houston Miller, N., Hubbard, V. S., Lee, I.-M., Lichtenstein, A. H., Loria, C. M., Millen, B. E., Nonas, C. A., Sacks, F. M., Smith, S. C. Jr, Svetkey, L. P., Wadden, T. A., & Yanovski, S. Z. (2014). 2013 AHA/ACC guideline on lifestyle management to reduce cardiovascular risk: A report of the American College of Cardiology/American Heart Association Task Force on Practice Guidelines. *Journal of the American College of Cardiology, 63*(25, 25 Part B), 2960–2984. doi:10.1016/j.jacc.2013.11.003 PMID:24239922

FDA. (2020). *What is Digital Health?* https://www.fda.gov/medical-devices/digital-health-center-excellence/what-digital-health

Flores-Mateo, G., Granado-Font, E., Ferré-Grau, C., & Montaña-Carreras, X. (2015). 2015/11/10). Mobile Phone Apps to Promote Weight Loss and Increase Physical Activity: A Systematic Review and Meta-Analysis. *Journal of Medical Internet Research, 17*(11), e253. doi:10.2196/jmir.4836 PMID:26554314

Fogel, A. L., & Kvedar, J. C. (2018). Artificial intelligence powers digital medicine. *NPJ Digital Medicine, 1*(1), 1–4. doi:10.103841746-017-0012-2 PMID:31304291

Gardner, H. (2002). *Frames of Mind: The Theory of Multiple Intelligences*. Basic Books.

Ghose, A., Guo, X., Li, B., & Dang, Y. (2021). *Empowering patients using smart mobile health platforms: Evidence from a randomized field experiment*. Forthcoming at MIS Quarterly.

Green, B. B., Cook, A. J., Ralston, J. D., Fishman, P. A., Catz, S. L., Carlson, J., Carrell, D., Tyll, L., Larson, E. B., & Thompson, R. S. (2008). Effectiveness of home blood pressure monitoring, Web communication, and pharmacist care on hypertension control: A randomized controlled trial. *Journal of the American Medical Association, 299*(24), 2857–2867. doi:10.1001/jama.299.24.2857 PMID:18577730

Guo, C., Ashrafian, H., Ghafur, S., Fontana, G., Gardner, C., & Prime, M. (2020). Challenges for the evaluation of digital health solutions—A call for innovative evidence generation approaches. *NPJ Digital Medicine, 3*(1), 1–14. doi:10.103841746-020-00314-2 PMID:32904379

Harrington, R. A., Califf, R. M., Balamurugan, A., Brown, N., Benjamin, R. M., Braund, W. E., Hipp, J., Konig, M., Sanchez, E., & Joynt Maddox, K. E. (2020). Call to action: rural health: a presidential advisory from the American Heart Association and American Stroke Association. *Circulation, 141*(10), e615–e644. doi:10.1161/CIR.0000000000000753 PMID:32078375

Heijmans, M., Waverijn, G., Rademakers, J., van der Vaart, R., & Rijken, M. (2015). Functional, communicative and critical health literacy of chronic disease patients and their importance for self-management. *Patient Education and Counseling, 98*(1), 41–48. doi:10.1016/j.pec.2014.10.006 PMID:25455794

IQVIA. (2017). *Grows as Innovation, Evidence and Adoption of Mobile Health Apps Accelerate*. https://www.iqvia.com/newsroom/2017/11/impact-of-digital-health-grows-asinnovation-evidence-and-adoption-of-mobile-health-apps-accelerate/

Krathwohl, D. R. (2002). A revision of Bloom's taxonomy: An overview. *Theory into Practice, 41*(4), 212–218. doi:10.120715430421tip4104_2

Krebs, P., & Duncan, D. T. (2015). Health app use among US mobile phone owners: A national survey. *JMIR mHealth and uHealth, 3*(4), e4924. doi:10.2196/mhealth.4924 PMID:26537656

Lloyd-Jones, D. M., Hong, Y., Labarthe, D., Mozaffarian, D., Appel, L. J., Van Horn, L., Greenlund, K., Daniels, S., Nichol, G., Tomaselli, G. F., Arnett, D. K., Fonarow, G. C., Ho, P. M., Lauer, M. S., Masoudi, F. A., Robertson, R. M., Roger, V., Schwamm, L. H., Sorlie, P., ... Rosamond, W. D. (2010). Defining and setting national goals for cardiovascular health promotion and disease reduction: The American Heart Association's strategic Impact Goal through 2020 and beyond. *Circulation, 121*(4), 586–613. doi:10.1161/CIRCULATIONAHA.109.192703 PMID:20089546

Magid, D. J., Olson, K. L., Billups, S. J., Wagner, N. M., Lyons, E. E., & Kroner, B. A. (2013). A pharmacist-led, American Heart Association Heart360 Web-enabled home blood pressure monitoring program. *Circulation: Cardiovascular Quality and Outcomes, 6*(2), 157–163. doi:10.1161/CIRCOUTCOMES.112.968172 PMID:23463811

Magnani, J. W., Mujahid, M. S., Aronow, H. D., Cené, C. W., Dickson, V. V., Havranek, E., Morgenstern, L. B., Paasche-Orlow, M. K., Pollak, A., & Willey, J. Z. (2018). Health literacy and cardiovascular disease: fundamental relevance to primary and secondary prevention: a scientific statement from the American Heart Association. *Circulation, 138*(2), e48–e74. doi:10.1161/CIR.0000000000000579 PMID:29866648

Margolis, K. L., Asche, S. E., Bergdall, A. R., Dehmer, S. P., Groen, S. E., Kadrmas, H. M., Kerby, T. J., Klotzle, K. J., Maciosek, M. V., Michels, R. D., O'Connor, P. J., Pritchard, R. A., Sekenski, J. L., Sperl-Hillen, J. A. M., & Trower, N. K. (2013). Effect of home blood pressure telemonitoring and pharmacist management on blood pressure control: A cluster randomized clinical trial. *Journal of the American Medical Association*, *310*(1), 46–56. doi:10.1001/jama.2013.6549 PMID:23821088

Miller, W. R., & Rollnick, S. (2002). *Motivational interviewing: Preparing people for change*. Book Review.

Monaco, A., Palmer, K., Faber, N. H. R., Kohler, I., Silva, M., Vatland, A., van Griensven, J., Votta, M., Walsh, D., & Clay, V. (2021). Digital health tools for managing noncommunicable diseases during and after the COVID-19 pandemic: Perspectives of patients and caregivers. *Journal of Medical Internet Research*, *23*(1), e25652. doi:10.2196/25652 PMID:33464206

Morrison, L. G. (2015). Theory-based strategies for enhancing the impact and usage of digital health behaviour change interventions: A review. *Digital Health*, *1*. doi:10.1177/2055207615595335 PMID:29942544

National Institute for Standards and Measures. (2021). *Malcolm Baldridge National Quality Award*. https://www.nist.gov/baldrige/baldrige-award

Nutbeam, D. (2008). The evolving concept of health literacy. *Social Science & Medicine*, *67*(12), 2072–2078. doi:10.1016/j.socscimed.2008.09.050 PMID:18952344

PatientBond. (2021). *Psychographics: The Key to Motivating Healthcare Consumer Behaviors*. https://www.patientbond.com/psychographics

Patrick, K., Hekler, E., & Estrin, D. (2016). Rapid rate of technological development and its implications for research on digital behavior change interventions. *American Journal of Preventive Medicine*.

Paul, M., & Das, A. (2017). Service Level Agreements for Smart Healthcare in Cloud. *International Journal of Grid and High Performance Computing*, *9*(4), 57–70.

Paul, M., & Das, A. (2017). Health informatics as a service (HIAAS) for developing countries. In Internet of Things and big data technologies for next generation healthcare (pp. 251–279). Springer. doi:10.1007/978-3-319-49736-5_11

Prochaska, J. O., & DiClemente, C. C. (1983). Stages and processes of self-change of smoking: Toward an integrative model of change. *Journal of Consulting and Clinical Psychology*, *51*(3), 390–395. doi:10.1037/0022-006X.51.3.390 PMID:6863699

Prochaska, J. O., Redding, C. A., & Evers, K. E. (2008). The transtheoretical model and stages of change. In K. Glanz, B. K. Rimer, & K. Viswanath (Eds.), *Health behavior and health education: Theory, research, and practice*. Jossey Bass.

Ratz, T., & Lippke, S. (2021). Health Behavior Change. In *Reference Module in Neuroscience and Biobehavioral Psychology*. Elsevier. doi:10.1016/B978-0-12-818697-8.00068-6

Richard-Amato, P. A. (2003). *Making it happen: From interactive to participatory language teaching: Theory and practice*. Pearson.

Riegel, B., Moser, D. K., Buck, H. G., Dickson, V. V., Dunbar, S. B., Lee, C. S., Lennie, T. A., Lindenfeld, J., Mitchell, J. E., Treat-Jacobson, D. J., & Webber, D. E. (2017). Self-care for the prevention and management of cardiovascular disease and stroke: A scientific statement for healthcare professionals from the American Heart Association. *Journal of the American Heart Association*, *6*(9), e006997. doi:10.1161/JAHA.117.006997 PMID:28860232

Ritchey, M. D., Maresh, S., McNeely, J., Shaffer, T., Jackson, S. L., Keteyian, S. J., Brawner, C. A., Whooley, M. A., Chang, T., Stolp, H., Schieb, L., & Wright, J. (2020). Tracking cardiac rehabilitation participation and completion among Medicare beneficiaries to inform the efforts of a national initiative. *Circulation: Cardiovascular Quality and Outcomes*, *13*(1), e005902. doi:10.1161/CIRCOUTCOMES.119.005902 PMID:31931615

Roane, H. S., & Betz, A. M. (2012). Behavior Analysis. In V. S. Ramachandran (Ed.), *Encyclopedia of Human Behavior* (2nd ed., pp. 267–273). Academic Press. doi:10.1016/B978-0-12-375000-6.00059-8

Roger, V. L., Sidney, S., Fairchild, A. L., Howard, V. J., Labarthe, D. R., Shay, C. M., Tiner, A. C., Whitsel, L. P., Rosamond, W. D., & Committee, A. H. A. A. C. (2020). Recommendations for cardiovascular health and disease surveillance for 2030 and beyond: A policy statement from the American Heart Association. *Circulation*, *141*(9), e104–e119. doi:10.1161/CIR.0000000000000756 PMID:31992050

Roth, G. A., Mensah, G. A., Johnson, C. O., Addolorato, G., Ammirati, E., Baddour, L. M., Barengo, N. C., Beaton, A. Z., Benjamin, E. J., Benziger, C. P., Bonny, A., Brauer, M., Brodmann, M., Cahill, T. J., Carapetis, J., Catapano, A. L., Chugh, S. S., Cooper, L. T., Coresh, J., ... Fuster, V. (2020). Global burden of cardiovascular diseases and risk factors, 1990–2019: Update from the GBD 2019 study. *Journal of the American College of Cardiology*, *76*(25), 2982–3021. doi:10.1016/j.jacc.2020.11.010 PMID:33309175

Rowlands, G., Protheroe, J., Winkley, J., Richardson, M., Seed, P. T., & Rudd, R. (2015). A mismatch between population health literacy and the complexity of health information: An observational study. *The British Journal of General Practice*, *65*(635), e379–e386. doi:10.3399/bjgp15X685285 PMID:26009533

Rudolph, M., Barr, M. S., Kuhn, T., Hersh, W. R., & McDonald, C. J. (2008). *E-health and its impact on medical practice*. https://www.acponline.org/advocacy/where_we_stand/policy/ehealth.pdf

Santo, K., Richtering, S. S., Chalmers, J., Thiagalingam, A., Chow, C. K., & Redfern, J. (2016). Mobile phone apps to improve medication adherence: A systematic stepwise process to identify high-quality apps. *JMIR mHealth and uHealth*, *4*(4), e6742. doi:10.2196/mhealth.6742 PMID:27913373

Shabani, K., Khatib, M., & Ebadi, S. (2010). Vygotsky's zone of proximal development: Instructional implications and teachers' professional development. *English Language Teaching*, *3*(4), 237–248. doi:10.5539/elt.v3n4p237

Smith, B., & Magnani, J. W. (2019). New technologies, new disparities: The intersection of electronic health and digital health literacy. *International Journal of Cardiology*, *292*, 280–282. doi:10.1016/j.ijcard.2019.05.066 PMID:31171391

Solberg Nes, L. (2020). Digital Health in Cardiology: Time for Action. *Cardiology*, *145*(2), 106–109. doi:10.1159/000504797 PMID:31825946

Spring, B., Ockene, J. K., Gidding, S. S., Mozaffarian, D., Moore, S., Rosal, M. C., Brown, M. D., Vafiadis, D. K., Cohen, D. L., Burke, L. E., & Lloyd-Jones, D. (2013). Better population health through behavior change in adults: A call to action. *Circulation, 128*(19), 2169–2176. doi:10.1161/01.cir.0000435173.25936.e1 PMID:24100544

Strauss, V. (2013). *Howard Gardner: 'Multiple intelligences' are not 'learning styles'*. https://www.washingtonpost.com/news/answer-sheet/wp/2013/10/16/howard-gardner-multiple-intelligences-are-not-learning-styles/

Thomas, K. L., Shah, B. R., Elliot-Bynum, S., Thomas, K. D., Damon, K., Allen LaPointe, N. M., Calhoun, S., Thomas, L., Breathett, K., Mathews, R., Anderson, M., Califf, R. M., & Peterson, E. D. (2014). Check it, change it: A community-based, multifaceted intervention to improve blood pressure control. *Circulation: Cardiovascular Quality and Outcomes*, *7*(6), 828–834. doi:10.1161/CIRCOUTCOMES.114.001039 PMID:25351480

Topol, E. J. (2015). *The patient will see you now: The future of medicine is in your hands*. Basic Books.

Topol, E. J. (2019). High-performance medicine: The convergence of human and artificial intelligence. *Nature Medicine*, *25*(1), 44–56. doi:10.103841591-018-0300-7 PMID:30617339

Vest, J. R., & Gamm, L. D. (2009). A critical review of the research literature on Six Sigma, Lean and StuderGroup's Hardwiring Excellence in the United States: The need to demonstrate and communicate the effectiveness of transformation strategies in healthcare. *Implementation Science; IS*, *4*(1), 1–9. doi:10.1186/1748-5908-4-35 PMID:19570218

Virtanen, L., Kaihlanen, A. M., Laukka, E., Gluschkoff, K., & Heponiemi, T. (2021). Behavior change techniques to promote healthcare professionals' eHealth competency: A systematic review of interventions. *International Journal of Medical Informatics*, *149*, 104432. doi:10.1016/j.ijmedinf.2021.104432 PMID:33684712

Vos, T., Abajobir, A. A., Abate, K. H., Abbafati, C., Abbas, K. M., Abd-Allah, F., Abdulkader, R. S., Abdulle, A. M., Abebo, T. A., Abera, S. F., Aboyans, V., Abu-Raddad, L. J., Ackerman, I. N., Adamu, A. A., Adetokunboh, O., Afarideh, M., Afshin, A., Agarwal, S. K., Aggarwal, R., ... Murray, C. J. L. (2017). Global, regional, and national incidence, prevalence, and years lived with disability for 328 diseases and injuries for 195 countries, 1990–2016: A systematic analysis for the Global Burden of Disease Study 2016. *Lancet*, *390*(10100), 1211–1259. doi:10.1016/S0140-6736(17)32154-2 PMID:28919117

WHO. (2019). *WHO guideline: recommendations on digital interventions for health system strengthening*. World Health Organization.

WHO. (2021). *Global strategy on digital health 2020–2025*. World Health Organization. https://www.who.int/docs/default-source/documents/gs4dhdaa2a9f352b0445bafbc79ca799dce4d.pdf?sfvrsn=f112ede5_38

Wisniewski, H., Liu, G., Henson, P., Vaidyam, A., Hajratalli, N. K., Onnela, J.-P., & Torous, J. (2019). Understanding the quality, effectiveness and attributes of top-rated smartphone health apps. *Evidence-Based Mental Health*, *22*(1), 4–9. doi:10.1136/ebmental-2018-300069 PMID:30635262

ADDITIONAL READING

Banerjee, A. (2017). Bridging the global digital health divide for cardiovascular disease. *Circulation: Cardiovascular Quality and Outcomes*, *10*(11), e004297. doi:10.1161/CIRCOUTCOMES.117.004297 PMID:29133470

Dunn, P., & Hazzard, E. (2019). Technology approaches to digital health literacy. *International Journal of Cardiology*, *293*, 294–296. doi:10.1016/j.ijcard.2019.06.039 PMID:31350037

Foraker, R. E., Benziger, C. P., DeBarmore, B. M., Cené, C. W., Loustalot, F., Khan, Y., Anderson, C. A. M., & Roger, V. L. (2021). Achieving optimal population cardiovascular health requires an interdisciplinary team and a learning healthcare system: A scientific statement from the American Heart Association. *Circulation*, *143*(2), e9–e18. doi:10.1161/CIR.0000000000000913 PMID:33269600

Leopold, J. A., Davis, R. B., & Antman, E. M. (2021). Data from Digital Health Devices Informs Ideal Cardiovascular Health. *Journal of Personalized Medicine*, *11*(3), 189. doi:10.3390/jpm11030189 PMID:33801949

McConnell, M. V., Turakhia, M. P., Harrington, R. A., King, A. C., & Ashley, E. A. (2018). Mobile health advances in physical activity, fitness, and atrial fibrillation: Moving hearts. *Journal of the American College of Cardiology*, *71*(23), 2691–2701. doi:10.1016/j.jacc.2018.04.030 PMID:29880130

Roger, V. L., Sidney, S., Fairchild, A. L., Howard, V. J., Labarthe, D. R., Shay, C. M., Tiner, A. C., Whitsel, L. P., & Rosamond, W. D.American Heart Association Advocacy Coordinating Committee. (2020). Recommendations for cardiovascular health and disease surveillance for 2030 and beyond: A policy statement from the American Heart Association. *Circulation*, *141*(9), e104–e119. doi:10.1161/CIR.0000000000000756 PMID:31992050

Sarwar, C. M., Vaduganathan, M., Anker, S. D., Coiro, S., Papadimitriou, L., Saltz, J., Schoenfeld, E. R., Clark, R. L., Dinh, W., Kramer, F., Gheorghiade, M., Fonarow, G. C., & Butler, J. (2018). Mobile health applications in cardiovascular research. *International Journal of Cardiology*, *269*, 265–271. doi:10.1016/j.ijcard.2018.06.039 PMID:29921516

Saxon, L. A. (2016). Mobile health application solutions. *Circulation: Arrhythmia and Electrophysiology*, *9*(2), e002477. doi:10.1161/CIRCEP.115.002477 PMID:26810595

Key terms and definitions

Cardiovascular Health: All disorders that affect the health and the blood vessels.

Care Plan: A collection of evidence-based content designed to assist a patient in their self-management care.

Digital Health: The use of information and communication technology in health and health-related services.

Health Behavior Theories/Models: Theories and models designed to understand the biological, behavioral, sociocultural, economic, and ecological determinants of health behaviors and the process of health behavior change.

Health Education: Field of education that educates people about health, promotes health and encourage behavioral change.

Intelligent Health Solutions: A content management system and digital coaching platform developed by the American Heart Association that gives digital platforms an easy way to provide science-based content and evidence-based practice from a trusted source and to deliver a comprehensive health management solution.

Life's Simple 7: A strategy developed by the American Heart Association that proposes 7 criteria to achieving ideal cardiovascular health.

ENDNOTE

1 Health literacy is defined by the Center for Disease Control and Prevention (CDC) as is the degree to which individuals have the ability to find, understand, and use information and services to inform health-related decisions and actions for themselves and others (CDC, 2021).

Chapter 7
Predictive Healthcare Web Analytics Using Machine Learning

Anjali Agarwal
Amity University, Kolkata, India

Ajanta Das
Amity University, Kolkata, India

Ravish Kumar Bansal
https://orcid.org/0000-0002-5588-7177
St. Martinus University, Curaçao

ABSTRACT

Data analytics reflects trends on the particular subject based on comparison with historical dataset and present dataset. With the advancement of technology, healthcare predictive analytics at periodic intervals affords insights into diseases collectively, identifying risk of the patients' health in the future. The novelty of this project is to analyze symptoms and healthcare datasets, to predict the risk of the mentioned diseases using machine learning algorithms to better time management and convenience for physicians and the general population. Hence, the proposed model provides the provision to save patients directly from risk to the particular disease based on the periodic trend analysis. On the contrary, the hospital will utilize the proposed model to control future disease outbreaks.

INTRODUCTION

The medical care field has been for a long while an early adopter of innovative technological advances and benefitting massively from them (Food and Drug Administration, 2020). The current COVID-19 epidemic has highlighted the need for digital health technologies, with lockdowns and public health measures forcing health care providers to use various remote tactics and ehealth platforms to offer healthcare

DOI: 10.4018/978-1-7998-9490-2.ch007

to their patients (Monaco et al., 2021). The United Nations Agenda for sustainable development has also emphasized the potential of health technology to speed progress toward meeting health-related sustainable development goals (World Health Organization, 2021). Since 2005, the recognition of eHealth services resulted in a growing global consensus in the health community on the use of digital health tools to help ensure people's access to universal health coverage and improved protection from health emergencies. These days, machine learning, a subset of artificial intelligence plays an essential part in various medical care areas, including the advancement of new operations, overseeing patient information and records, and foreseeing the continuous illnesses as well as its therapy. In layman's words, machine learning is an application of artificial intelligence that allows computers to think and learn on their own and make judgments based on trial and error. Its core concept lies in the collection and analysis of data, then in "learning" how to utilize them to create plans to improve customer experience based on the quantity of data available. Without being explicitly programmed, it is a type of algorithm that allows computers to learn from data, anticipate events, and even improve themselves (Yarabarla et al., 2019). For example, it has been seen that obese persons are more likely to get heart disease, therefore they decide to attempt to maintain their weight to avoid heart disease. Furthermore, current advancements in artificial intelligence (AI) and machine learning (ML) may enable the creation of novel treatments as well as more precise outcome prediction (Fogel & Kvedar, 2018; Santo et al., 2016; Topol, 2019).

This chapter describes the prototype of a novel web application which is a multi- disease Prediction System that can be deployed in cloud and accessed through proper authorization. Using languages like Python, Hypertext Markup Language, cascading style sheets, and machine learning algorithms, we have prepared a prototype that can predict whether a person is suffering from a specified disease or not and that can be launched and made available for global usage in the future. An evolving world and evolving medicine lead to the discovery of new diseases and treatments that are very hard to compile in a small-scale web application. However, such compilation can be achieved with more research and resources.

Currently, the web application development is at its initial stage. It is aimed at helping physicians, medical students, and the general population. Physicians and medical students will be able to determine the symptoms and risk factors they want to focus on for specific diseases (Fahad & Pallavi, 2018). On the other hand, the general population will be able to identify common symptoms of certain diseases, and to recognize their risks of developing the significant diseases. Important features of the web application are its ease of use, simplicity, and cost-efficiency.

The web application targets the following diseases: COVID-19, diabetes, lung diseases, heart diseases, liver diseases, and kidney diseases, which are the most occurring diseases and ones that could lead to significant damage to the human body, with life-threatening potentials, if not addressed appropriately and promptly. The lungs, the heart, the liver, and the kidneys are a few of the most vital organs of the human body, therefore any issues with them would affect a person's overall health.

HOW DOES MACHINE LEARNING WORK?

Assume someone is attempting to throw a ball into a tub. The person could overshoot the target the first time because they used too much force. They may lower the force on the second try, but they will miss the ideal angle of their throw. Likewise, they might be able to land the ball in the tub in their third attempt. This is because the brain is always learning and adapting to new experiences, resulting in a better end product. In machine learning, the same concept can be applied to a machine. Data analytics and artificial intelligence are now capable of accomplishing this type of learning and adaptation.

Web health applications are dynamically being utilized to perform undertakings that are routinely carried out by medical professionals engaged in promoting health, forestalling sickness, determining therapy, and checking support for health services (Grampurohit & Sagarnal, 2020). For example, medical check-ups are very expensive and not everyone is capable of undergoing unaffordable tests. In order to address this issue, this application is designed to provide correct information to the general population, compactly and conveniently, to inform them about their health. This medical web application is assembled utilizing machine learning algorithms that will be able to foresee the risk of the six significant medical conditions presented earlier. Consequently, the medical personnel and general individuals would be able to use it to handle future sickness outbreaks.

Since its inception in the year 2000, the notion of digital health tools has been fast growing (Guo et al., 2020). The use of digital health technology attempts to increase efficiency, improve access and quality of health services while lowering costs and ensuring that patient care is more individualized (Food and Drug Administration, 2020). The current COVID-19 epidemic has highlighted the need for digital health technologies, with lockdowns and public health measures forcing health care providers to use various remote tactics and ehealth platforms to offer healthcare to their patients. Mobile applications, health information technology, smart wearable devices, remote monitoring, health platforms, telehealth, and telemedicine are all examples of digital health tools (Guo et al., 2020). According to recent research, the number of these instruments is steadily expanding. Huge number of health apps are presently accessible on the App Store, with more than 200 new apps being uploaded every day (IQVIA, 2017). Promoting healthy behaviors (for example, computerized cognitive behavioral therapy for mental health and somatic problems) are all examples of how digital health tools have been used in healthcare (Ghose et al., 2021; Murray et al., 2016). Taber et al. (2015) reported three primary sorts of motivations for refusing medical treatment. First, more than a third of those surveyed (33.3%) had negative feelings about obtaining medical help, citing variables such as physicians, healthcare institutions, and emotional worries. Second, a subset of individuals (12.2%) indicated a low perceived need for medical treatment, owing to the expectation that their sickness or symptoms would improve with time (4.0%). Third, many individuals (58.4%) mentioned typical obstacles to medical treatment, such as excessive costs (24.1%), lack of health insurance (8.3%), and time restrictions (15.6%). Thus, web health applications are being utilized by everyone and has proved to be beneficial for the society.

INSPIRATIONS AND INSIGHTS FOR THIS MEDICAL WEB APPLICATION

The medical application presented in this chapter has several advantages listed below:

1. It can reach a large number of individuals and is not restricted by borders. It is especially useful in developing countries like India, Pakistan, and Bangladesh, where a large section of the population faces poverty that prevents it from getting proper and unbiased treatment (Kaplan, 1990). Additionally, this section of the population suffers from a lack of awareness and correct information, which leads it to get defrauded without the ability to make use of advanced knowledge, science, and technology.

2. It can support individuals with incomes below the poverty line, who cannot stand to go through costly tests by giving them a foresight of their health at their fingertips. People below the poverty line have access to smartphones and will ultimately be served and benefit.
3. The medical care application will permit the patients to screen their well-being at an individual level and help them take convenient actions, hence, subsiding the rumors on wrong or uninformed symptoms for certain diseases (Lee et al., 2018). While social networking sites have advantages such as freedom of speech, they can sometimes be used to spread rumors that can have harmful effects on people. Every individual has a right to receive correct information, especially when it pertains to their health and life.
4. It is a benefit for individuals in remote regions where medical help is lacking. In developing countries such as India and Pakistan, health and many other services are not available in every region. There are still many villages and large sections of the population that are distant from proper health services and awareness about healthy lifestyles, despite advancement in health and technology.
5. This application cannot take over the knowledge and expertise of medical professionals. The main goal is to counter the prevalent misinformation and to provide accurate information in an easily accessible manner. This application only contains the most common symptoms and risk factors associated with significant diseases and predicts if the user is at risk of developing such disease or not, therefore it does not diagnose. The parameters used in this application are not sufficient to diagnose the user with the disease. Hence, even if the patient is at risk they should go to a medical professional for further and proper evaluation.

Apart from the above ideas, what inspired this web application was the opportunity of different fields of sciences to collaborate to make a better and improved product to help people improve their health. In this case, Medicine and Technology are working symbiotically to help each other grow so that it could be easily accessible by everyone. Medicine-Technology symbiosis has been going on for a very long period, nowadays there is robotic machinery for medical procedures, improved screening tools, modern treatments, etc. (Panch, et al., 2018). This advancing symbiosis has been proved to be immensely beneficial for humanity and will continue to do so (Guo et al., 2020).

BACKGROUND

Prediction of disease based on patient treatment history and health data by using data mining and machine learning approaches has been a real challenge for decades. Many studies have used data mining approaches to forecast particular diseases using pathology data or medical profiles. These methods attempted to predict illness recurrence. In addition, several techniques attempted to forecast illness management and progression. The recent success of deep learning in a variety of machine learning applications has prompted a move toward models that can learn rich, hierarchical representations of raw data with little pre-processing and provide more accurate results. Below is an overview of recent research done in this domain.

Kaur et al. (2017) presented a broad framework for customized healthcare that considers the benefits of remote monitoring, cloud computing, big data, and reactive machine learning. The framework provided a systematic approach to support fast-growing data of people with severe diseases. It also simplified the tasks of physicians by not overwhelming them with false alerts. The architecture proposed in the framework has the potential of supporting artificial intelligence-based healthcare analytics by providing batch and stream computing, extendable storage solution, and query management. In the future? The system will be able to extract useful knowledge that helps in decision making and monitoring real-time medical data through intelligent process analysis and big data processing.

Likewise, Panch et al. (2018) examined the direct influence of machine learning on health systems. The authors looked at how artificial intelligence (AI) might be used to improve the efficiency, effectiveness, equality, and responsiveness of public health and health care services, as well as how AI may be used to change health systems to attain universal health coverage.

On the other hand, Mustafa et al. (2021) conducted a thorough survey and an analytic study on Automated Machine Learning (AutoML) for clinical notes. To that aim, their article presented the basics of AutoML and its many tools and approaches. It also went over the difficulties of dealing with clinical notes and the advantages of building AutoML for medical note processing. Moreover, the article provided recommendations for future studies and discussed the problems and possibilities that this new subject presented. Mustafa et al. hoped to develop an AutoML platform for medical notes, which, if successful, may change patient outcomes.

Specific to disease prediction, Grampurohit and Sagarnal (2020) developed a disease prediction system using machine learning algorithms such as *decision tree*, *random forest*, and *naïve bayes* classifier. They presented a comprehensive comparative study of these three algorithms' performance on a medical record, each yielding an accuracy up to 95 percent. The performance was analyzed through a confusion matrix and accuracy score.

Similarly, Shah et al. (2020) defined various data mining techniques useful for effective heart disease predictions. Efficient and accurate predictions with a lesser number of attributes and tests were done. Fourteen essential attributes and four data mining classification techniques were considered. The data pre-processing stage was done and then utilized in the respective model. Naïve Bayes and random forests were the algorithms that showed the best results in that model. The accuracy after implementing four algorithms was found to be highest in K-nearest neighbors (k = 7).

Ankita et al. (2020) addressed the problem of classifying cancer genomic profiles. They developed a technique based on using the support vector machine learning algorithm that achieved a 73 percent accuracy rate for classifying hospital data. As the sample size increased, model output also improved, showing a positive aspect towards the model's robustness and adaptability.

Chauhan et al. (2017) proposed a disease prediction system using three machine learning algorithms, Gaussian Naïve Bayes, decision tree, and random forest. They found that after comparing the output of these three algorithms in terms of accuracy, random forest outperformed the best with 97.04% of accuracy after pre-processing.

Yarabarla et al. (2019) introduced breast cancer detection and prediction using the random forest algorithm. Its best detection accuracy was 70%, using both classifying and regression methods. The authors aimed at pre-training the system by providing numerous datasets so that when the user inputs data, it will run through the attributes, check the values, and present the result.

On the other hand, Fahad and Pallavi (2018) proposed a backpropagation algorithm based on convolutional neural networks in which the hospital data was taken and analyzed and in which structured and unstructured types of data were used. A neural network (also known as an artificial neural network or ANN) is a computer system made up of virtual neuron cells. Neural networks, which are based on the human brain, are used to solve computational issues by simulating the way neurons fire or activate in the brain. Fahad and Pallavi were able to achieve a prediction rate of 96.4%, aiming at improving the prediction rate in future work.

Moreover, Lee et al. (2018) proposed a disease prediction system using neural networks and machine learning algorithms. According to the different prediction algorithms applied to the data set, neural networks seemed to have the highest accuracy for the test data. The accuracy for the training data was 82.3% and the accuracy for the test data set was 80.2%. Artificial neural networks were able to handle non-linear and complex relationships efficiently, which is important because, in real life, most of the relationships between inputs and outputs can be non-linear and complex. The accuracy shown by neural networks was 80.2% for the data set used, which is a good performance for real-time applications.

From the above studies, we can observe that by using a machine learning approach, we can implement a web application and thus, we are proposing to present a multi-disease prediction system which can detect the above-mentioned diseases. We can forecast illnesses based on a patient's treatment history and health information.

Problem Statement

The healthcare industry has grown into a multibillion-dollar industry. The healthcare sector generates huge volumes of healthcare data regularly, which may be utilized to extract information for forecasting sickness that may occur in the future, based on patients' treatment history and health data. This concealed yet informative healthcare data can be used to make impactful decisions about patients' future health and to make improvements to the health sector in general. Thus, the prototype of the multi- disease Prediction System described in this chapter was developed to 1) help users predict the risk of acquiring a particular disease, such as COVID-19, diabetes, lung diseases, heart diseases, liver diseases, and kidney diseases; 2) offer early treatment to patients based on prediction of diseases; 3) reduce the chance of death and saving lives, and; 4) lower the cost of disease treatment to some extent.

The increased use of electronic health records has resulted in a plethora of fresh patient data, which is a goldmine for gaining knowledge of better human health. Data mining and machine learning approaches come into the picture here. The approach described above is used to forecast illnesses based on a patient's treatment history and health information.

Because the amount of data is so vast, the main difficulty is figuring out how to extract information from the raw dataset. This process is explained in further details under Data Collection and Pre-Processing. Furthermore, the intended objective and scope of this research were to find the data from the patients for the parameters in the dataset mentioned in Table 1 to 6 below.

PROPOSED WEB APPLICATION

As mentioned earlier in the chapter, the proposed multi- disease Prediction System is a prototype at an initial stage that can be deployed in cloud and accessed through proper authorization. As such, the prototype raises important privacy and security guidelines. At this stage of the project, the privacy of the data is maintained using a public key and a private key during launching. The public key is shared with the doctors who can review the information while the private key is shared with the users. Further privacy and security guidelines will be investigated and set in place with the broader dissemination of the application.

This application is a hybrid blend of six different machine learning models which when combined into one hybrid model will anticipate whether an individual is at risk of the referenced sicknesses or not. The model foresees the result of the referenced infections based on the analytic diagnostic test and health parameters utilized by the physicians to break down the presence or absence of specific signs and symptoms that will be given by the user to the web application. For instance, parameters utilized inside the dataset to find the diabetes are age, sex, body mass index, fasting blood sugar, HbA1c (a diabetes specific test), and family history of diabetes. This dataset can be easily provided by both physicians and patients, making it user-friendly and cost-efficient. The primary goal of this dataset is to prepare the model to know whether the patient is at risk for a specific disease or not, principally found in the health measurements and symptoms in the dataset. After information assortment, data pre-handling follows to change over the crude information into an arranged and clean information for viable preparation and working of the model. At that point, the model will be worked by parting the whole dataset into train and test data which can be additionally used to quantify the exhibition and precision of the model.

The model will be prepared to utilize different machine learning calculations and deep learning algorithms like decision trees, random forest, logistic regression, K-Nearest Neighbor (KNN), and support vector machines, which will be discussed later. After the model has been assembled, we have performed hyperparameter tuning procedures to improve the productivity of the model. Accordingly, we can serialize the model and afterward deploy it utilizing Heroku, a container-based cloud platform as a service (PaaS) that will empower it to convey it into a web application for end clients.

METHODOLOGY

The development of the model goes into various phases described in Fig. 1. These phases are 1) data collection, a stage where we collect information to train the model from medical practitioners; 2) data processing to clean the data from any arbitrary values; 3) splitting the dataset into two parts namely training data and testing data; 4) training the model from the information we already have gathered and followed by the test for efficiency of the model's performance, a classification which will help to distinguish whether the user is suffering from a particular disease or not, then followed by the pre-processing steps with Python programming language using the scikit-learn library (Machine Learning in Python, n.d.) and (Matplotlib Library in Python, n.d.); and finally 5) prediction

Data Collection and Pre-Processing

This section briefly presents the symptoms of the six chosen diseases used for proper identification, followed by a tabular presentation of sample data set with certain important parameters of each specific disease. These diseases are coronavirus disease, diabetes mellitus, lung disease, heart diseases, liver diseases, and kidney diseases. The data set was collected from patients' interaction through survey forms with prior consent and the parameters were identified by the physicians. The surveys have been collected amongst the colleagues and family members and they were aware of the data usage in the research work.

Figure 1. Proposed architecture of predictive healthcare system

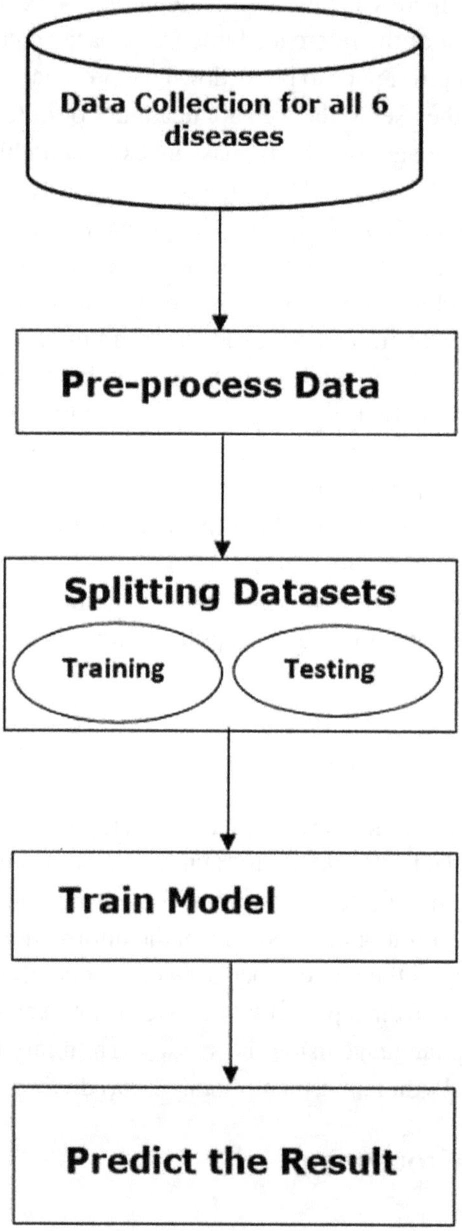

Coronavirus Disease (COVID-19)

*Corona*Virus Disease (COVID-19) is an infectious disease caused by the virus named SARS-CoV-2, which is a new strain of the already discovered SARS-CoV-1 responsible for causing Severe Acute Respiratory Syndrome (SARS). COVID-19 was declared a pandemic on March 11, 2020, due to the sudden outbreak of the new strain of coronavirus in Nov 2019 in Wuhan, China. Underestimating of responsible organizations lead to a major spread worldwide, causing a pandemic. As of 15th January 2022, 3.69

Table 1. Dataset sample for Coronavirus (COVID-19)

Parameters	Patient 1 Data	Patient 2 Data	Patient 3 Data	Patient 4 Data
Fever	100.0	98.4	99.9	102.6
Cough	1	0	0	1
Loss of Smell / Taste	0	1	1	1
Difficulty in Breath	1	1	0	0
Recent exposure to COVID-19 patient	1	0	1	0

Crore people have been infected and near about half a million people have died due to COVID-19 and still adding up. The newness and insufficient knowledge about the disease lead to a tremendous number of rumors and misconceptions, causing a chaotic state in every part of the world. The goal of selecting coronavirus disease was to provide accurate information about symptoms and a handy diagnostic tool in order to avoid confusion.

SARS-CoV-2 affects people differently. The majority of infected people develop mild to moderate symptoms and do not need hospitalization, but a significant number of them develop severe symptoms, needing hospitalization (Singh et al., 2021). Mildly to moderately infected people commonly develop fever, cough, fatigue, and loss of taste or smell. Difficulty in breathing or chest pain signifies increasing severity.

In this project, the authors gathered a few important symptoms and risk factors relevant for COVID-19 from medical practitioners. This dataset consisted of 7105 corona patients of all ages and both sexes. It contained five major symptoms and risk factors that play a significant role in COVID-19 and can help the model distinguish whether the user is at risk of suffering from COVID-19 or not. These parameters help the model to further predict if the user is at risk of developing the specific disease based on the data the user enters. The following parameters were chosen based on the most common symptoms and risk factors that physicians use to diagnose the disease and on the ease of identification by the general population. The sample dataset is provided below in Table 1.

In the following dataset, value "1" stands for "Yes" and value "0" stands for "No" for the parameters of cough, loss of smell/taste, difficulty in breath, and recent exposure to COVID-19 patient, whereas the value data recorded for fever is the thermometer reading in °C.

Diabetes Mellitus

Diabetes mellitus (DM) is a metabolic disease characterized by elevated blood glucose levels due to insufficient insulin production (Type 1) or increased insulin resistance (Type 2). Type 1 DM is most seen in children or adolescents while Type 2 DM affects middle-aged and older adults. The most common and major risk factor for DM is a sedentary or unhealthy lifestyle, which in turn causes prolonged high blood sugar levels.

Beta cells or Islets of Langerhans in the pancreas are responsible for insulin production in the human body (Sapra & Bhandari, 2021). In Type 1 DM, beta cells produce insufficient or no insulin at all due to genetic factors. Whereas in Type 2 DM, beta cells do produce insulin, which is unable to act on the specific receptors on the cells (insulin resistance) to break down glucose, causing hyper-glycemia. Stress,

Table 2. Dataset sample for Diabetes Mellitus

Parameters	Patient 1 Data	Patient 2 Data	Patient 3 Data	Patient 4 Data
Age (in years)	50	31	32	21
Gender	1	0	1	0
BMI	33.6	22.6	23.3	28.1
Fasting Blood Glucose Levels	158	85	132	93
HbA1c	7.2	6.6	5.4	8.6
Family History of Diabetes	1	0	0	1

obesity, unhealthy diet, and family history of diabetes are some of the major risk factors for developing diabetes. Fasting blood glucose levels and HbA1c (a diabetes specific test) are the gold standard tests done to diagnose it.

In this project, the authors collaborated with medical professionals to identify a few important indicators linked to diabetes. This dataset included 769 diabetes patient records from people of all ages and both sexes. It contained six critical symptoms and risk factors that can help the algorithm determine if a user is at risk of developing diabetes or not. The significant parameters were chosen based on the most common symptoms and risk factors physicians use to diagnose the disease and on the ease of identification by the general population. The authors have included an example dataset below in Table 2.

In the following dataset, value "1" logged for sex stands for "Male" and value "0" stands for "Female", whereas value "1" for family history of diabetes stands for "Yes" and value "0" stands for "No". Data recorded for BMI is the calculated Body Mass Index in kg/m^2. Data recorded for fasting blood glucose levels is the measured blood glucose before eating via glucometer in mmol/L. Data recorded for HbA1c is the calculated value of the blood glucose attached to hemoglobin in mmol/mol.

Lung Disease

Lungs are one of the vital organs and epicenter of the respiratory system, susceptible to many diseases affecting a healthy lifestyle. Every cell of the human body needs oxygen to survive and do its work, and the main function of the lungs is to provide oxygen to the human body via the gaseous exchange process at the level of alveoli. Lungs exchange waste carbon dioxide from the body with oxygen from the environment. Every time human beings breathe; they inhale oxygen and exhale carbon dioxide.

Considering the importance of the function of the lungs, any issue or hurdle in this process can disrupt normal body functions affecting health. Bronchitis, chronic obstructive pulmonary disease (COPD) (Gentry & Gentry, 2017), and asthma are some of the most common lung disorders noted in different regions of the world. Lung diseases can be temporary acute or long-term chronic illnesses. Lung diseases are generally caused by foreign particles or pathogens present in the air, leading to inflammation or allergic reactions, causing difficulty in breathing. Cough is the most common initial symptom of any lung disease. Exposure to industrial or tobacco smoke plays a principal role in the development of any lung disease. Family history of any lung disease or any history of allergies is also a risk factor for significant lung disorders.

Table 3. Dataset sample for lung diseases

Parameters	Patient 1 Data	Patient 2 Data	Patient 3 Data	Patient 4 Data
Age (in years)	17	57	36	24
Sex	1	1	0	1
Fever	100.8	101.9	98.8	102.4
Cough	0	1	0	1
Sputum Production	0	0	0	1
Shortness of Breath	1	1	1	1
History of Lungs Disease	0	1	0	0
Family History of Lungs Disease	1	0	0	1
Smoking	1	1	0	1

In this model, medical specialists helped to select a few key symptoms and risk factors for lung diseases. There were 570 records for patients suffering from lung disease in this collection, including people of various ages and both sexes. This dataset comprised nine key symptoms and risk factors that might aid the algorithm in determining whether a user is at risk of suffering from any lung disease. The reasoning behind choosing these specific parameters was to include the symptoms and risk factors most common between varying lung diseases that physicians use to diagnose the disease, in addition to the ease of identification by the general population. An example dataset is shown below in Table 3.

In the following dataset, value "1" recorded for cough, sputum production, shortness of breath, history of lung disease, family history of lungs disease, and smoking equals "Yes" whereas a value of "0" equals "No". Moreover, a value of "1" recorded for sex equals f "Male" and a value of "0"' equals for "Female". Data recorded for fever is the thermometer reading in °C.

Heart Disease

The heart is the second most vital organ in the human body as it pumps blood to all the body parts, which carries all the essential nutrients, oxygen, and everything the human body needs to be alive. Any obstruction in this pump would lead to significant damage to various cells in the human body (Ballard & Jan, 2018). Stress, smoking, unhealthy diet, alcohol, recreational drugs, and genetics are some of the most common risk factors that may lead to any heart disease. Other diseases such as diabetes, hypertension are also major risk factors for a cardiac event.

Chest pain is the initial presentation or symptom seen in any heart disease. It is the first and the most important organ to monitor for chest pain although it might indicate other problems as well. Endocarditis, rheumatic heart disease, coronary artery disease, and conduction abnormalities are a few of the most common heart diseases worldwide. Coronary artery disease is the obstruction of blood flow to the heart due to plaque formation in coronary arteries. It is the most common heart disease worldwide and could be life-threatening if not treated in time. Instead of predicting current heart disease, this web application in turn predicts the risk of a future cardiac event or heart disease occurrence.

Table 4. Dataset sample for heart disease

Parameters	Patient 1 Data	Patient 2 Data	Patient 3 Data	Patient 4 Data
Age (in years)	63	23	37	49
Sex	1	1	0	0
Smoking	1	1	0	1
Alcohol	0	1	0	0
Blood Pressure	1	0	1	1
Diabetes	0	1	0	1
Palpitations	0	1	1	0
Total Cholesterol	194	155	202	122
Shortness of Breath on Exertion	1	1	1	0
History of Cardiac Event	1	1	0	0
Family History of Heart Disease	1	1	0	0

In this project, medical experts helped to identify a few key symptoms and risk factors associated with heart disease. This dataset contained 304 heart disease patient records, including individuals of various ages and both sexes. This dataset comprised eleven key symptoms and risk factors that can assist the algorithm in determining whether or not a user has a risk for having heart disease. The following parameters are the most crucial symptoms and risk factors responsible for a cardiac event and important for physicians in diagnosing the disease. Concurrently, they can certainly be provided by the general population. An example dataset is shown below in Table 4.

In the following dataset, value of "1" recorded for smoking, alcohol, blood pressure, diabetes, palpitations, shortness of breath on exertion, history of cardiac event, and family history of heart disease equals "Yes" whereas a value of "0" equals "No". On the contrary, a value of "1" recorded for sex equals "Male" and Value "0" equals "Female". Data recorded for cholesterol is the calculated cholesterol levels in mg/dL via lipid panel test.

Liver Disease

The liver is one of the body's most important organs. The main function of the liver is to eliminate toxins, bilirubin, and break down fat by producing and secreting bile juice (Sharma & John, 2021). The liver also helps in the metabolism of drugs, poisons, and metabolism of glucose, amino acids, proteins, and all the essential nutrients that occur in the liver (Antunes et al., 2021). The liver is also responsible for producing clotting factors and immune factors. The liver excretes harmful substances and their by-products via bile and blood.

Liver diseases are much more common and could be life-threatening if not given proper attention. As mentioned earlier, the liver is very important in excreting out toxins and producing clotting or immune factors. Any obstruction in these processes could lead to further damage to various parts of the human body. Some of the most important risk factors for developing liver diseases are age, sex, alcohol intake,

Table 5. Dataset sample for liver disease

Parameters	Patient 1 Data	Patient 2 Data	Patient 3 Data	Patient 4 Data
Age (in years)	45	26	62	39
Sex	0	1	1	1
Alcohol Intake	1	1	0	1
BMI	18.4	25.5	34.1	22.4
Loss of Appetite	1	0	0	1
Changes in Urine Color	1	1	0	1
Changes in Stool Color	1	1	1	0
Yellowish Skin	1	0	1	0
Family History of Liver Disease	0	0	1	1

and obesity. Nausea/vomiting, loss of appetite, yellow skin changes (jaundice), dark urine, and pale or black stools are some of the most common and early symptoms of liver diseases (Qasim & Patel, 2021).

In this project, the authors asked medical specialists to provide a few important symptoms and risk factors posing risks of liver illness. This dataset comprised 584 patient records for liver illness, with patients of all ages and both sexes represented. This dataset contained nine conventional symptoms and risk factors that are important in assessing whether a user has a risk of experiencing liver illness and can help the model determine whether or not the user has it. Below mentioned parameters are the most conventional symptoms and risk factors correlated with liver disease that physicians use in their diagnosis and that can conveniently be provided by the general population. An example dataset is provided below in Table 5.

In the following dataset, value "1" recorded for alcohol intake, loss of appetite, changes in urine color, changes in stool color, yellowish skin, and family history of liver disease equals "Yes" and value "0" equals "No". Whereas value "1" recorded for sex equals "Male" and value "0" equals for "Female". Data recorded for BMI is the calculated Body Mass Index in kg/m^2.

Kidney Disease

The kidney is one of the most vital organs, acting as a purifier to filter out waste products, excess water, and other impurities from the blood. The kidney is also responsible for regulating electrolytes such as potassium, sodium, and pH levels in the body. The core function of the kidney is to manage blood pressure and control red blood cell production (Bindroo et al., 2021). Kidneys are also responsible for excreting the toxins and the waste products metabolized by the liver.

Hypertension is the most underrated disease as it could affect multiple organs in the human body and the kidney is the sole regulator for blood pressure. People with a history of hypertension, heart disease, diabetes, and kidney disease need to be very careful in maintaining proper kidney function. Kidney diseases do not cause symptoms in the kidney, symptoms are to be noted in the part or organ affected by it. Age, sex, diabetes, hypertension, history of kidney stones, and family history of kidney diseases, are some of the major risk factors for any kidney illness. Some commonly used drugs such as non-steroidal anti-inflammatory drugs (NSAID) have side effects on the kidney, therefore overuse of some drugs also affects kidney function.

Similarly, the authors have obtained a few key symptoms and risk factors related to kidney disease from medical professionals for the model. This dataset contained 583 kidney disease patient records, of all ages and both sexes. This dataset comprised eleven key symptoms and risk factors that play a crucial part in kidney disease and can aid the model in determining whether the user has it. Selected parameters are the most typical symptoms and risk factors for kidney disease used by physicians for diagnosis and are easily identified by the general population. Below is a sample dataset in Table 6.

In the following dataset, value "1" recorded for diabetes, hypertension, NSAIDs use, flank pain, changes or difficulty in urination, history of kidney disease, history of heart disease, family history of kidney disease equals "Yes" and Value "0" equals "No". Similarly, value "1" recorded for sex equals "Male" and Value "0" equals "Female".

Table 6. Dataset sample for kidney disease

Parameters	Patient 1 Data	Patient 2 Data	Patient 3 Data	Patient 4 Data
Age (in years)	48	27	62	82
Sex	1	0	0	0
Diabetes	1	0	1	0
Hypertension	1	1	1	1
NSAIDs Use	1	1	1	1
Flank Pain	1	1	1	0
Changes or Difficulty in Urination	0	0	1	1
History of Kidney Disease	0	1	1	0
History of Heart Disease	0	0	1	1
Family History of Kidney Disease	0	1	1	1

Splitting Dataset

Splitting the dataset in machine learning is utilized to assess the exhibition of the proposed model. In this procedure, the dataset is partitioned into two sections, regularly known as training data set and testing data set. The training set is an initial set of data where the authors train and let the model analyze and learn, whilst test data is simply used to evaluate the model's performance. The output of training data is accessible for modeling, but testing data is unseen data for which predictions must be generated. Test data is a last, real-world verification of an unknown dataset to ensure that the machine learning algorithm is properly trained. The model is worked to foresee future objectives that are obscure. Therefore, to check the precision of model forecasts, the authors need some obscure information for the model to anticipate which is essentially named as testing dataset. The dataset is separated haphazardly in the ratio

80:20 respectively for training and testing, utilizing the train-test split capacity which is accessible in scikit-learn library (n.d.) work as demonstrated in Figure 1.

Classification

It might be difficult to determine which machine learning algorithm would perform best for a given data collection because there are many different algorithms to choose from. Therefore, it is important to understand the advantages and disadvantages of each before selecting the one that is ideal for the model. As a result, the most effective approach for aiding in designing the most efficient algorithm is trial and error. In the context of machine learning, classification is a subset of supervised machine learning techniques in which a result is categorized into two or more categories, such as whether a person is suffering from a certain disease or not. A classifier may also be thought of as a mathematical computational function that maps incoming data into the appropriate category. The following list shows examples of different algorithms.

1. *Gaussian Naïve Bayes.* Gaussian Naive Bayes is a type of naive bayes algorithm that follows a normal or Gaussian distribution and continuous data values consistently. It is especially useful when the data's characteristics have continuous values. A Gaussian Naive Bayes model is constructed by assuming that the data follow a normal distribution with no covariance, i.e., an independent distribution. To define a distribution, the Gaussian model may be easily fitted by simply calculating the standard deviation and mean of the data points.
2. *Random Forest.* Random forest is a supervised machine learning method that can classify and predict data. It consists of a mixture of numerous separate decision trees that are directly proportionate to the intended conclusion, as the name implies. Each internal node in the tree represents a specific feature or characteristic, whereas each leaf node represents a class label. The most successful model is random forest, which relies on many decision trees being based on balloting.
3. *Decision Tree.* A decision tree is a graphical representation of an outline chart that a person uses to select an activity progression or to display a likelihood. It molds the shape of a woody plant, which is mostly upright but occasionally lies on its sides. Every branch of the decision tree represents a probability of making a decision, getting a consequence, having a reaction, or making a choice. Every node in the decision tree refers to a specific test case for certain characteristics and descending down the edges leads to the test cases' probable outcomes. A recursive decision tree is the same for every subtree since it is rooted at the new nodes.
4. *Support Vector Machine.* The support vector machine (SVM) is a supervised machine learning method that can classify and predict data. The support vector machine is generally used to divide data into categories. Based on the recognition of patterns, the algorithm creates a model that will produce distinct hyperplanes to isolate or separate the data. The hyperplane with the greatest distance between the data points and the hyperplane itself will be the most effective.

Performance Evaluation Metrics

A confusion matrix is a technique used for evaluating and analyzing the performance of a model that has been created based on its predictions. The model divides the issue statement into two or more categories, positive class and negative class, to help readers understand if the model is appropriately categorizing the test and training the data. The authors of this work evaluated the accuracy of the confusion matrix by using the confusion matrix function from the scikit-learn package. The confusion matrix is evaluated using the values of precision, recall value, and accuracy values that are achieved from the equations shown below. The confusion matrix and all other metrics are e discussed in Das et al. (2021).

- *Recall* - Recall addresses how much data is anticipated correctly out of all the positive classes. The higher the number, the better the model.

$$\text{Recall} = \frac{TP}{\left(TP + FN\right)}$$

- *Precision* - Precision represents how much data are positive out of all the positive classes the model has predicted correctly.

$$\text{Precision} = \frac{TP}{\left(TP + FP\right)}$$

- *Accuracy* - Out of the total classes, based on the probability the model predicts correctly. The higher the number, the better the model.

$$\text{Accuracy} = \frac{\left(TP + TN\right)}{\left(TP + TN + FP + FN\right)}$$

- *Training accuracy* - It represents the accuracy the model achieves when it is applied to the training data.
- *Testing accuracy* - It represents the accuracy the model achieves when it is applied to the testing data which is unseen to the model.
- *Accuracy gap percentage* – It represents the difference percentage between training accuracy and testing accuracy.

Accuracy Gap = Training Accuracy – Testing Accuracy

*True Positive (TP) = The predicted value corresponds to the actual value. The model anticipated a positive value, and the actual result was positive.

*True Negative (TN) = The anticipated value is identical to the actual value. The model anticipated a negative value, and the actual value was negative.

*False Positive (FP) = Also known as Type 1 error, the predicted value was incorrectly anticipated. Although the actual result was negative, the model projected that it would be positive.

*False Negative (FN) = Also known as Type 2 error, the predicted value was incorrectly anticipated. Although the actual number was positive, the model predicted that it would be negative.

EXPERIMENTAL RESULTS AND DISCUSSIONS

The Confusion Matrix is represented below for each disease in Fig. 2 to Fig. 7.

Coronavirus (COVID-19)

Here, in COVID 19, there are 736 True Negative and 0 False Positive. While 685 False Negative and 0 True Positive.

Figure 2. Confusion matrix of COVID-19

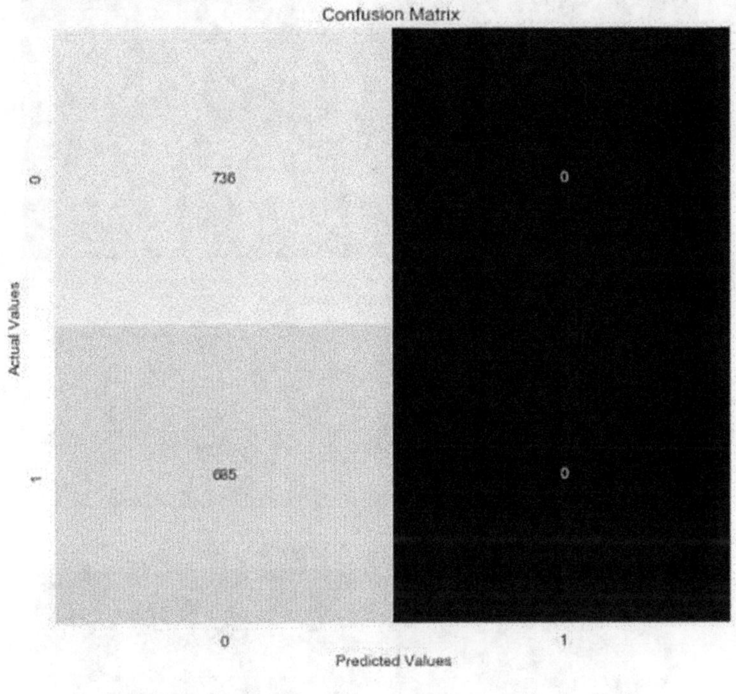

Diabetes

Here, in Diabetes, there are 272 True Negative and 0 False Positive. While 4 False Negative and 124 True Positive.

Lung Disease

Here, in Lung Disease, there are 21 True Negative and 6 False Positive. While 2 False Negative and 32 True Positive.

Figure 3. Confusion Matrix of Diabetes

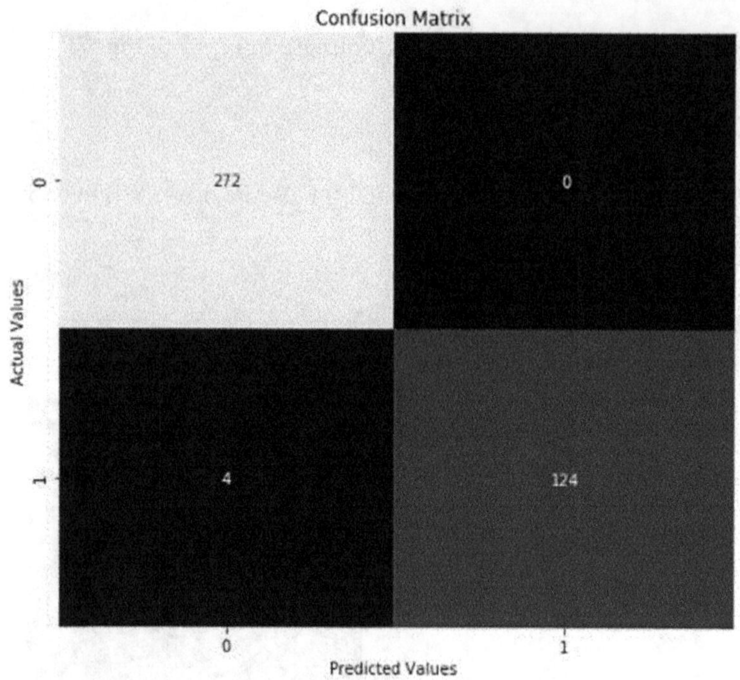

Figure 4. Confusion Matrix of Lung Diseases

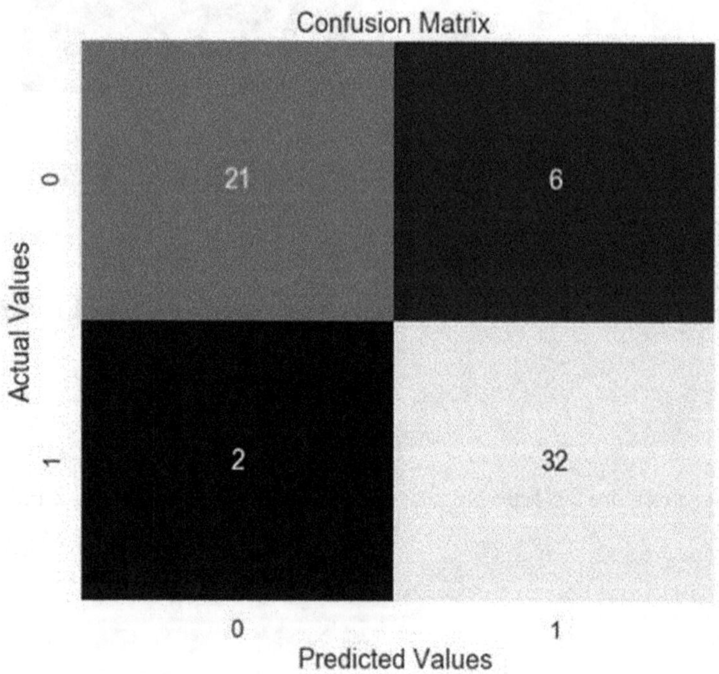

Figure 5. Confusion matrix of heart diseases

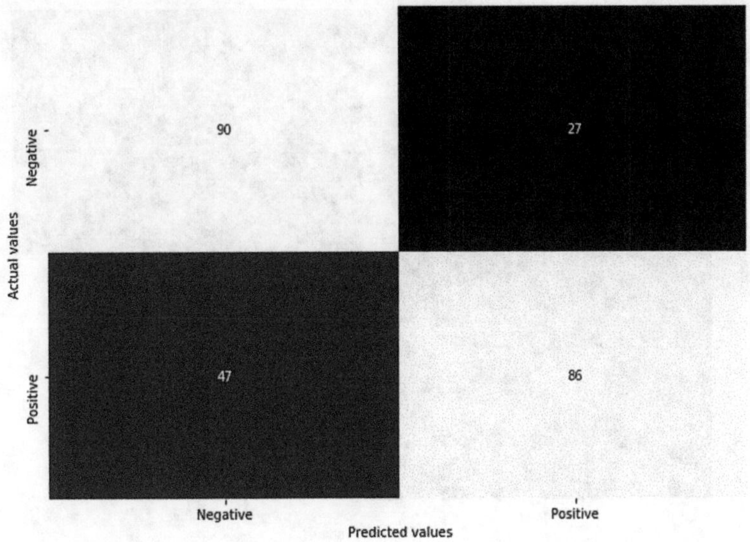

Heart Disease

Here, in Heart Disease, there are 90 True Negative and 27 False Positive. While 47 False Negative and 86 True Positive.

Liver Disease

Here, in Liver disease, there are 69 True Negative and 48 False Positive. While 39 False Negative and 94 True Positive.

Kidney Disease

Similarly, for Kidney disease, there are 83 True Negative and 34 False Positive. While 38 False Negative and 95 True Positive.

The authors can depict from the above six confusion matrix that the values for true positive, true negative, false positive, and false negative are not very high, indicating that the model has performed quite well. The values for lung disease are extremely low, denoting that the lung disease model outperformed the others.

The training accuracy and the testing accuracy of respective algorithms are shown in Table 7 and in the graphical representation in Fig. 8. The minimum the accuracy gap, the better the model. The table explains that there is the least difference between the performance of the model trained and the performance of the model tested. A high difference between the training and test errors suggests that the model is overfitted, which can generally be corrected by training with more data. When a model learns the information and noise in the training data to the point that it degrades the model's performance on fresh data, this is known as overfitting. This implies that the model picks up on noise or random fluctuations in the training data and learns them.

Figure 6. Confusion matrix of liver diseases

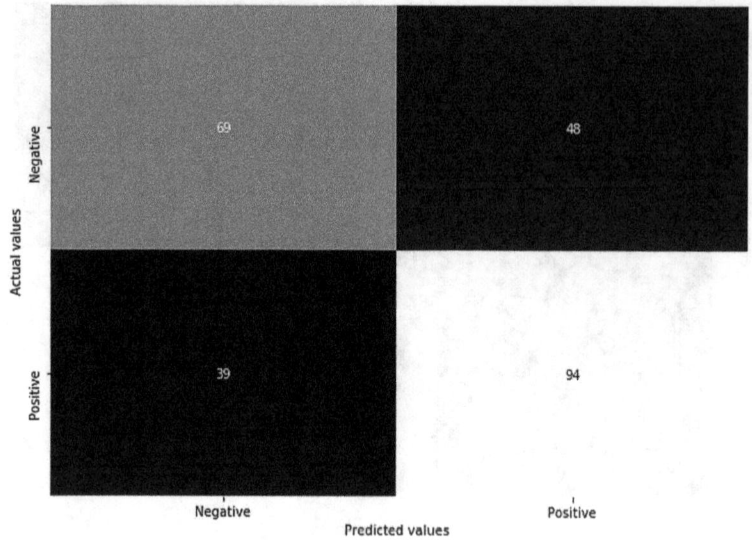

While the maximum accuracy gap is for diabetes, the training accuracy of 100% and testing accuracy of 99% are very high. The accuracy gap is highest that is 0.34 in the case of liver disease which depicts that the model is not efficient enough. The model built for COVID-19 has an accuracy gap of 0.08 which proves to be the least efficient as training and testing accuracy achieved is also low.

Figure 7. Confusion matrix of kidney diseases

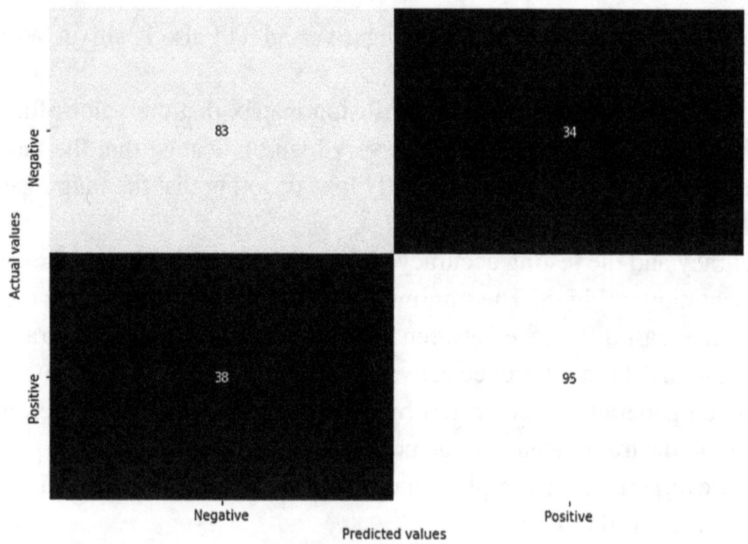

Table 7. Comparative analysis of all six diseases

Algorithm	Training Accuracy	Testing Accuracy	Accuracy Gap %
COVID-19	0.59	0.51	0.08
Diabetes	1	0.99	0.1
Lungs Diseases	0.90	0.80	0.1
Heart Diseases	0.99	0.7	0.29
Liver Diseases	0.99	0.65	0.34
Kidney Diseases	0.95	0.7	0.25

Figure 8. Graphical representation of training and testing accuracy

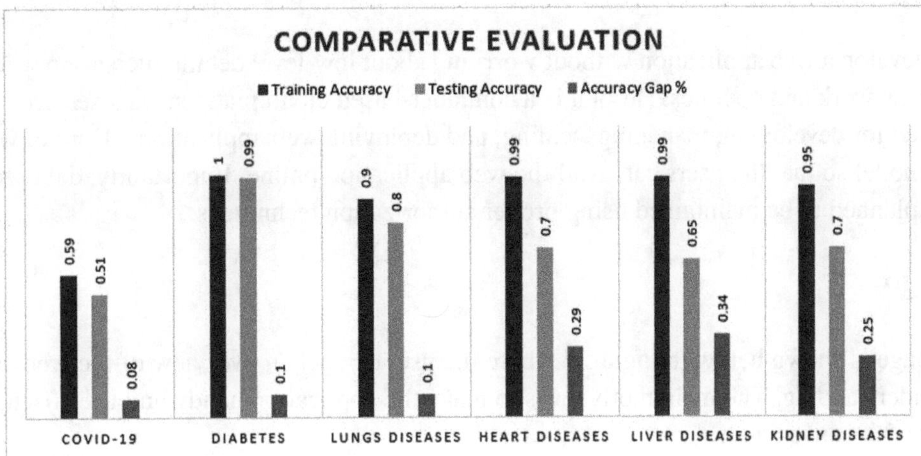

EXECUTION OUTCOME OF WEB APPLICATION

The development, adoption, and implementation of a wide range of new ehealth applications (such as online health information websites, interactive electronic health records, health decision support programs, tailored health education programs, health care system portals, mobile health communication programs, and advanced telehealth applications) have huge potentials to improve consumer and provider access to relevant health information, improve care quality, and reduce costs (Kreps et al., 2020). In its current state, the model described in this chapter is a web application prototype. In the future, it can be developed further to become freely available to users on a wide scale.

The web application has three pages: a Home page that gives an overview of the application, an About page that provides a brief introduction about each disease, and a Result page where the user can input the relevant information and retrieve the desired output. Currently, the prototype of the web application uses local storage, but in the future, it can be deployed to cloud storage where it can be used globally.

The web templates were rendered using Flask. Flask is an application programming interface of Python, basically, a micro web framework that helps in building web applications thus rendering web templates and managing HTTP requests. It is developer-friendly and easy to use and code. It also helps

Figure 9. Home page of web application

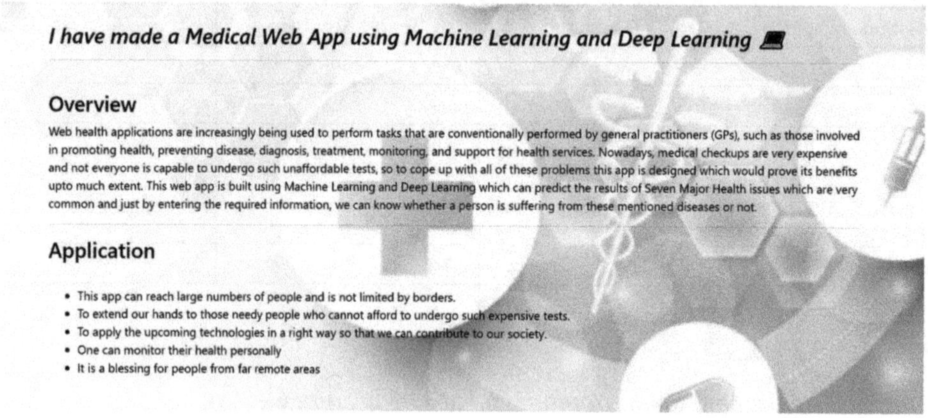

the user to develop a web application without worrying about low-level details such as how does underlying functions work and operates. Heroku is a container-based cloud platform as a service (PaaS) that is mostly used for developing, managing, scaling, and deploying web applications. Heroku was used to deploy the model so that the users can avail the web application online. Importantly, data security and privacy are planned to be maintained using proper authorization techniques.

Home Page

The home page is shown below in Figure 9 where the user can get an overview of the web application for better understanding. The main motive was to make the application handy and user-friendly for the users to use with convenience.

About Page

The about page is shown below in Figure 10 where the user can get a brief introduction about the disease, its symptoms, and root causes.

Result Page

This is the result page as shown below in Figures 11 and Figure 12 where the user can choose a particular disease amongst all the six diseases as mentioned they might be suffering from. The user needs to enter the values of the symptoms and then click on the predict button. It will show whether the user has a risk of suffering from the disease or not.

FUTURE RESEARCH DIRECTIONS

In the future, the authors would like to expand this project to develop a stronger disease detection method capable of detecting the majority of critical diseases. Future work can also be done by making an ad-

Figure 10. About Page of Web Application

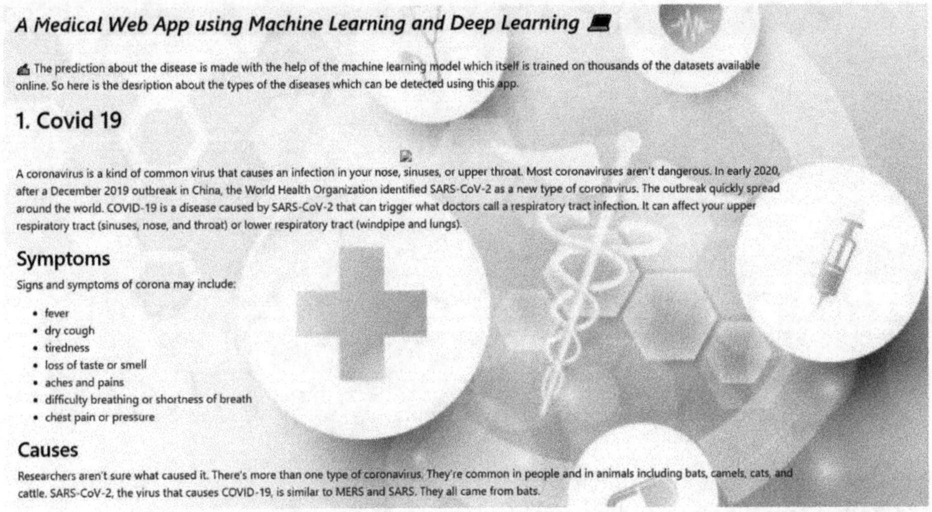

ministrative account that can handle all the medical databases to organize state data. Health administrators from various hospitals can directly track their patients. This application can provide a countrywide platform for storing and maintaining people's medical databases using Aadhar card verification and linkage for personal identification, e.g. social security number for USA.

Advancing medicine and technology creates a lot of potential for new and creative ideas to provide awareness and information about health via new-age technology. In this paper, the authors aspire to create awareness about a healthy lifestyle and address rumors that spread incorrect information. But this is just the first step towards the big picture when health services will become easily accessible by every human being with widespread awareness about a healthy lifestyle. At the moment, the authors

Figure 11. User input page of web application

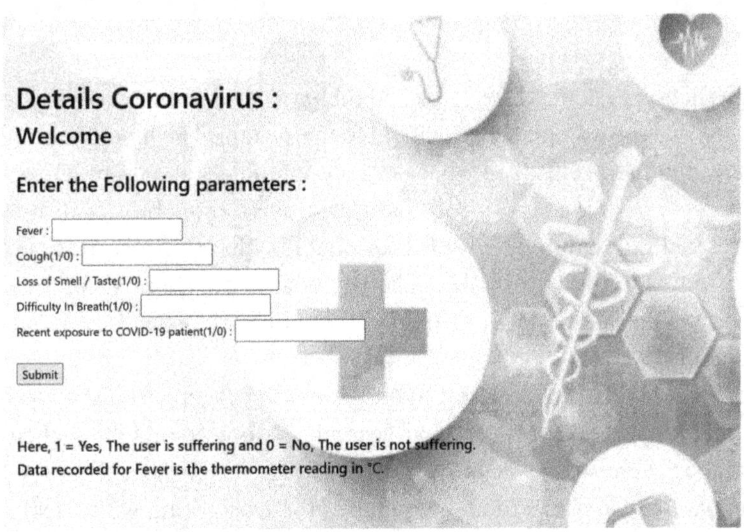

Figure 12. Output page of web application

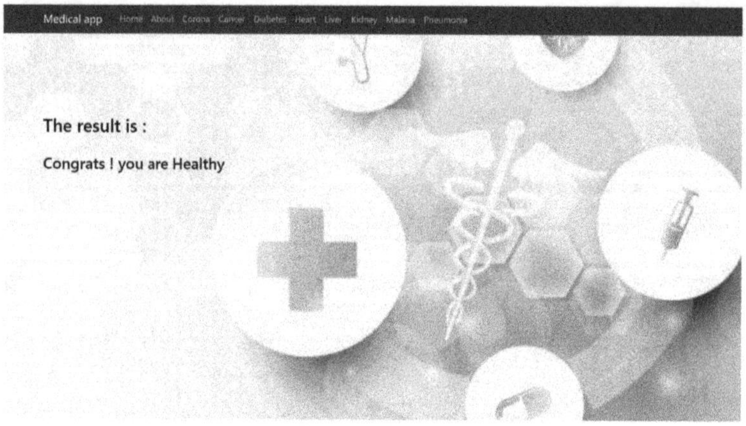

have included only a few diseases and generalized many diseases into one category. Further research and data could be collected to discover easily available and cost-efficient diagnostic criteria, which then could be used to evaluate the risk.

In developing and overpopulated countries like India, it is very important to collect and analyze health data to avoid misuse of medications and conclude incorrect treatment. The first step towards a healthy community is to spread awareness about the importance of monitoring and rightfully treating health instead of following superstitions and rumors. The web application describes in this chapter needs more detailed evaluation and research to categorize various symptoms and risk factors which could be easily used to distinguish and diagnose various diseases.

Now, diagnosing diseases correctly needs tests or studies which makes health services expensive and inaccessible for people with financial issues. Hence, more research and resources could help to discover cheap and easily accessible ways to provide proper health care and awareness to everyone because everybody has a right to get proper treatment.

CONCLUSION

The multi- disease prediction system is focused on predictive modeling which forecasts the user's disease based on the symptoms that the user presents as input to the system. The machine analyses the symptoms given by the patient as input and returns the disease's probability as an output. Disease prediction is accomplished using machine learning algorithms that measure the probabilities of the disease.

The multi-disease prediction system is useful for people who are concerned about their health and want to know what is going on in their bodies. The key goal in developing this system is to help them become aware of their wellness. They will overcome these difficulties and go about their everyday life with ease.

Four machine learning algorithms are used in the proposed system: Gaussian Naive Bayes, decision tree, random forest, and support vector machine. The analysis showed that the diabetes model is the best out of all as the training accuracy achieved is 100% and testing 99% with an accuracy gap of just 1%. The least efficient model was the Covid 19 model which had the least training and testing accuracy of 59%

and 51% with an accuracy gap of 0.08. The accuracy gap is highest that is 0.34 in case of liver disease which depicts that the model is not efficient enough. The authors observed that the accuracy percent difference between training and the testing accuracy is lowest in cases of liver and kidney diseases after analyzing the outputs of these four algorithms.

ACKNOWLEDGMENT

This Chapter is an outcome of the collaborative inter discipline research work between Amity Institute of Information Technology, *Amity University Kolkata, India,* and Medical School in Willemstad, *St. Martinus University, Curacao.* Significant contribution of this chapter is presented from Major Project work of Anjali Agarwal and Medical Internship of Ravish Kumar Bansal. Anjali Agarwal has carried out her major project under the supervision of Ajanta Das. Both, Anjali Agarwal, and Ravish Kumar Bansal have contributed to some extent equally with respect to the research credentials and datasets.

REFERENCES

Antunes, C., Azadfard, M., Hoilat, G. J., & Gupta, M. (2020). Fatty Liver. StatPearls Publishing.

Ballard, B. D., & Jan, A. (2018). *Cardiovascular Disease.* StatPearls Publishing. https://www.ncbi.nlm.nih.gov/books/NBK535419/

Belte, A., Suryawanshi, V., Sharma, R., & Deore, M. (2020). Cancer Disease Prediction Using Machine Learning Over Big Data. International Research Journal of Engineering and Technology, 7(3).

Bindroo, S., Quintanilla Rodriguez, B. S., & Challa, H. J. (2021, August 13). Renal Failure. StatPearls Publishing.

Chauhan, R. H., Naik, D. N., Halpati, R. A., Patel, S. J., & Prajapati, M. A. (2008). Disease Prediction using Machine Learning. *Clinical Reports*, 783-7.

Das, A., Agarwal, A., & Das, R. (2021). *Evaluation of Social Human Sentiment Analysis using Machine Learning Algorithms.* Presented in the 2nd International Conference on Computer Engineering & Communication Systems (ICACECS 2021).

Fahad, P. K., & Pallavi, M. S. (2018, April). Prediction of human health using machine learning and big data. In *2018 International Conference on Communication and Signal Processing (ICCSP)* (pp. 195-199). IEEE. 10.1109/ICCSP.2018.8524352

Fogel, A. L., & Kvedar, J. C. (2018). Artificial intelligence powers digital medicine. *NPJ Digital Medicine*, *1*(1), 1–4. doi:10.103841746-017-0012-2 PMID:31304291

Food and Drug Administration. (2020). *What is Digital Health?* https://www.fda.gov/medical-devices/digital-health-center-excellence/what-digital-health

Gentry, S., & Gentry, B. (2017). Chronic obstructive pulmonary disease: Diagnosis and management. *American Family Physician*, *95*(7), 433–441. PMID:28409593

Ghose, A., Guo, X., Li, B., & Dang, Y. (2021). *Empowering patients using smart mobile health platforms: Evidence from a randomized field experiment*. Forthcoming at MIS Quarterly.

Grampurohit, S., & Sagarnal, C. (2020, June). Disease prediction using machine learning algorithms. In *2020 International Conference for Emerging Technology (INCET)* (pp. 1-7). IEEE.

Guo, C., Ashrafian, H., Ghafur, S., Fontana, G., Gardner, C., & Prime, M. (2020). Challenges for the evaluation of digital health solutions—A call for innovative evidence generation approaches. *NPJ Digital Medicine*, *3*(1), 1–14. doi:10.103841746-020-00314-2 PMID:32904379

IQVIA. (2017). *Grows as Innovation, Evidence and Adoption of Mobile Health Apps Accelerate*. https://www.iqvia.com/newsroom/2017/11/impact-of-digital-health-grows-asinnovation-evidence-and-adoption-of-mobile-health-apps-accelerate/

Kaplan, R. M., & Simon, H. J. (1990). Compliance in medical care: Reconsideration of self-predictions. *Annals of Behavioral Medicine*, *12*(2), 66–71. doi:10.120715324796abm1202_2

Kaur, J., & Mann, K. S. (2017, December). AI based healthcare platform for real time, predictive and prescriptive analytics using reactive programming. *Journal of Physics: Conference Series*, *933*(1), 012010.

Kreps, G. L., & Neuhauser, L. (2010). New directions in eHealth communication: Opportunities and challenges. *Patient Education and Counseling*, *78*(3), 329–336. doi:10.1016/j.pec.2010.01.013 PMID:20202779

Lee, R., & Chitnis, C. (2018, December). Improving Health-Care Systems by Disease Prediction. In *2018 International Conference on Computational Science and Computational Intelligence (CSCI)* (pp. 726-731). IEEE. 10.1109/CSCI46756.2018.00145

Machine Learning in Python. (n.d.). https://scikit-learn.org/

Matplotlib Library in Python. (n.d.). https://matplotlib.org/

Monaco, A., Palmer, K., Faber, N. H. R., Kohler, I., Silva, M., Vatland, A., van Griensven, J., Votta, M., Walsh, D., & Clay, V. (2021). Digital health tools for managing noncommunicable diseases during and after the COVID-19 pandemic: Perspectives of patients and caregivers. *Journal of Medical Internet Research*, *23*(1), e25652. doi:10.2196/25652 PMID:33464206

Mustafa, A., & Rahimi Azghadi, M. (2021). Automated Machine Learning for Healthcare and Clinical Notes Analysis. *Computers*, *10*(2), 24. doi:10.3390/computers10020024

Panch, T., Szolovits, P., & Atun, R. (2018). Artificial intelligence, machine learning and health systems. *Journal of Global Health*, *8*(2), 020303. doi:10.7189/jogh.08.020303 PMID:30405904

Qasim, A., & Patel, J. (2021). *ANCA Positive Vasculitis*. StatPearls Publishing. https://www.ncbi.nlm.nih.gov/books/NBK554372/

Sapra, A., Bhandari, P., & Wilhite Hughes, A. (2021). Diabetes Mellitus (Nursing). StatPearls Publishing.

Scikit-Library. (2021). https://scikit-learn.org/

Shah, D., Patel, S., & Bharti, S. K. (2020). Heart disease prediction using machine learning techniques. *SN Computer Science*, 684-687.

Sharma, B., & John, S. (2020). Hepatic Cirrhosis. StatPearls Publishing.

Shetty, V. (2016, November 22). *Machine Learning in layman's terms*. Academic Press.

Singh, A., Avula, A., & Zahn, E. (2021). *Acute bronchitis*. StatPearls Publishing. https://www.ncbi.nlm.nih.gov/books/NBK448067/

Stone, P., Brooks, R., Brynjolfsson, E., Calo, R., Etzioni, O., Hager, G., ... Teller, A. (2016). *Artificial intelligence and life in 2030: the one hundred year study on artificial intelligence*. Academic Press.

Taber, J. M., Leyva, B., & Persoskie, A. (2015). Why do people avoid medical care? A qualitative study using national data. *Journal of General Internal Medicine*, *30*(3), 290–297. doi:10.100711606-014-3089-1 PMID:25387439

WHO. (2021). *Global strategy on digital health 2020–2025*. World Health Organization. https://www.who.int/docs/default-source/documents/gs4dhdaa2a9f352b0445bafbc79ca799dce4d.pdf?sfvrsn=f112ede5_38

Yarabarla, M. S., Ravi, L. K., & Sivasangari, A. (2019, April). Breast cancer prediction via machine learning. In *2019 3rd International Conference on Trends in Electronics and Informatics (ICOEI)* (pp. 121-124). IEEE. 10.1109/ICOEI.2019.8862533

ADDITIONAL READING

Blumenthal, D., & Tavenner, M. (2010). The "meaningful use" regulation for electronic health records. *The New England Journal of Medicine*, *363*(6), 501–504. doi:10.1056/NEJMp1006114 PMID:20647183

Darcy, A. M., Louie, A. K., & Roberts, L. W. (2016). Machine learning and the profession of medicine. *Journal of the American Medical Association*, *315*(6), 551–552. doi:10.1001/jama.2015.18421 PMID:26864406

Gordis, L., Markowitz, M., & Lilienfeld, A. M. (1969). The inaccuracy in using interviews to estimate patient reliability in taking medications at home. *Medical Care*, *7*(1), 49–54. doi:10.1097/00005650-196901000-00006 PMID:5804663

Iuga, A. O., & McGuire, M. J. (2014). Adherence and health care costs. *Risk Management and Healthcare Policy*, *7*, 35. PMID:24591853

Jha, S., & Topol, E. J. (2016). Adapting to artificial intelligence: Radiologists and pathologists as information specialists. *Journal of the American Medical Association*, *316*(22), 2353–2354. doi:10.1001/jama.2016.17438 PMID:27898975

Lafleur, J., & Oderda, G. M. (2004). Methods to measure patient compliance with medication regimens. *Journal of Pain & Palliative Care Pharmacotherapy*, *18*(3), 81–87. doi:10.1080/J354v18n03_09 PMID:15364635

Robinson, R. L., Long, S. R., Chang, S., Able, S., Baser, O., Obenchain, R., & Swindle, R. W. (2006). Higher costs and therapeutic factors associated with adherence to NCQA HEDIS antidepressant medication management measures: Analysis of administrative claims. *Journal of Managed Care Pharmacy*, *12*(1), 43–54. doi:10.18553/jmcp.2006.12.1.43 PMID:16420107

Santo, K., Richtering, S. S., Chalmers, J., Thiagalingam, A., Chow, C. K., & Redfern, J. (2016). Mobile phone apps to improve medication adherence: A systematic stepwise process to identify high-quality apps. *JMIR mHealth and uHealth*, *4*(4), e6742. doi:10.2196/mhealth.6742 PMID:27913373

Toy, E. L., Beaulieu, N. U., McHale, J. M., Welland, T. R., Plauschinat, C. A., Swensen, A., & Duh, M. S. (2011). Treatment of COPD: Relationships between daily dosing frequency, adherence, resource use, and costs. *Respiratory Medicine*, *105*(3), 435–441. doi:10.1016/j.rmed.2010.09.006 PMID:20880687

Key terms and definitions

Classification: Categorizing into different groups accordingly.

Confusion Matrix: A confusion matrix is a table that shows how well a classification model (or “classifier”) performs on a set of test data for which the real values are known.

COPD: Chronic Obstructive Pulmonary Disease is a term for a group of disorders that obstruct the airways and make it difficult to breathe.

COVID-19: A viral infection that results in severe acute respiratory failure.

eHealth: Information and communication technology (ICT) is being used in health and health-related services.

Heroku: Heroku is a cloud-based platform as a service (PaaS) that allows developers to create, run, and maintain applications entirely in the cloud.

Hypertension: Blood pressure that is unusually high, particularly arterial blood pressure.

Outbreaks: An undesirable event, like as war or sickness, that occurs unexpectedly.

Symbiosis: A partnership between two or more persons or groups that is mutually beneficial.

Web Application: An application software that operates on a web server.

Chapter 8
Implementing Social–Emotional Learning in the Virtual Environment for K–12 Classrooms

Erika L. Patterson
York School District One, USA

ABSTRACT

The COVID-19 pandemic precipitated several mental health effects on people such as stress, depression, irritability, anger, and confusion. Especially affected were school-aged children whose daily routines were disrupted by school closure and isolation. Hamilton et al. reported that the social-emotional health of 30-40% of students in the USA was impacted negatively, especially those learning remotely and historically marginalized. The virtual learning environment for students needed an intervention to help alleviate the impacts of isolation during remote and virtual learning. Social emotional learning curriculum was implemented in the virtual learning environment for students in a seventh grade English class. Theories of mindfulness and social emotional learning are addressed to show the academic and mental health benefits for implementing social emotional learning in the classroom for adolescents learning in the virtual environment.

INTRODUCTION

The COVID-19 pandemic precipitated several mental health effects on people such as stress, depression, irritability, anger, and confusion (Pfefferbaum & North, 2020). Especially affected were school-aged children whose daily routines were disrupted by school closure and isolation (Bartlett et al., 2020). Hamilton et al. (2021) reported that the social-emotional health of 30-40% of students in the USA was impacted negatively, especially those learning remotely and historically marginalized. The World Health Organization (2022) defines health as "a state of complete physical, mental and social well-being and not merely the absence of disease or infirmity" (para. 1). Furthermore, it stresses the importance of mental

DOI: 10.4018/978-1-7998-9490-2.ch008

health in children and adolescents because of the rapid brain growth and development that shape the formation of cognitive and social emotional skills during this stage of life. Similarly, Greenberg et al. (2015) posit that building social and emotional skills helps students with stress management that will ultimately improve their overall health. Moreover, research shows that the healthier the students, the better their academic achievement (Ickovics et al., 2013; Puskar & Bernando, 2007; Ride et al., 2010).

Although the need to address the social emotional well-being of students was exacerbated by the pandemic, awareness about it emerged years earlier, with the expressed need for social emotional learning (SEL) in schools, due to the demands for preparing students for life and work and not only academically, the increased racial and cultural diversity in schools, and the need to target students' different abilities (Weissberg et al., 2015). To date, thousands of schools have adopted SEL programs with promising results (Gueldner et al., 2020; Weissberg et al., 2015). SEL programs have shown positive influences on students' self-esteem (Papadopoulos, 2020), their school engagement (Yang et al., 2018), the development of social and emotional skills, and improved behavior (Durlak et al. 2011).

To address the emotional stressors caused by the pandemic and the resulting disruption, many schools focused on SEL to support their communities (Cipriano, 2020). Moreover, Hauge (2020) determined that by moving classrooms to the virtual environment, "screens have become the portal through which many… children learn and experience relationships," increasing the need for connection at this crucial developmental stage (p. 55).

SEL THEORETICAL FRAMEWORK

While there is no consensus on the definition of SEL (DeArmond et al. 2021; Gueldner et al., 2020), Weissburg et al. (2015) concluded its framework involves the "personalization of the education process and engaging pedagogies and relevant curricula that offer opportunities for deeper learning and connection to the world beyond school" (p. 11). Brackett et al. (2015) claimed that more than one theory frames SEL because on one hand it involves content related to the connections between emotional skills and students' development and on the other, it addresses instructional strategies that engage students. Consequently, SEL theoretical framework might include systems theories that explain the dynamics between students and their environment, learning theories that inform the design of instruction, theories of child development that guide age-appropriate design, information processing theories that address processing and retainment of information in memory, and theories of behavior change that focus on motivation and sustainment of behavior (Brackett et al., 2015). Similarly, Gueldner et al. (2020) asserted that many frameworks are used to design SEL activities such as developmental psychology, public health, neuroscience, and teaching and learning.

One approach that has been successfully combined with SEL programs is mindfulness (Coholic et al., 2020; Lemberger-Truelove et al., 2018; Sapthiang et al., 2019). Mindfulness has shown positive effects in SEL like reducing aggressive behavior and promoting emotional regulation, self-compassion, and social connectedness (Gómez-Olmedo et al., 2020). Positive results have also emerged from integrating mindfulness in comprehensive health education interventions (Klainin-Yobasa et al., 2019; Salmoirago-Blotchera et al., 2018).

MINDFULNESS

Mindfulness practice aims at calming the mind (Karunamuni & Weerasekera, 2020). It is rooted in Buddhist psychology in which a person is immersed in awareness of their engagement with the world and their conscious interactions within their environment. Bishop et al. (2004) proposed two mindfulness components. One is self-regulation of attention to bring "awareness to ... thoughts, feelings, and sensations from moment to moment" (p. 232). The other is orientation to experience to make "a commitment to maintain an attitude of curiosity about where the mind wanders" (p. 233). Similarly, Brown et al. (2007) defined mindfulness as a "receptive attention to and awareness of present events and experience" (p. 212). On the other hand, Morris (2020) argued that mindfulness is integral to transformative learning that plays a role in "chang[ing] one's frames of reference" (p. 50) and enhancing awareness to thinking by focusing on the present attention and regulating one's emotion.

While mindfulness originated in Buddhist psychology, the adoption of the practices in Western psychology differs based on the theoretical approach and usage mindfulness practice incorporates. Brown et al. (2007) pointed to the many theoretical and conceptual descriptions of mindfulness, the diversity of its definitions, and the nuanced meanings. Nevertheless, they reported on the research evidence that showed "links between mindfulness and enhanced executive attention, including more effective behavioral regulation and self-control in healthy and clinical populations" (p. 228).

Shapiro et al. (2006) proposed three axioms for mindfulness: attention, intention, and attitude, stating:

With intentional training, one becomes increasingly able to take interest in each experience as it arises and also allow what is being experienced to pass away (i.e., not be held on to). Through intentionally bringing the attitudes of patience, compassion and non-striving to the attentional practice, one develops the capacity not to continually strive for pleasant experiences, or to push aversive experiences away. (p. 377)

This chapter presents a social emotional intervention based on mindfulness and aimed at addressing the needs of middle school students during the COVID-19 pandemic. It describes the instructional design process. Additionally, it shows the alignment with the social cognitive theory developed by Bandura (1998, 2004), a theoretical framework widely used and applicable in the disciplines of education and health, specifically in academic achievement and emotional and mental health, the cornerstones of this intervention (Luszczynska, & Schwarzer, 2005).

THE INSTRUCTIONAL DESIGN PROCESS

The design process of the intervention as described below illustrates the elements of the generic instructional design model ADDIE model that stands for Analysis, Design, Development, Implementation, and Evaluation (Molenda, 2003).

Analysis

The analysis phase highlights the need that drove the design and implementation of the virtual SEL intervention. Bradshaw (1972) classified needs into different types, identifying expressed needs as needs turned into action by the demands of people. Moreover, the World Health Organization (2020) described initial needs assessment as the type of assessment "undertaken promptly at the outset of a crisis or following a new event or sudden change" (p. 321). The changes imposed by the pandemic and the needs expressed by teachers, administrators, parents, and students exemplify these types of needs.

During the 2020-2021 school year, school districts in South Carolina in the United States of America implemented virtual programs, due to the COVID-19 pandemic. Students eligible to apply for the virtual program addressed in this SEL intervention were those who needed to be enrolled in the program for medical reasons, with at-risk family members, and whose families stated they had Internet services that were reliable and/or did not want their children to wear masks in the schools or be exposed to other students that may have contracted COVID-19. Teachers in the district applied to teach in the virtual program, attended scheduled interviews, and were chosen to teach in the program based on skills, their own at-risk needs, and the positions available. As a teacher in the district trained in technology instruction, having experience teaching in an online platform, being at-risk with medical diagnoses, and having at-risk family members, I was hired to teach middle school English in this program, as a solution for my school district to address the needs of the local community and to keep their children safe during the pandemic.

Teachers hired for the virtual program were provided Edgenuity®, an online platform to provide instruction for grades seven through twelve. Prior to the COVID-19 pandemic, Edgenuity® was used for credit recovery units for students failing due to absences, who needed to be homebound for medical reasons, or who were attending the district alternative school. The district found the program effective for these students. Therefore, they selected it for the virtual program in order to ensure a smooth transition for teachers.

Problems with the online curriculum began with students not having access to Wi-Fi with the bandwidth to stream the lessons. The school district is in a rural agricultural community with a small town as its center. Most of the district wealth resides within the town limits with a few outlying communities and farms that have been able to financially sustain the impacts of the pandemic. Many families in locations not receiving higher Wi-Fi bandwidths could not afford the cost of the cable and Internet providers. Moreover, some providers would not offer service in the rural areas. However, one solution for the lack of Internet connection was the availability of Wi-Fi hotspots through cell phone providers that were funded by the South Carolina Department of Education (2021a). While families received hotspots to provide Internet service, the hotspots did not have sufficient bandwidth to support streaming videos in Edgenuity® for multiple student users in a single household. So, students living in these areas and initially enrolled in the virtual program were transferred back to the face-to-face environment and the program was limited to student with reliable Internet access. This digital divide is common in rural areas around the world and was compounded by the pandemic when schools were forced to move learning online (Khlaif & Salha, 2021; Rodriguez et al., 2021).

Challenges to the Virtual Program

The curriculum implemented through Edgenuity® as the primary instruction for virtual students led to gaps in learning due to the abbreviated 2019-2020 school year. Students received emergency lessons issued by the district in March 2020 that failed to address the curriculum students were expected to learn by the end of that current school year. Fortunately, English Language Arts contains circular standards that provide instruction that incorporates the same content across sixth, seventh, and eighth grades, which helped seventh grade students focus on skills they missed during the prior abbreviated 2019-2020 school year (South Carolina Department of Education, 2015). Learning involved strengthening what they already understood, while introducing new concepts in the English Language Arts classroom through eighth and seventh grade content. Edgenuity® provided higher reading Lexiles in the material than in the school curriculum for seventh grade English Language Arts, so strategies to address the reading slide due to the prior school year were implemented in instruction.

Reading Lexile levels are determined by the student's level of reading and the ability to understand what they are reading, based on standardized test scores that provide the Lexile reading level of a student (Booksource, 2022). Booksource (2022), an online resource that teachers use to categorize their classroom libraries and track books that students have borrowed, states that a proficient reading Lexile for seventh grade students is between 970L-1120L. Edgenuity (2018) realigned their reading Lexile levels for their curriculum for grades six through eight to be 955L-1155L, which puts a proficient seventh grade reader in an appropriate reading level (p. 19). The seventh-grade merit class had Lexile levels from 915L-1065L at the lowest score to 1495L-1645L at the highest score. These students received the eighth-grade curriculum that would have the highest Lexile level to meet their educational needs. The seventh-grade non-merit class had Lexile levels from 50L-200L for the lowest scorer to 1150L-1300L for the highest scorer. Twenty-seven of the sixty-six seventh grade students had a Lexile level that was below the starting Lexile of 955L in Edgenuity curriculum. Only twenty-nine of the sixty-six seventh grade students had a starting Lexile level of 955L, therefore over half of the seventh-grade students from both the merit and non-merit courses were not prepared for the Edgenuity curriculum and the expected reading Lexiles.

The reading slide, originally termed the summer reading slide, refers to a student's loss of reading levels. Booksource (2018) stated, "Students who lack books to read at home during the summer can fall months, and eventually years, behind their peers" (booksourcebanter.com). Typically, the summer is between two to three months, but when students were told they were going remote in March 2020, they ended up having five months out of school. While teachers sent books home for them to read, the students no longer had access to the school library, the public library, or new books they could choose to read. The summer slide for students without access to books shows an average loss of two to three months, the six months out of school became an overall reading slide with a loss of five to eight months. With the higher reading Lexile levels of Edgenuity, over half the students were not ready to read at 955L or higher, and in a new virtual environment, students struggled in the 2020-2021 school year.

Moreover, students in the district typically were introduced to the digital content in Canvas© and Microsoft 365® in seventh and eighth Grades. Canvas© is the Learning Management System (LMS) the school district used for the delivery of digital content for students, providing an online platform for instruction. Teachers design lessons and lesson activities, upload them into the LMS, and organize the instruction for student access and assessment. Canvas© hosts digital and interactive applications for students to use, providing them with lessons, activities, assignments, and quizzes in one location for each of their courses. Microsoft 365® for students and faculty gives them access to Microsoft applications like: Word, Excel, PowerPoint, OneDrive, and Class Notebooks. Teachers set up Class Notebooks for the virtual program courses to provide students with handouts, interactive lessons, note-taking, and feedback online. Since the district had yet to implement one-to-one for middle and high school (one computer for every student), the rising seventh grade students did not have the skills required to use the digital applications used for the lessons. Additionally, some students had never operated a Chromebook and needed direct instruction for using the device, saving their assignments, and accessing them to upload into Canvas©. Seventh grade students were not versed in navigating Canvas©, had never used Microsoft 365® applications, and found navigating Edgenuity® difficult. Their parents became the primary support for their students' learning but needed assistance and resources to navigate the technology their children would be using. The district and the virtual program offered training throughout the school year but there was low attendance at those training, due to parents' work conflicts, transportation, and childcare coverage.

Students and parents expressed feeling overwhelmed by the multiple digital platforms and asked for direct instruction from teachers. At the start of Fall 2020, teachers, parents, and students were instructed to use Edgenuity® as the primary curriculum for seventh grades students as asynchronous learning with teacher support. After a month into school, some parents complained that their students were not receiving one-on-one interactions with their teachers and stated that was a need. Teachers were told to begin implementing live class meetings with curriculum that scaffolded the materials students were introduced to in the Edgenuity® curriculum to help improve their success in the courses, essentially making their classes. When the virtual program teachers provided online class meetings, the change from asynchronous (flexible schedules) to synchronous (teacher determined schedules) learning confused the virtual students and disrupted their schedules. Students expressed frustration and some began falling behind in the lessons, resulting in lower grades. They fell behind on work, showed a lack of motivation, and stopped attending the live class meetings. These observations were also reported in the literature. The lack of connectivity and technology skills results in negative feelings about learning, diminished engagement, and delayed communication (Khlaif & Salha, 2021; Rodriguez et al., 2021).

The Substance Abuse and Mental Health Services Administration (2021) stated, "Emotional distress can happen before and after a disaster. Coping strategies include preparation, self-care, and identifying support systems" (para. 1). Students in the virtual program who had no prior behavioral or academic problems were beginning to display behavior and emotions of children who were in a traumatic event. According to the National Alliance on Mental Health (2021), "The coronavirus (COVID-19) has resulted in an unprecedented crisis that affects not only our physical health and daily lives, but also our mental health" (para. 1). The impact of mental health due to the pandemic emerged in student responses to virtual learning as they navigated "uncertainty, change in routine, social isolation, and fears" (nami.org, 2021, para. 4). Therefore, I designed strategies to help students cope with the demands of Edgenuity® and the digital environment and implemented a predesigned social emotional learning curriculum to help students incorporate self-care into their learning.

The South Carolina Department of Education SEL Mandates

The South Carolina Department of Education Services whose goal is to meet student needs for positive outcomes and to support their development socially, emotionally, and academically, determined that students need various skills to develop conflict resolution, decision making, and teamwork (ed.sc.gov, 2021). Each of these skills adds to the employability, self-esteem, and success of students upon graduation. They stated:

The mission of [the] social emotional learning team is to provide consistent, collaborative, proactive direction and support focused in the areas of social emotional learning, by using data-based decision making, quality instruction, family and community engagement and fidelity of implementation to meet the profile of the South Carolina graduate. (South Carolina Department of Education, 2021b)

Teachers in South Carolina are expected to address the emotional and psychological needs of their students to help mitigate trauma that children may experience in their communities, school, or home. The COVID-19 pandemic exacerbated trauma responses in students after they were sent home in March 2020, students did not return to a normal school year in August 2020, and the district continued to have masking and quarantining guidelines from the state impact the 2021-2022 school year.

After the prior year of school closures due to COVID-19, the South Carolina Department of Education projected an increase in mental health needs and decided that providing SEL resources would be an initial step towards meeting the needs of students and teachers in the state. Consequently, the South Carolina Department of Education launched a plan to support SEL in August 2020. The state launched its initiative for schools to start implementing social-emotional learning based on the Collaboration for Academic, Social and Emotional Learning (CASEL) competencies of self-awareness, self-management, responsible decision-making, relationship skills, and social awareness (CASEL, 2022). The South Carolina Department of Education began to provide resources and guidelines to schools to direct teachers to implement social and emotional learning lessons in the classroom.

Resources provided for teachers included a website devoted to social emotional learning and links to three organizations for addressing social emotional learning initiatives, at-risk students, and mental health training to serve student needs. First, Collaboration for Academic, Social and Emotional Learning (CASEL) whose mission is to promote evidence based SEL integration in education and who developed a framework of five competencies that students should develop and graduate with for success in the world after high school (CASEL, 2022). Second, PromotePrevent provided services for schools to help navigate challenges in students' environments and aimed to make schools safer through programs that address cyberbullying, mental health, and substance abuse (PromotePrevent, 2013). Third, Mental Health First Aid trainings provided skills-based training courses for teachers to learn about mental health and substance-use issues (Mental Health First Aid, 2022). Additionally, the South Carolina Department of Education's Social Emotional Learning Portal (SCDE SEL Portal) provided educators with a curriculum specific to the students they teach. This portal outlined how the five competencies of SEL from CASEL align and complement the Profile of a South Carolina Graduate (PSCG) competencies (South Carolina Department of Education, 2021c). CASEL identified five competencies that are critical for a student: self-awareness, self-management, social awareness, relationship skills, and responsible decision-making (PersonlizedSC.ed.gov). According to SCDE (2021c), the following competencies of a South Carolina graduate give students the opportunity to integrate the five competencies of social emotional learning (South Carolina Department of Education, 2021d):

- Self-Awareness: Navigate Conflict, Learn Independently, Sustain Wellness, and Develop Networks.
- Self-Management: Navigate Conflict, Learn Independently, Sustain Wellness, and Lead Teams.
- Social Awareness: Navigate Conflict, Lead Teams, Engage as a Citizen, and Develop Networks.
- Relationship Skills: Express Ideas, Navigate Conflict, Lead Teams, and Develop Networks.
- Responsible Decision-Making: Navigate Conflict, Learn Independently, Sustain Wellness, Engage as a Citizen, and Lead Teams.

The CASEL and PSCG competencies aligned should develop a graduate who is ready for the world of either college or the work force that helps them remain in tune with their interactions in their environment; who is able to manage their time, understand how to plan for projects, and show leadership in either college or a career; who is socially aware and uses their social awareness to acknowledge others and build a community to better their community to promote equity in their society; who promote effective communication skills as they navigate college course and their work environments; and who enters their world able to make choices that not only better their lives and the life of their immediate family but also improves their community and the world (PSCG & CASEL Competency Crosswalk, 2021). Therefore, based on the needs discussed above and the SEL mandates by the South Carolina Department of Education, I designed a virtual SEL intervention for my seventh-grade English students.

Design and Development

The design phase of the instructional process consists of determining objectives and outcomes, sequencing the learning material, and selecting instructional and assessment strategies (Morrison et al., 2013). The SEL lessons needed to be aligned with South Carolina English 7 and 8 standards, stating what they addressed, what a student was expected to be able to do at the end of the lesson, and how to know the lesson was effective via formative or summative assessment. The SEL lessons were always assessed via formative assessment to address and determine the students' social and emotional needs. Accordingly, objectives and assessment strategies were set. The challenge remained in sequencing and selecting appropriate instructional strategies in addition to developing the materials needed for the virtual learning environment.

When the South Carolina Department of Education instructed school districts to begin incorporating SEL lessons in the middle of the 2020-2021 school year, the provided lessons were developed for elementary-aged students, to which middle school students did not respond positively. Therefore, with the administrator's permission, I incorporated the *30 Days of Mindfulness in the Classroom* program I had been offered for free as a teacher, prior to the COVID-19 pandemic. The benefit of the *30 Days of Mindfulness in the Classroom* curriculum was the provision of lessons for different age groups. Each of the lessons has directions and videos that are specialized for elementary, middle school, and high school students' age groups, and interests for each age group. The program consists of 30 mindfulness lessons focused on "breathing exercises… meditations…[and] relaxation activities" that help students "discover new practices to help improve focus, manage stress, regulate emotions and develop compassion" (Calm Schools, 2020, p.3). The lessons encourage reflective thoughts, journaling, and use active engagement of the body and mind together of both the teacher and students to practice mindfulness and acceptance of everyone in the classroom (Calm for Schools, 2020). Since mindfulness has shown positive effects on SEL (Coholic et al., 2020; Gómez-Olmedo et al., 2020; Lemberger-Truelove et al., 2018; Sapthiang et al., 2019), incorporating *30 Days of Mindfulness in the Classroom* aimed at supporting the SEL curriculum. Therefore, we hoped that students would begin to attend virtual classes more often, show a decrease in stress, improve their academic achievement in their courses, and show an improvement in MAP and SCReady standardized test scores at the end of the year.

The *30 days of Mindfulness in the Classroom* was originally designed for a face-to-face classroom environment, though the lessons were recorded lessons in the online Calm© application. However, the virtual environment and virtual classroom required students to be motivated to attend class when they have the distractions of video games, siblings, and slower Internet speeds to prevent them from attending class at the scheduled times. The additional frustration many students experienced about the reality of the virtual environment diminished their motivation. Therefore, it was important to determine a way to implement the *30 Days of Mindfulness in the Classroom* in the virtual classroom.

Planning interactive lessons for SEL, though already created and structured in the *30 Days of Mindfulness in the Classroom*, required additional steps to implement them virtually. First, while many of the lessons were applicable, some involved tactile and sensory activities that could not work with equity in the virtual environment, since they would require students to have resources not easily available in their homes. Therefore, I had to determine that the ones that required face-to-face interaction or materials and supplies parents needed to provide would not be applicable for the virtual environment. The goal was to alleviate stress and not to add an additional burden on the students' families. As a result, eleven lessons were selected out of the available thirty. Then, I focused on building each of these lessons into the Module of the Week that incorporated an SEL page. Each Monday was dedicated to SEL, which gave students a chance to destress and learn new ways to reconnect with mindfulness strategies for the week.

Second, implementing the *30 Days of Mindfulness in the Classroom* into the virtual learning environment via the Canvas© LMS, required daily tasks to provide students with access to materials and videos. Students were not only required to listen and view the lesson but also to respond to the lesson. The goal was to build a system that students could navigate on the Canvas© LMS that would allow them to respond and interact with their peers, but also provided a safe environment that was stress-reducing and gave them tools to use through the week to manage their stress. These tasks included recording directions, sharing the Calm® application videos and recording the lessons, and creating assignments in the form of a discussion board post.

1. Recording Directions: I prerecorded the directions for what students needed to complete each week. Recording the video lesson required additional work and multiple retakes due to background noise, technical difficulties, and interruptions in the middle of the lesson. So, that time needed to be scheduled to meet the needs of the virtual environment.
2. Sharing the Calm® application videos and recording the lessons: I uploaded the mindfulness videos via the Microsoft 365® Teams application for students to view and experience within the weekly modules. However, the Teams application would not share the sound of the video as it shared the computer screen, so the first few lessons required links from the Calm® application to be embedded into a Canvas© page. Later, I was able to embed the videos using Canvas Studio©. Canvas Studio© provided a way for recording videos from the *30 Days of Mindfulness in the Classroom* and embedding them into a Canvas© page, which allowed students to download the video and watch it later. This gave them the ability to go to a school campus or to one of the provided buses in the community that provided WiFi, download all the videos they needed for their lessons, and then work on their assignments on their Chromebooks without streaming the provided video lessons. Moreover, while many students attended the live class sessions and attendance improved as time passed, there were still some students who were unable to attend for various reasons. To address their needs and to assure that the virtual classroom provided them with a safe and equitable environment, I needed to provide the same lesson offline. However, recording the live sessions proved to be problematic. Some students would log in to the class late and ask questions in the middle of the activity, others struggled with remaining muted during the mindfulness exercise or silencing their notifications in Microsoft 365© Teams. These caused distractions that impacted the recording. So, recording a clean version of the lesson without students present proved more effective and provided all the students with a clear recording.
3. Discussion post assignments: The discussion board posts were designed for students to respond to reflection questions via the virtual platform. While expectations were that students would will-

ingly participate, the current emotional distress of students required the activity to be meaningful and worthwhile for them. Each post students responded to gave them extra credit points towards a minor grade in the class. The discussion boards required brief responses to provided questions, were low risk with no right or wrong answers, and allowed for students to be honest in their answers. While many students liked individual lessons, they were hesitant to say they did not like some lessons. With reinforcement during instruction and positive feedback that praised their honest answers, students began to feel at ease with providing their honest feedback on whether they found the lessons helpful. Virtual students were told that not all the lessons would be a good fit for everyone, and that it was acceptable for them to say it was not helpful to them. This allowed for students to have the freedom to assess the mindfulness activity and to determine if they could use it in the future. The discussion board post responses were graded and assessed as formative assessments to address and determine the students' social and emotional needs. The discussion questions listed below aimed at encouraging student responses, increasing their engagement, and serving as formative assessment. Based on their responses, they received feedback on strategies they could use to improve their activity.

a. What did you like/dislike about the activity?
b. What did you find helpful with the activity?
c. How do you plan to use this activity this week?
d. If you did not like the activity, explain what you struggled with.

In addition to the tasks, the SEL lessons needed to be designed and strategically sequenced to achieve the best outcomes (English & Reigeluth, 1996)

Lessons From 30 Days of Mindfulness in the Classroom

Three stages of lessons occurred to introduce students to mindfulness and social-emotional learning in the virtual classroom. The first stage was an introduction lesson to share with students the things I use to alleviate stress in my life. The second stage included four lessons that introduced the students to the elements of mindfulness practices and acclimated them to the concepts and strategies of mindfulness. The third stage consisted of seven lessons that addressed different strategies of mindfulness from which students could choose what worked best for them to manage stress during the school year. The lessons for the second and third stages were selected from the Calm® app's *30 Days of Mindfulness in the Classroom* (Calm.com 2020).

- *Stage 1: Introduction to Stress Relief Activities.* This stage consisted of an introductory lesson on social emotional learning followed by five sessions. The introductory lesson revolved around hobbies and interests that I used to decrease stress while attending graduate school. The five sessions were: meditation, planting seedlings, building LEGOs, developing a craft or hobby, and a step into nature. Students could attend three out of five sessions for attendance and a grade.
    - Meditation: In the first session, I introduced the participating students to various applications on their phones that were free and could help them find breathing and meditation exercises that they liked. This session provided the opportunity to introduce students to the Calm® app that I planned to use in the classroom with them.

  - Planting seedlings: The second session consisted of showing my students how to plant seeds in a germinating tray. I talked with them about how getting your hands in soil is relaxing since it reconnects you to the earth. I took them through the process of following a process for planting seeds and how it was a relaxing process since it is repetitive and can be a form of meditation. Students were able to ask questions and talk about how they connected it to their own lives.
  - Building LEGOs: The third session guided students through the process of building LEGOs. I talked with them about how when I was writing papers and got stuck, I would take a break and go build with LEGOs since they activated a different part of my brain. I shared with them how the process of building and following a design allowed my mind to relax, which frequently led to new ideas and ways of thinking for the projects I worked on. I talked with them about how it unlocked the creativity part of my brain in an organized way that led to clearer ideas that I could implement in my projects.
  - Developing a craft or hobby: The fourth session was introducing my students to the idea of using a hobby or craft to destress and take a break. I used my table loom and showed my students the process of weaving and how it was meditative for me, since it follows a specific pattern, provides for sensory stimulation through the yarn and fibers used in weaving, and results in the visual patterning and immediate reward of seeing the project emerge as you weave. During the session, students were given the chance to ask questions about how the loom worked and began sharing their own hobbies and what they do to relax.
  - A step into nature: In the final session, I took my phone, and the present students on a walk into nature. The goal was to get the students to go on a walk with me in their own areas. Many of the students went outside and explored their environment. We talked about the things we saw and what we noticed in our surroundings. We discussed how walking in general makes the body feel energized. The goals of these sessions were to introduce the students to social emotional learning and to become aware of the benefits it provides to overall wellbeing. Since it was different from the class lessons on Edgenuity®, the students viewed this Monday as an opportunity to participate in something new.
- *Stage 2. First Series of Introduction to Mindfulness Lessons***.** I used four introductory lessons from Calm® app's *30 Days of Mindfulness in the Classroom* to introduce students to the basics of mindfulness: *Finding Calm, Breathe Bubble, Moving with Music,* and *Resting with Music*.
  - *Finding Calm.* The lesson introduced the students to the idea of relaxation and mindfulness. Through it I aimed to help my students become aware of their surroundings and to determine how to best set them up for implementing social emotional learning exercises from their homes in the virtual environment. This lesson directed students to begin a relaxation exercise, to scan their environment, and to find an object that they liked and helps them feel calm. The focus of this lesson was to help students connect to an item or a person that could help them feel calmer when they have higher moments of stress.
  - *Breathe Bubble.* This lesson introduced students to a breathing exercise that helped them count their breath in and out with pauses in between. Using a breathing exercise of this type helped students to slow down and just focus on their breathing. By practicing ways to slow down, students could become more aware of how they were feeling emotionally and physically.

- *Moving with Music*. In contrast to the first two lessons, the third introductory lesson required students to move their bodies to the music that I played. The music was slow and strange sounding to the students, unusual to what they are used to listening to. They were instructed to move their body in any way they wanted as the music changed. This was a moment they could just be silly. Middle school students and teenagers need to be able to move in a classroom for blood flow and creativity but may feel self-conscious of moving around in front of their peers or have a fear that if they get out of their seat they will get in trouble. Even though students in the virtual environment have the freedom to move around, they tend to sit all day long in front of a computer screen, only giving themselves short breaks to go to the restroom and get snacks.
- *Resting with Music*. It helped students find ways they could meditate in a relaxing location and position. This led students through their first actual meditation exercise. The strategy was to give students a moment where all they had to do was lay there or sit and listen to the music. The purpose was to impress that it is okay to just take time to listen to music and do nothing more. This exercise taught them how to be comfortable with not having an active task to complete, that all they had to do was just be in the moment. I let them know it was okay if they dozed off and that however their body and mind needed to relax was okay. They were nervous about the possibility that they could fall asleep, so I had to reinforce the idea that falling asleep was perfectly normal and acceptable.

- Stage 3. *Second Series of Introduction to Mindfulness Lessons* Seven lessons from the Calm® app's *30 Days of Mindfulness in the Classroom* were incorporated to guide students through mindfulness activities: *The Senses, Mental Fitness, Meditation, Morning Wake Up, Squeeze and Release; Soundscapes,* and *Feelings*. Each lesson was followed by reflections activities.
  - *The Senses* helped students identify items using their five senses to help them connect with the present moment. They identified items they can see, touch, hear, smell, and taste in a countdown of five items to one item. This lesson asked them to reflect on their favorite sense, what they noticed with each sense, and which sense they would feel drawn to use the next time they felt stressed.
  - *Mental Fitness* incorporated LeBron James as part of the mindfulness lesson and addressed how the brain is a muscle that needs exercise as much as the rest of the body. In this lesson, they listened to LeBron James talk about getting prepared mentally for his basketball games. Then he led them through the mindfulness meditation he uses for his pre-game preparation. The reflection questions addressed how mental focus has helped them with important moments in life, the things that make focus difficult, what they learned from LeBron James's exercise, and what they want to bring more focus to in their lives.
  - *Meditation* incorporated the first guided meditation to help students begin to incorporate it to help them alleviate stress. The purpose of this lesson was to help students build the start to a meditation practice to help them deal with the impact of stress from schoolwork, expectations, and struggles from the pandemic. It helped them focus on the present moment and find a place of compassion for themselves. In the reflection, they discussed what they learned about themselves, what they enjoyed, and what they found challenging.
  - *Morning Wake Up* incorporated stretching and releasing tension in the body to help students re-energize. The goal was to give students a way to use movement that is relaxing to help them re-energize, address moments where they struggle with sitting still for long periods of

time, and improve their mental state with light stretching. The reflections addressed how they felt before and after the stretching, the movement and stretches that released tension, and what they learned about their bodies and where they hold the most tension.

- *Squeeze and Release* used a series of tensing different muscle groups as tight as you can and then releasing them completely. The focus of this session was to help students become aware of the tension they hold in the different parts of their bodies. By doing this exercise students became aware of how their bodies felt and where they tend to hold tension when they become stressed or placed in a stressful situation. The reflections they responded to included how they felt before and after the lesson, identifying where they hold tension, how it felt to relax the different muscle groups, and what part of their bodies they found it hard to relax.
- *Soundscapes* was the penultimate lesson that students participated in. This lesson used the sounds of crickets chirping, Humpback whale songs, a campfire crackling, and rain falling. Students quietly listened to the sounds and took note of which sounds were relaxing for them. They also took note of which sounds they did not like. The focus of this lesson was to help students identify relaxation sounds they could listen to for help with getting to sleep, listening to when they are stressed, or having a moment of quiet that helps them relax. After listening to the four soundscapes, they reflected on which sounds helped them relax the most and why, while also noting the other things they noticed, which is when they responded with the sounds they did not like.
- Feelings was the final lesson. It addressed the feelings that students deal with and how emotions were perceived in their home and family. It focused on the habits we have of pushing our emotions away instead of accepting them. The goal of this lesson was to help students face their emotions and accept them honestly and openly. At the end of the lesson students were expected to reflect on the expectations about feelings and emotions they face in their family, home, and friendships, and to then address their own judgements about expressing feelings and emotions.

Theoretical Links to the Design

This intervention so designed and sequenced aligns with the social cognitive theory (SCT) proposed by Bandura (1998, 2004) who discussed the reciprocity between behavior, personal characteristics, and the environment. He added that behavioral change is influenced by beliefs in self-efficacy, outcome expectations, cognized goals, and barriers preventing behavior. Furthermore, Bandura (1998) asserted that self-efficacy is enhanced by mastery experience (the experience of mastering a behavior), vicarious experiences (modeling), social persuasion, and emotional states.

This first stage aimed at introducing students to stress-relief strategies. Sharing my personal strategies with them, provided them with instances of observational learning, modeling, and focusing attention, all parts of building vicarious experiences, in addition to triggering emotional arousals that set the stage for changes in attitudes. Moreover, it helped connect to prior knowledge and experiences. In the second stage, the first lesson on scanning the environment and finding calm underscored the importance of the environment on behavior; the second lesson on breathing enhanced mastery experiences; the third lesson fostered positive emotions through moving with music, and the fourth lesson also focused on mastery experiences, practicing relaxation. Once these introductory lessons were completed and mindfulness self-efficacy began building, the students were ready for the next series of lessons. Lessons in the third stage focused more heavily on mastery experiences. The exercises helped them to self-regulate their attention and be aware of their minds wandering and to focus on the present moment (Bishop et al., 2004; Brown et al., 2007). Additionally, the reflection activities helped students envision outcome expectations, form cognized goals, and identify barriers preventing the calming behavior (Bandura, 1998, 2004).

Implementation

Each week I developed daily modules in the Canvas© LMS. The Monday curriculum became Mindfulness Mondays. Students were expected to either participate in the live lesson or to access the embedded lesson and discussion board if they were unable to attend. Each lesson consisted of an introduction, a mindfulness exercise, and reflection and feedback.

Introduction

I introduced the lesson we would participate in together. Then, to model what was expected, I completed the mindfulness activity with the students and discussed how it impacted me. I would explain how they needed to be situated in their personal space and give them time to prepare their space for the activity. Additionally, I gave them options that allowed them to sit in chairs, lay on the floor, or sit on the floor so they were relaxed in their environment. These options helped them in assessing their environment to determine if it would function for them as they participated in the activity.

Mindfulness Exercises

After the introduction and giving the students time to arrange their environment and get comfortable, I started the Calm® app video for the lesson of that Monday.

Reflection and Feedback

At the end of the lesson, I asked the reflection questions that were posted in the discussion board post to the live sessions. I also asked students to determine if the SEL activity of the day was beneficial or helpful for them. If their answers indicated it was not helpful, I directed the students to revisit a prior activity that helped them relieve or reduce stress. If the activity was helpful, then I directed the students to try using the activity for the week and take note of how they felt after they used the activity. The goal was to give students a new activity each week that could help them reduce stress, with the hope that they would discover a few that they could use throughout the school year and in the future to help them reduce stress. The students responded to how they felt and decided on the effectiveness, which had them actively practicing self-reflection. It made them self-aware and allowed them the chance to see that their peers may have a different perspective, which helped them practice social awareness and relationship skills. So, these middle school students were already practicing what CASEL and PSCG promote for SEL in the 2021-2022 school year.

Eventually, SEL Mondays became live lessons with video support if students missed the lesson or needed to rewatch the videos for quiet moments of reflection. The lessons became the live implementation where students would experience the social emotional lessons each Monday morning with me. I participated in the activities with them, as is appropriate for modeling what is expected of them, and then we had a discussion on how they felt after the lessons. Then I would open the SEL lesson of the day for their class after the initial class lesson. This allowed for students who were actively participating to receive their discussion board points during the live session and not have to respond to the discussion board module assignment, which promoted participation and class attendance. The improvement in attendance gave us the chance to interact with students that we needed contact with for weekly check-ins and to know that the students were safe and receiving what they needed.

Evaluation

Evaluating SEL outcomes is challenging on what and how to measure even when aligned with CASEL competencies. Ecological factors such as classroom and community as well as students' factors such as academic competence, interpersonal and intrapersonal skills play a role in the impact of SEL (Gueldner et al., 2020). Among the outcomes that can be used in SEL evaluation are academic skills and students' experiences and perspectives about the program (Gueldner et al., 2020). In this intervention, students' reflections and student achievement in seventh grade English were selected as assessment measures and discussed below.

Overall, the seventh-grade students that received the program were those taking the English 7 and English 7 Merit classes. Participation and response rates were high but diminished at the end of the school year due to state standardized testing.

Student's Reflections

The Senses. Students varied in their identification of their favorite senses, giving reflective statements such as:

- "Tasting my favorite tea is calming; feeling [a] hot shower water is relaxing."
- "What I noticed while I explored each sense was how vital they are. When I feel stressed I [look at] trees, and the sky."
- "The next time I feel stressed I might look at our bird feeder, where we can occasionally see a cardinal or some blue jays."
- "I really like to eat and try new things. I am like my mom, when she gets stressed she likes to cook and bake new things." (Seventh-grade students, Spring 2021)

Mental Fitness. All the students except one perceived the lesson as beneficial, giving reflecting statements such as:

- "When I get mad and wanna say something but use my mental focus to calm down."
- "[Mental fitness] help[s] me pay attention in your head and outside of it, so you can put your brain on the one thing in front of you."
- "It has helped me be more aware of my surroundings and think about what I want to say before I say it.... I learned that I have to be more calm about situations. I want meditation to bring more focus into my life."
- "It help[ed] me pay attention to surroundings. Having electronics around me distract me. I learned that the best thing in life is experience. I want to bring more focus in my body."

- "It has helped me get through struggles throughout the year like school and not being able to see my family."
- "Mental focus helps me just to focus on what going on before I do it and think positive, but sometimes when it gets hard I just start to think so many negative thoughts.... I want to bring more focus to my life by getting calm and think more positively than negatively."
- "My mental focus helped me when I was doing my N.A.G.A. (North American Grappling Association). What can make it hard to focus is all the energy and excitement and also all the fear." (Seventh-grade students, Spring 2021)

Meditation. All the students except one perceived the lesson as beneficial, giving reflecting statements such as:

- "What I learned about myself is that I struggle to let go, the part I really enjoyed about meditating is the calmness that surrounds me."
- "It's easy for me to focus and get things done if I meditate before."
- "I learned to appreciate the calm moments in this world with so much going on."
- "It's okay to calm down and just take a breathe [*sic*]."
- "It helps with relaxing after a stressful day, you can also do it to help with sleeping like if you have too much energy you can do it to calm yourself down for bed."
- "I learned that I can do this activity to relieve tension headaches."
- "I learned that when I'm calm I can think a lot more clearly."
- "I learned that there are a lot of noises that I usually tune out that are around me. I enjoyed being able to do and think about nothing." (Seventh-grade students, Spring 2021)

Morning Wake Up. All of the students found the stretching beneficial and stress relieving, with some stating that they were difficult to complete. They gave reflecting statements such as:

- "Before the session, I felt tired and sleepy. After the session I became more woke and alive."
- "He felt] more energized and not as sleepy."
- "Before the meeting I was a little restless and distracted but after the session I was calm, tired, and also I felt peaceful. My mind felt good."
- "I learned that my body [gains] a huge value when it come[s] to being calm [and] knowing what to do to be calm."
- "Before I was stressed out about work, as usual, and afterward I'm still a little stressed, but I feel more relaxed." (Seventh-grade students, Spring 2021)

Squeeze and Release. All of the students except one perceived the lesson as beneficial, another student found the exercise difficult to complete. They gave reflecting statements such as:

- "It felt like weight was being lifted off my shoulders."
- "I felt stressed before the session...I tend to store a lot of tension in my neck. Relaxation is like a moment of peace for me."
- "Before I [was] tense and aggravated then after I was calm.... I was a little shocked. Like I just had the best spa day."

- "I felt very peaceful… It felt like I was in the most peaceful place in the world."
- "I felt ready to go and start my day after… I felt the tension in my body just leave and feel more relaxed." (Seventh-grade students, Spring 2021)

Soundscapes. Most students perceived the lesson as beneficial; some did not like it; others found the sounds spooky or disturbing. They gave reflecting statements such as:

- "The soundscape with the rain falling on the leaves made me feel very relax[ed]. It has always been something about the sound of rain that always relaxes me."
- "Makes me feel like I'm at the pond fishing. This is the quietest and peaceful and relaxing feeling ever."
- "It's just so mesmerizing to hear their calls, and I could just listen to it on loop."
- "It made me feel like I was outside hanging out with my family at night." (Seventh-grade students, Spring 2021)

Feelings. The students that attended the lesson live responded openly in class but found this a difficult lesson to respond to. All of the students except one perceived the lesson as beneficial, giving reflecting statements such as:

- "I learned that no matters what you were taught about feelings, whether it's wrong or right, go with what you feel is the right feelings or emotions."
- "[He] was told that it is best to express your feelings. Especially if you are feeling sad or upset."
- "Feelings should always be expressed when you feel them, and you don't need to hide them."
- "It [is] okay to cry and let everything out…. It is not healthy to not express or tell how you feel. (Seventh-grade students, Spring 2021)

Student Achievement

The impact of SEL was measured by looking at the students' semester averages, comparing the first semester (when they did not have SEL lessons) and the second semester (when students had SEL lessons). Choosing semester averages to determine impact allowed attendance rates in classes to be tracked, where the students who participated in SEL lessons tended to also attend the other live class sessions during the week. Semester averages were a constant and ongoing program of assessment that data could be easily gathered and evaluated for ongoing student growth. The goal was to improve student stress, increase student attendance, and to help students improve academically.

Did SEL impact student achievement? Social emotional learning did appear to impact student achievement in the English 7 course. Thirty-three students in the English 7 course participated in SEL, while thirty-two students did not participate. All but five of the students who participated in SEL from the English 7 course improved their course averages from Semester 1 to Semester 2. The average grade for Semester 1 for the participants in SEL was 66%, and the average grade for Semester 2 was 76%. The average grade for Semester 1 of the non-participants was 57.34% and the average grade for Semester 2 was 56.81%. While the average for this group showed they were failing English 7 on average, ten of the students improved their averages from Semester 1 to Semester 2 and nine students were passing the course with a 60% or higher.

Did SEL help students who were high achievers function better? The English 7 Merit course had the same trend as the English 7 course. Eleven students participated in SEL, while twelve students did not participate in SEL. All but two students who participated in SEL improved their grades from Semester 1 to Semester 2. The average grade for Semester 1 for the participants was 75.82%, and the average grade for Semester 2 was 82.45%. The average grade for Semester 1 of the non-participants was 56.42% and the average grade for Semester 2 was 54.08%. Two of the students in the non-participants did improve their averages from Semester 1 to Semester 2. Therefore, SEL impacted the achievement by at least a letter grade or more for the participants in the English 7 Merit course.

While an official measurement of social emotional health was not gathered, the attendance rates of the English 7 Merit group improved after the SEL lessons began. The students that attended the SEL lessons on Mondays increased their class participation and attendance by two to three days each week. Some students increased their class participation by three to four days per week. Therefore, the increase in attendance may have also impacted the students' averages for Semester 2 since they were more present and participating in live class lessons.

Did SEL help students who had a history of lower achievement function better? Twelve of the students in the English 7 course who were low achievers and participated in SEL, with a Semester 1 grade between 50%-68% improved their Semester 2 grade by 7-25 points. Their Semester 2 grades were between 63%-87%. All twelve of those students had an average improvement for Semester 2 that was at least one, if not two letter grades higher. These increases in scores show that SEL improved their overall achievement.

Like the English 7 Merit students, the English 7 students' attendance for class lessons improved after implementing SEL lessons. Many of the students that attended the SEL lessons improved their class participation and attendance rates by two to four days each week. Some students improved their attendance rates by five to six days each week. Their increase in attendance may have impacted their averages for Semester 2 since they were more present and participating in live class lessons.

Due to the average increases in semester averages for the participants in SEL, it appears that SEL does impact student achievement. The focus of SEL is to teach the whole child, not just the curriculum they need to know for the course. Students need to have emotional support and the advantage of skills to improve their overall mental health, which impacts how they perform in school and interact in their world.

FUTURE RESEARCH DIRECTIONS

A longitudinal study of students who receive SEL from early ages in K-12 needs to be conducted to determine if SEL impacts students in the long term. Additionally, a survey of students as they progressed through school from the March 2020 impact of the COVID-19 pandemic to the end of the 2021-2022 school year should be conducted to determine if they received SEL in their schools and how it may have helped them manage these precedented years of education. Hearing the voices of our students and their experiences with learning should be the focus in education as we navigate the new normal in our schools.

CONCLUSION

The COVID-19 pandemic forced schools to shut down and isolate students in March of the 2019-2020 school year. When the 2020-2021 school year started, a virtual program for students with at-risk needs and at-risk family members was offered. The students that attended the virtual school showed signs of disengaging with their learning as attendance rates dropped and student averages for Semester 1 suffered. Implementing social emotional learning in the virtual classroom helped students regain and maintain a connection with not only their teacher, but also with their peers. Additionally, their Semester 2 grades improved in seventh grade English. Relationship building in the virtual environment through social emotional lessons helped students begin to decrease stress, overcome challenges in the curriculum, and communicate more effectively as they reflected on the SEL lessons. The result of SEL lessons for those students who participated showed their attendance rates improved, class participation improved, and the Semester 2 averages increased in comparison to Semester 1.

REFERENCES

Bandura, A. (1998). Health promotion from the perspective of social cognitive theory. *Psychology & Health, 13*(4), 623–649. doi:10.1080/08870449808407422

Bandura, A. (2004). Health promotion by social cognitive means. *Health Education & Behavior, 31*(2), 143–164. doi:10.1177/1090198104263660 PMID:15090118

Bartlett, J. D., Griffin, J., & Thomson, D. (n.d.). *Resources for supporting children's emotional well-being during the COVID-19 pandemic*. https://aisa.or.ke/wp-content/uploads/resources/health-and-wellbeing/wellbeing-resources/resources-for-supporting-childrens-emotional-well-being-during-the-covid-19-pandemic-290320.pdf

Booksource. (2018). Summer brain drain: Surprising statistics on summer slide. *Booksource Banter Blog*. https://www.booksourcebanter.com/2018/05/04/summer-brain-drain-statistics-summer-slide/

Booksource. (2022). *Reading level chart*. Booksource. https://www.booksource.com/reading-level-chart

Brackett, M. A., Elbertson, N. A., & Rivers, S. E. (2015). Applying theory to the development of approaches to SEL. In J. A. Durlak, C. E Domitrovich, R. P., Weissberg, & T. P. Gullotta (Eds.), Handbook of social and emotional learning: Research and practice (pp. 20-32). Guilford Publications.

Bradshaw, J. (1972). Taxonomy of social need. In G. McLachlan (Ed.), *Problems and progress in medical care: Essays on current research, 7th series* (pp. 71–82). Oxford University Press.

Brown, K. W., Ryan, R. M., & Creswell, J. D. (2007). Mindfulness: Theoretical foundations and evidence for its salutary effects. *Psychological Inquiry, 18*(4), 211–237. doi:10.1080/10478400701598298

Calm for Schools Lesson Plan. (2020). *30 days of mindfulness in the classroom*. https://www.calm.com/schools/resources

Coholic, D., Schwabe, N., & Lander, K. (2020). A scoping review of arts-based mindfulness interventions for children and youth. *Child & Adolescent Social Work Journal, 37*(5), 511–526. doi:10.100710560-020-00657-5

Collaboration for Academic, Social and Emotional Learning. (2022). *Our mission and work*. https://casel.org/about-us/our-mission-work/

Collaborative for Academic, Social, and Emotional Learning (CASEL). (2021). *Fundamentals of SEL: What Is the CASEL Framework?* https://casel.org/fundamentals-of-sel/what-is-the-casel-framework/#self-awareness

Durlak, J. A., Weissberg, R. P., Dymnicki, A. B., Taylor, R. D., & Schellinger, K. B. (2011). The impact of enhancing students' social and emotional learning: A meta-analysis of school-based universal interventions: Social and emotional learning. *Child Development, 82*(1), 405–432. doi:10.1111/j.1467-8624.2010.01564.x PMID:21291449

Edgenuity. (2018). *Edgenuity Courseware: Reviewer's guide.* Edgenuity, Inc.

Eide, E. R., Showalter, M. H., & Goldhaber, D. D. (2010). The relation between children's health and academic achievement. *Children and Youth Services Review, 32*(2), 231–238. doi:10.1016/j.childyouth.2009.08.019

English, R. E., & Reigeluth, C. M. (1996). Formative research on sequencing instruction with the elaboration theory. *Educational Technology Research and Development, 44*(1), 23–42. doi:10.1007/BF02300324

Gómez-Olmedo, A. M., Valor, C., & Carrero, I. (2020). Mindfulness in education for sustainable development to nurture socioemotional competencies: A systematic review and meta-analysis. *Environmental Education Research, 26*(11), 1527–1555. doi:10.1080/13504622.2020.1777264

Greenberg, M. T., Domitrovich, C. E., Weissberg, R. P., & Durlak, J. A. (2017). Social and emotional learning as a public health approach to education. *The Future of Children, 27*(1), 13–32. doi:10.1353/foc.2017.0001

Gueldner, B. A., Feuerborn, L. L., & Merrell, K. W. (2020). Social and emotional learning in the classroom, second edition: Promoting mental health and academic success. Guilford Publications.

Hamilton, C.-C. L., Gross, C.-C. B., Adams, D., Bradshaw, C. P., Cantor, P., Gurwitch, R., Jagers, R., Murry, V. M., & Wong, M. (n.d.). *How has the pandemic affected students' social- emotional well-being? A review of the evidence to Date.* https://files.eric.ed.gov/fulltext/ED614131.pdf

Ickovics, J. R., Carroll-Scott, A., Peters, S. M., Schwartz, M., Gilstad-Hayden, K., & McCaslin, C. (2014). Health and academic achievement: Cumulative effects of health assets on standardized test scores among urban youth in the United States. *The Journal of School Health, 84*(1), 40–48. doi:10.1111/josh.12117 PMID:24320151

Karunamuni, N., & Weerasekera, R. (2019). Theoretical foundations to guide mindfulness meditation: A path to wisdom. *Current Psychology (New Brunswick, N.J.), 38*(3), 627–646. doi:10.100712144-017-9631-7

Khlaif, Z. N., Salha, S., Fareed, S., & Rashed, H. (2021). The hidden shadow of coronavirus on education in developing countries. *Online Learning, 25*(1), 269–285. doi:10.24059/olj.v25i1.2287

Klainin-Yobas, P., Kowitlawakul, Y., Lopez, V., Tang, C. T., Hoek, K. E., Gan, G. L., Lei, F., Rawtaer, I., & Mahendran, R. (2019). The effects of mindfulness and health education programs on the emotional state and cognitive function of elderly individuals with mild cognitive impairment: A randomized controlled trial. *Journal of Clinical Neuroscience, 68*, 211–217. doi:10.1016/j.jocn.2019.05.031 PMID:31303397

Lemberger-Truelove, M. E., Carbonneau, K. J., Atencio, D. J., Zieher, A. K., & Palacios, A. F. (2018). Self-regulatory growth effects for young children participating in a combined social and emotional learning and mindfulness-based intervention. *Journal of Counseling and Development*, *96*(3), 289–302. doi:10.1002/jcad.12203

Luszczynska, A., & Schwarzer, R. (2005). Social cognitive theory. In M. Conner & P. Norman (Eds.), Predicting health behaviour: Research and practice with social cognition models (pp. 127-169). Open University Press.

Mental Health First Aid. (2022). *About MHFA*. https://www.mentalhealthfirstaid.org/about/

Molenda, M. (2003). In search of the elusive ADDIE model. *Performance Improvement*, *42*(5), 34–36. doi:10.1002/pfi.4930420508

Morgan, H. (2020). Best practices for implementing remote learning during a pandemic. *The Clearing House: A Journal of Educational Strategies, Issues and Ideas*, *93*(3), 135–141. doi:10.1080/00098655.2020.1751480

Morris, T. H. (2020). Transformative learning through mindfulness: Exploring the mechanism of change. *Australian Journal of Adult Learning*, *60*(1), 44–65.

Morrison, G. R., Ross, S. M., Kalman, H. K., & Kemp, J. E. (2013). *Designing effective instruction*. Wiley & Sons, Inc.

National Alliance on Mental Illness. (2021). *COVID-19 resource and information guide*. https://nami.org/Support-Education/NAMI-HelpLine/COVID-19-Information-and-Resources/COVID-19-Resource-and-Information-Guide#q18

Padilla Rodríguez, B. C., Armellini, A., & Traxler, J. (2021). The forgotten ones: How rural teachers in Mexico are facing the COVID-19 pandemic. *Online Learning*, *25*(1), 253–268. doi:10.24059/olj.v25i1.2453

Papadopoulos, D. (2020). Effect of a social-emotional learning-based program on self-esteem and self-perception of gifted kindergarten students: A pilot study. *Journal for the Education of Gifted Young Scientists*. doi:10.17478/jegys.779438

Pfefferbaum, B., & North, C. S. (2020). Mental health and the Covid-19 pandemic. *The New England Journal of Medicine*, *383*(6), 510–512. Advance online publication. doi:10.1056/NEJMp2008017 PMID:32283003

PromotePrevent. (2013). *Who we are*. http://www.promoteprevent.org/about

Puskar, K. R., & Bernardo, L. M. (2007). Mental health and academic achievement: Role of school nurses. *Journal for Specialists in Pediatric Nursing*, *12*(4), 215–223. doi:10.1111/j.1744-6155.2007.00117.x PMID:17956370

Salmoirago-Blotcher, E., Druker, S., Frisard, C., Dunsiger, S. I., Crawford, S., Meleo-Meyer, F., Bock, B., & Pbert, L. (2018). Integrating mindfulness training in school health education to promote healthy behaviors in adolescents: Feasibility and preliminary effects on exercise and dietary habits. *Preventive Medicine Reports*, *9*, 92–95. doi:10.1016/j.pmedr.2018.01.009 PMID:29527459

Sapthiang, S., Van Gordon, W., & Shonin, E. (2019). Health school-based mindfulness interventions for improving mental health: A systematic review and thematic synthesis of qualitative studies. *Journal of Child and Family Studies*, *28*(10), 2650–2658. doi:10.100710826-019-01482-w

South Carolina Department of Education. (2015). *College- and career-ready standards for English language arts*. https://ed.sc.gov/scdoe/assets/file/programs-services/59/documents/ELA2015SCCCRStandards.pdf

South Carolina Department of Education. (2021a). *Free and lower-cost Internet response to Covid-19*. https://ed.sc.gov/districts-schools/shared-services/free-and-lower-cost-internet-in-response-to-covid-9/

South Carolina Department of Education. (2021b). *Social emotional learning*. https://ed.sc.gov/districts-schools/special-education-services/social-emotional-learning/

South Carolina Department of Education. (2021c). *PersonalizeSC: Social and emotional learning*. https://personalizesc.ed.sc.gov/pscg-competencies/social-and-emotional-learning/

South Carolina Department of Education. (2021d). *PSCG & CASEL competency crosswalk PDF*. https://personalizesc.ed.sc.gov/competencies-based-ed/sc-competencies-prototype/casel-competencies-pscg-competencies-crosswalk/

Substance Abuse and Mental Health Services Administration. (2021). *Coping tips for traumatic events and disasters*. https://www.samhsa.gov/find-help/disaster-distress-helpline/coping-tips

Weissberg, R. P., Durlak, J. A., Domitrovich, C. E., & Gullotta, T. P. (2015). Social emotional learning: Past, present, and future. In J. A. Durlak, C. E Domitrovich, R. P., Weissberg, & T. P. Gullotta (Eds.), Handbook of social and emotional learning: Research and practice (pp. 3-19). Guilford Publications.

World Health Organization. (2020). *Health Clusters*. https://healthcluster.who.int/publications/i/item/9789240004726

World Health Organization. (2022). *Constitution of the World Health Organization*. https://www.who.int/about/governance/constitution

World Health Organization. (2022). *Improving the mental and brain health of children and adolescents*. https://www.who.int/activities/improving-the-mental-and-brain-health-of-children-and-adolescents

Yang, C., Bear, G. G., & May, H. (2018). Multilevel associations between school-wide social–emotional learning approach and student engagement across elementary, middle, and high schools. *School Psychology Review*, *47*(1), 45–61. doi:10.17105/SPR-2017-0003.V47-1

ADDITIONAL READING

Creswell, J. D. (2017). Mindfulness interventions. *Annual Review of Psychology*, *68*(1), 491–516. doi:10.1146/annurev-psych-042716-051139 PMID:27687118

Durlak, J. A., Domitrovich, C. E., Weissberg, R. P., & Gullotta, T. P. (Eds.). (2015). *Handbook of social and emotional learning: Research and practice*. Guilford Publications.

Gueldner, B. A., Feuerborn, L. L., & Merrell, K. W. (2020). Social and emotional learning in the classroom, second edition: Promoting mental health and academic success. Guilford Publications.

Zenner, H.-K., Herrnleben-Kurz, S., & Walach, H. (2014). Mindfulness-based interventions in schools-a systematic review and meta-analysis. *Frontiers in Psychology*, *5*, 603–603. doi:10.3389/fpsyg.2014.00603 PMID:25071620

KEY TERMS AND DEFINITIONS

High Achievers: Students that are identified as Gifted and Talented and are placed in accelerated classes.

Lower Achievement: Low grades that suggest a student is at risk of failing.

Mindfulness: To engage in sensory and physical experiences that build upon releasing stress and tension and help build a mindset for growth to promote educational and social development.

Online Curriculum: Curriculum and lessons that are instructor created or provided through a curriculum program.

Social Emotional Learning: The interrelated concepts of social theory and experiential theory to help address the emotions and stress students experience in their homes and school environments.

Stress or Tension: The emotional or physical pressures of a person's environment that negatively impact their ability to function in their world. It typically is held in the body, impacting large muscle groups, causing headaches, and affecting emotional and behavior responses to outside stimuli.

Virtual Learning: And online learning environment with an instructor and a group of students.

Section 3

eHealth and mHealth Education Interventions: Exemplars in Higher Education

Chapter 9
mHealth, Data, and Privacy: The Case of the Higher Education Community

Stephanie J. Blackmon
William and Mary School of Education, USA

Tiera J. Lanford
Milken Institute School of Public Health, George Washington University, USA

ABSTRACT

The intersection between higher education, technology, and mHealth is growing at a rapid pace, bringing with it an array of implications for data privacy. It is important for instructional designers to attend to these new and constantly shifting data privacy considerations when developing mHealth interventions. Therefore, with a connection to both extant instructional design literature and sociocultural theory, the authors of the current work provide strategies for developing more privacy-conscious mHealth interventions for the higher education community.

INTRODUCTION

Although health-related interventions can involve the community at large, there are also times when these interventions are directly related to a higher education campus community. Also, there have been numerous uses for applications (apps) and mobile technology in higher education (France et al., 2016; Ibacache, 2019), and some of those uses have included information sharing and engagement related to individual health, such as apps for stress, anxiety, or time management, as well as community health—without much information on how the privacy components of those interactions align with pre-existing university policies or users' perspectives on the implications for their privacy. However, the quickly converging landscape of public health and United States (U.S.) higher education necessitates interventions that address the implications of app integration and what that means for prospective app users and mHealth overall, especially as it relates to data privacy. Therefore, the current chapter explores using

DOI: 10.4018/978-1-7998-9490-2.ch009

sociocultural learning theory to develop instructional design interventions that support using mHealth in ways that are more transparent, inclusive, and attentive to users' data privacy.

BACKGROUND

Growth of mHealth in U. S. Higher Education

While apps were already widely used in higher education for learning and engagement purposes, apps used for monitoring health related information were fairly novel for many campuses. In response to the COVID-19 pandemic, for example, campuses across the country began working closely with internal risk management staff and local public health departments to attempt to contain the spread of the virus in what is typically a high-density environment. Together, the organizations developed management methods that most often involved some level of prevalence and population surveillance testing. Higher education has consistently collected student data with minimal active consent; however, collecting health related data at the population level presents new privacy concerns, especially as vaccines become widely available. Student uptake of COVID-19 apps, specifically, have become critical to the successful prevention of community spread. Features range from symptom monitoring to voluntary COVID-19 test result sharing. Many institutions have developed institution specific mobile applications allowing members of the campus community to record any COVID-19 related symptoms. However, as students began using the apps, security vulnerabilities were discovered, and some campus apps required constant access to students' real-time location.

Even though COVID-19 apps provide an immediate example of the incorporation of health-related apps, the focus of this work is not just on COVID-19, as these concerns related to data privacy pre-date the pandemic (Blackmon, 2018; Blackmon & Moore, 2020). Prior to COVID-19, it was not uncommon for higher education institutions to explore and study apps for other mHealth purposes, such as helping students to manage symptoms associated with depression and anxiety (Lattie et al., 2019). Higher education institutions have struggled to manage the demand for behavioral and mental health programs and services (National Council on Disability, 2017; Watkins et al., 2012). Professional counselors and wellness professionals have developed creative ways to promote health and well-being across campuses at both individual and collective levels. In order to meet demand, colleges and universities have begun providing self-service alternatives to individual and group counseling. Among those alternatives, as noted by several subsequent examples, mHealth apps have been a popular solution to address space and employment constraints colleges and universities face, allowing them to serve more students with fewer resources. mHealth technologies that can leverage ecological momentary interventions are even more valuable to universities as they provide real-time risk intervention strategies that are designed to encourage behavior change.

One university explored mHealth outcomes on college student behaviors by developing an app called *SmarTrek* to reduce risky alcohol use (Kazemi, 2019). Researchers split participants into two groups, the first group using the app for one week, while the second group used the app for two. They also used various forms of testing and focus groups to better conceptualize the user experience and evaluate the app's effectiveness. Ultimately, 90% of participants found the app easy to use, and 60% reported that the app positively impacted their drinking habits (Kazemi, 2019). This research suggests that apps may be able to significantly impact individual behavior change, and perhaps even campus culture.

Popular consumer-based apps promoted by many universities on their counseling resource and other behavioral health-related webpages include *Calm*, *CBT-i Coach*, *Headspace*, *Mindshift*, and *Nod*. *Nod* is a newer app, developed to assist college students transitioning to college that may have trouble making social connections, which can lead to heightened feelings of loneliness and depression. The app is designed to assist college students in developing cognitive and behavioral skills by suggesting activities designed to build social connections; providing cognitive framing exercises; and supporting a growth mindset towards social connection building. A recent randomized control trial evaluating the app's efficacy has determined the app to successfully help students cope with loneliness, build connections and social support, enhance sleep quality, and buffer against loneliness and depression (Bruehlman-Senecal et al., 2020). *SmarTrek* and *Nod* are just two examples of how institutions have been able to leverage mHealth to improve the behavioral health of their students. In both cases, the findings present examples of how universities can use mHealth to positively impact their campus communities.

The *Calm* app can be used by college students to help promote healthy stress management. The app guides users through mindful meditation sessions to improve stress management and self-compassion. In a randomized control trial conducted at a large university in the southwestern region of the United States (U.S.), researchers tested the efficacy of mindfulness meditation as a stress management intervention using the *Calm* app for 8 weeks. Participants were randomly assigned to the intervention or control group, with surveys delivered via Qualtrics at baseline, post-intervention, and follow-up, four weeks post-intervention. During the study, participants in the intervention group actively used the *Calm* app for eight weeks, while the control group was instructed to refrain from using the app or participating in mindfulness activities, such as meditation or yoga, for 12 weeks (Huberty et al., 2019).

Ultimately, 88 students participated in the study, with 41 participants randomly assigned to receive the intervention. Findings from survey data indicate about half of participants found the *Calm* app helpful for reducing stress, with roughly 85% reporting being somewhat to very satisfied with their experience. Ultimately, researchers found the *Calm* app to successfully reduce stress perception post-intervention, and significantly improve mindfulness and self-compassion among college students (Huberty et al., 2019). A study on a similar app, *Headspace,* also included a randomized control trial to evaluate the app's ability to reduce symptoms of depression among college students. Researchers reached similar conclusions to that of *Calm*, concluding *Headspace* to be an effective and appropriate intervention to improve symptoms of depression among college students (Fish & Saul, 2019). While additional research is recommended to support the efficacy of mHealth apps, Huberty et al. (2019), Fish and Saul (2019) and additional research about similar apps, provide strong evidence to suggest that the promotion of mHealth in higher education settings can have a positive impact on health outcomes for college students. However, even with controlled, experimental uses, it was not clear that colleges and universities always knew or discussed the privacy implications for using those apps.

MAIN FOCUS OF THE CHAPTER

The Urgency of Data Privacy

The ubiquity of digital data collection and use within higher education is evident in everything from students' university identification cards and learning analytics course data to the apps noted in the previous section of this chapter (Jivet et al., 2020; Jones et al., 2019). Even with the invocation of the Family

Educational Rights and Privacy Act (FERPA) to account for the myriad means of data collection across universities, that still does not address the murkiness of that policy as it relates to the operationalizing of digital data collection on university campuses. For example, apps that are used and suggested across universities have their own terms, conditions, and privacy policies, and it is not clear how these policies align with FERPA. Even with something like learning analytics data from students' courses, the data privacy and access trails are not usually discussed or addressed in ways that support students, and in some cases faculty and administrators, knowing how students' information will be access or used (Blackmon & Moore, 2020). Furthermore, the data can be used to track and monitor students in ways that they may not be fully informed about, appreciate, or want (Blackmon & Moore, 2020; Shum, 2012), teetering in the somewhat dangerous space between support and uninformed surveillance.

The lack of clarity regarding privacy issues is especially important for mHealth and instructional design because of the added layer of privacy necessary for aspects of health/mHealth data. It is not uncommon for instructors to use various apps as a part of course design and instruction; therefore, preparing instructional designers to not only address aspects of data privacy in their interventions but also to have conversations with instructors about the implications of data privacy on course design and delivery is imperative. Even the most well-intentioned initiatives can inadvertently infringe on students' data privacy rights, so the landscape of technology integration broadly must shift to one that is more aware, transparent, inclusive, and proactive when addressing data privacy. mHealth instructional design interventions are an excellent place to begin, as the incorporation of and possible interactions with mHealth data can heighten the all-important need for greater attention to data privacy.

Technology/STEM Integration and Instructional Design

Before merging the key components of data privacy, sociocultural theory, and mHealth in the case of higher education, it is important to discuss what the extant literature shares about instructional design and the connections to technology specifically and science, technology, engineering, and mathematics (STEM) generally, with a focus on what would be considered more traditional classroom settings as well as classroom settings such as libraries. Addressing these broader technology/STEM areas is a foundational aspect of the current chapter.

As the integration of technology in education settings has increased, so has the integration of technology into instructional design. Several studies have addressed some aspect of the growing technological components in courses and what that means for instructional design. For example, the integration of technology and instructional design methods extend to the education and development of health professions. Blended and online learning, virtual reality, and more traditional skill-building workshops have been shown to positively contribute to health profession education. Blended learning integrates online learning and traditional classroom teaching, and has been shown to improve independent learning, understanding, problem solving, and enhances learning efficacy (Chen et al., 2020). Chen et al. (2020) explored whether changing the instructional design of four medical school laboratory courses from traditional face-to-face lectures and experiments to a blended design that integrated online and in-person instruction would positively impact learning and perceptions of blended learning for lab courses among medical students at a university in China. One-hundred seventy-three students participating in the study received lectures and conducted experiments with a blended learning design. The researchers found that 75% of participants that were taught using a blended learning design felt the courses increased their enthusiasm for learning; 71% felt blended courses improved their understanding of concepts and theories; and the mean scores among students that participated in the blended lab courses were higher than the 168 for those who took the same courses with what the text discussed as traditional instructional design (Chen et al., 2020). Overall, blended learning resulted in better learning outcomes than traditional instructional design.

Rouleau et al. (2019) conducted a systematic review of 22 studies published between 2008 and 2018 exploring e-learning in nursing education and reached similar conclusions to that of Chen et al. (2020), with most findings describing positive learning outcomes and satisfaction among nurses. Nurses improved knowledge outcomes in 59% of studies and reported an improvement and increase in skills in 41% of studies. Where nurses were dissatisfied, researchers identified technical difficulties, digital literacy, slow information exchange, and preference for traditional learning formats as barriers to success (Rouleau et al. 2019).

Alharbi et al.'s (2020) exploration of three-dimensional virtual reality in the classroom (3D-VR) positively contributed to current literature on health profession education after the researchers conducted a study introducing 3D-VR in an anatomy course designed for medical students studying at a university in Saudi Arabia. The researchers considered 104 male and 66 female medical students for the mixed-method study and found that the introduction of 3D-VR resulted in higher overall knowledge scores compared with students who received traditional instruction. Performance differences between students with traditional instruction compared with those who received 3D-VR instruction were statistically significant in every case, though the strength varied by gender and retention time (Alharbi et al., 2020). While there are several concerns associated with using 3D-VR in medical education (i.e., digital literacy, technical operation, confidence, and preference for traditional teaching models), the study offers evidence of 3D-VR's successful integration into instructional design.

The COVID-19 pandemic introduced significant obstacles for most higher education institutions, and health profession programs were no exception. To reduce transmission of the infectious coronavirus disease, medical programs adhered to physical distancing and as a result, in-hospital training and activities were temporarily suspended. For many, the pandemic prompted the introduction of online education and training across health fields, and medical students in particular had the opportunity to use innovative instructional design that included virtual reality, virtual patients, and simulations (De Ponti et al., 2020; Seymour-Walsh et al., 2020).

In one study, a class of medical students completed their practical training (which is needed to qualify for residency programs) online with a virtual reality platform called Body Interact (De Ponti et al., 2020). The platform uses virtual patients with artificial intelligence to simulate scenarios and train medical students on taking patient clinical histories, giving physical exams, running labs and tests, administering medicine, and navigating intervention processes. After a student completes a simulated visit, the platform provides a report evaluating student performances based on current clinical guidelines. After participating in the study, 90% of participants responded positively to the training; more than 75% of participants considered the training realistic; and 84% considered the training useful when combined with a more traditional teaching method, such as an apprenticeship (De Ponti et al., 2020). The medical education community has been able to use the unfortunate circumstance of the pandemic to recognize more technology enhanced instructional design techniques as effective for health programs. Rhim and Han (2020) developed five pedagogical guidelines for instructional design for medical education. They recommend educators: design a structure and flow to embrace experiential learning; accommodate both synchronous and asynchronous learning; design and facilitate interactions; promote practice opportunities; and facilitate a community. Such concepts are meant to promote cognitive, social, and teaching presence; limit transactional distance between instructors and students; and promote independent learning. These guidelines are critical to overcoming educational challenges presented to medical students in online learning environments, but realistically can be extended to non-medical programs as well (Rhim & Han, 2020).

Even prior to the pandemic, medical students across the globe were introduced to novel instructional design that included virtual and simulation components. Isaza-Restrepo et al. (2018) used mixed-methods to evaluate how medical students use virtual patients (VPs) to develop history taking and clinical reasoning skills. In addition to finding VPs easy to use, medical students found using VPs to be less stressful than real patients, as they could focus on the learning process rather than the stress and consequences of an inappropriate interaction or diagnosis (Isaza-Restrepo et al.,2018). Kononowicz et al. (2019) conducted a systematic review to evaluate the effectiveness of VPs compared to traditional learning methods using studies published between 1990 and 2018. Ultimately, 51 individual studies were included in the review, and the researchers made similar conclusions to Isaza-Restrepo et al. (2018). Virtual patients were effective substitutes for training medical professionals, and students generally provided positive feedback about their experience with VPs. While most of their findings support the effectiveness of VPs, the researchers acknowledge that among students with exclusive VP experience, there was a reduction in confidence. Further, the researchers recommend continued methodically sound research grounded in educational theory to evaluate VPs impact on health profession education more thoroughly (Kononowicz et al., 2019).

Instructional design can encompass vastly different criteria and result in a multitude of experiences across institutions and student populations. One common but understated theme is the use of design thinking throughout instructional design recently introduced in health profession education, such as the previously discussed opportunities for blended learning, e-learning, and virtual simulations. Its increasing application in health profession education fosters creativity and critical thinking among both instructors and students, which can be used to develop multidisciplinary curricula and innovative instruction, as exemplified throughout the introduction of virtual realities and virtual patients in medical programs across the globe (Alharbi et al., 2020; Isaza-Restrepo et al., 2018; Kononowicz et al., 2019; McLaughlin et al., 2019). A systematic analysis of 23 studies that explored methods of developing patient history taking skills among medical students concluded that a variety of instructional design, including role-play, interviewing real patients, and using videotapes to enhance feedback, were effective in student engagement and skill development (Keifenheim et al., 2015). Ultimately, varying instructional design results in more creative and engaged students, which improves student learning, promotes inclusive classrooms, and encourages both instructors and students to engage in design thinking that promotes content mastery in addition to general student learning, success, and development (Goodman et al., 2018; Seymour-Walsh et al., 2020). Further, student involvement in instructional design not only promotes educational engagement, but also prepares more confident medical professionals and makes health profession education more accessible and sustainable, particularly for professionals in rural and remote environments (Seymour-Walsh et al., 2020). Blended learning and innovative instructional design in health profession education is not novel; the universal need to ensure continuous instruction during the COVID-19 pandemic has merely motivated the medical education community to introduce innovative instructional design more rapidly.

Researchers have also explored technology in instructional design for other types of courses, sometimes with very specific frameworks. Ritz and Buss (2016) discussed a framework that could be helpful in instructional design when using virtual reality. They focus on both the general aspects of virtual reality that provide immersion and the Cave Automatic Virtual Environment (CAVE) system specifically (Ritz

& Buss, 2016). The goal of the piece was to provide a framework that complemented and promoted learning when integrating CAVE and other IVRs so learners could manage both the systems and the learning content. Ritz and Buss's (2016) framework includes the following areas: content, engaging and interactive, differentiation by ability, presentation, physical and virtual environments, and technical knowledge.

Similarly, other researchers have shared instructional design frameworks to address the increasing opportunities for incorporating technology into learning. Reynolds (2016) described a "conceptual modular framework" specifically for 'social constructivist digital literacy' (p. 735). Furthermore, Reynolds (2016) uses both contructionism and constructivism, and highlights six "practice domains" (p. 741) that make up the framework: 'create, manage, publish, socialize/collaborate, research, and surf/play' (p. 741; Reynolds & Harel Caperton, 2009). Reynolds (2016) goes on to apply the framework in a research setting where the participants were teachers from criteria-specific schools in West Virginia. Barak (2017) explored what they refer to as 'cloud pedagogy' (p. 459) as a framework for integrating technology for the goal of social constructivist learning in science teacher education courses. Barak (2017) goes on to define social constructivism as:

A learning theory that contends that cognitive development is a social process derived from communication with people who are meaningful to the leader (e.g., parents, teachers, and friends) or from the use of mediator aids (e.g., books, physical models, computerized visualization, etc.). (p. 460)

Cloud pedagogy, then, "is an instructional framework designed to harness information and communication technologies (ICTs) for promoting social constructivism in science classrooms" (Barak, 2017, p. 462). It supports single and group learning in a variety of classroom settings. Furthermore, there are two layers for cloud pedagogy—social constructivism and techno-instructional (Barak, 2017). Barak (2017) notes that the social constructivism layer has four principles: exploring new venues, co-constructing contents, providing and receiving feedback, and increasing engagement. The exploring new venues principle includes actions that Barak (2017) refers to as "learning by investigating" and "discovering scientific principles" (p. 462) in various learning venues; co-constructing contents involves activities such as learning through developing science-related materials with peers via the production of writing, videos, and presentations; providing and receiving feedback includes tasks such as understanding through the process of giving others feedback; and the increasing engagement principle involves actions like "learning by interacting with close and distance peers," emphasizing the value of learners in community (p. 462). The techno-instructional layer focuses on social constructivism and shows how the elements of that theory are applied in various technological environments (Barak, 2017). Studio instruction is a teaching strategy that involves an interplay between brief sessions for instruction and longer sessions with active learning; embedded assessment includes formative and summative assessment for the duration of a learning experience; and cloud applications includes the use of Web 2.0 technologies on various mobile apparatuses to foster "real-time collaborative writing and editing" (Barak, 2017, p. 463). Barak (2017) also collected data on the use of cloud pedagogy and found, through participants' self-reporting, that although pre-service science teachers are expected to use these more advanced teaching techniques and technologies, there are not always opportunities for them to do so in their teacher preparation programs.

Frameworks for instructional design have also been incorporated in what could be considered non-traditional classroom settings as well. For example, Hess (2016) explores the integration of instructional design, thereby utilizing instructional design frameworks, in library settings because technology is a growing part of librarians' work. Campbell (2014) notes ways to expand the analysis, design, development, implementation, evaluation (ADDIE) framework to include technology. For example, what Campbell (2014) refers to as the "generic ADDIE" is "modified for the specific purpose of adding new technology in library instruction" (p. 141). In this case, the analysis involves understanding users' skillset with technology and the previously missed areas of learning that the technology would address; design includes locating novel technology to address the aforementioned skillset and gap; development includes the creation of modules for the library and the use of novel technology; implementation involves using the previously-noted modules in teaching; and evaluation includes ascertaining how well the novel technology works in teaching (Campbell, 2014). Campbell (2014) goes on to emphasize that the ADDIE model has historically been useful in instructional design and that the model's flexibility is a hallmark of its longstanding place in the instructional design area. Furthermore, Campbell (2014) notes that a design approach to the integration of technology in library instruction is absolutely necessary so that issues with technology do not detract from the content librarians are sharing via instruction. Hess (2016) specifically highlights Booth's (USER) model (understand, structure, engage, and reflect), which is an adjustment to the analysis, design, development, implementation, and evaluation (ADDIE) framework (Salas, 2018). Hess (2016) goes on to say that the USER model focuses on the experiences libraries have with technology in teaching.

Previous studies have explored frameworks for the integration of platforms connected to mobile learning (mLearning). Hyman et al. (2014), instead of providing an instructional design framework per se, focus on users' experiences with various digital libraries and other digital content through the use of mLearning in formal class settings. As a result of their findings, they discuss a research framework for using mLearning and how that research framework could potentially be helpful for instructional design.

Researchers have also investigated frameworks for instructional design and the integration of social media in courses. For example, Kazanidis et al. (2018) used the Community of Inquiry model (CoI) when exploring the use of Facebook™ and Moodle™ within instructional design. They note some of the challenges with CoI as an instructional design framework as well, stating that there have been questions about CoI's fit for, "learning outcomes based on different disciplines, as well as about whether the relationships between its constituent components among users' interactions (instructors and students) in blended and online instructional settings have merit in learning" (Kazanidis et al., 2018, p. 935). However, they used the "presence indicators" (p. 935) of CoI to create an instructional design framework for the integration of Moodle™ and Facebook™: "SP (interaction between members)," "TP (sharing roles and initiatives emanating from other peers in collaborative settings and from the instructor)," and "CP (content of messages, ideas, arguments and opinions or statements)" (Kazanidis et al., 2018, p. 935).

There are also earlier works that provide suggestions for how to develop instructional design models, particularly given the constantly shifting instructional design context. Lee and Jang (2014) analyzed 20 articles to develop what they referred to as "four critical dimensions and ten synthesized procedures" (p.743) for creating instructional design models. The four dimensions are function, origin, source, and analysis scheme (Lee & Jang, 2014). The function is the purpose of the instructional model, and the origin is the model's connection to theory, practice, or both of those elements. The source refers to the context and data collection location and process. The analysis scheme focuses on how developers use data to produce their instructional design models (Lee & Jang, 2014). The ten synthesized procedures involve a combination of scholars' and practitioners' contributions. The work does not reference technology specifically; however, the intent is to prepare framework developers for the changing environment of instructional design, and technology plays quite a large role in that regard.

Just as frameworks have been developed to address the integration of various technological tools, researchers have also developed frameworks to foster interaction. In Czerkawski and Lyman's (2016) article, for example, they offer an instructional design framework specifically for engagement in online courses: E-Learning Engagement Design (ELED). Like the work by Lee and Jang (2014), Czerkawski and Lyman (2016) also use synthesis in the creation of their instructional design framework but indicate that it is not meant to be static; they synthesize research related to students' interactions online. The ELED has four phases, and they are Identify Instructional Needs, Define Instructional Goals and Objectives, Develop Learning Environments, and Summative Assessment. For each phase, there are a series of questions to help designers during the development process. The Identify Instructional Needs phase includes questions such as: "Why is instruction needed? What performance problems exist in the current learning environment? What characteristics of the learners are most relevant to the instructional problem at hand?" (Czerkawski & Lyman, 2016, p. 535). The second phase, Define Instructional Goals and Objectives, includes questions like, "What is the purpose for this instruction? Are there any professional or content standards that should be considered?" (p. 536). Developing Learning Environments, the third phase, poses questions such as, "How will interaction and collaboration be structured to encompass diverse learners? How will learner misunderstandings, misconceptions and mistakes be identified and eliminated? What feedback strategies will be employed to increase learners' conceptualization of the course topic materials?" (p. 537). The fourth phase, Summative Assessment, includes questions like, "Do learning outcomes align with assessments? What types of assessments are most useful for identifying various levels of student learning and experiences?" (p. 537). Czerkawski and Lyman (2016) emphasize that these are guiding questions and are not meant to be limiting.

There are some works that explore ways to incorporate design-based strategies in STEM broadly, which of course includes technology along with other areas. Zhou et al. (2020) investigates this topic in an Australian context. Like previous works, they develop a conceptual framework that is guided by other frameworks, including those from instructional design. They use the distributed cognition theory coupled with the "four-component instructional design system (4C/ID-model)" (Zhou et al., 2020, p. 1) of instructional design, which includes the following four areas: learning tasks, supportive information, procedural information (which the original authors of the model, van Merriënboer et al., 2002, refer to as "just-in time (JIT) information, " p. 39) and part-task practice (van Merriënboer et al., 2002; Zhou et al., 2020). Because Zhou et al. (2020) discuss the integration of 3D printing specifically, the authors go on to indicate how distributed cognition, or facilitating knowledge across learners, works particularly well given that focus and the focus on student interactivity, and 4C/ID helps with the planning and instructional delivery. Similarly, Kahangamage and Leung (2020) also explore an area of STEM and instructional design—engineering. Kahangamage and Leung (2020) employ what they call the "scaffolded knowledge integration framework for instructional design" (p. 799) in their work to focus on redesigning an engineering exercise to maximize student learning. They use Linn's (1995) work on the "knowledge integration environment (KIE)" (Kahangamage & Leung, 2020, p. 802). Linn (1995) suggests four principles: "(1) identifying new goals for learning; (2) making thinking visible; (3) encouraging autonomous learning; (4) prodding social supports" (p. 105). Kahangamage and Leung (2020) describe those areas as "make content accessible, make thinking visible, help students learn from each other, promote lifelong learning" (p. 803). For their work, Kahangamage and Leung (2020) indicate the application of these principles by allowing students to immediately connect concepts from the course to new and previous content (making content accessible), having students engage with commonly-used tools and items to explore the designs of those objects (making thinking visible), providing students with opportunities to work with each other (helping students learn from each other), and supporting students in reflecting and applying what they were learning (promoting lifelong learning). In addition to developing a redesigned exercise using an instructional design framework, Kahangamage and Leung (2020) also collected data on students' experiences with the exercise. The results showed that students made improvements in areas connected to technology-related skills and understanding (Kahangamage & Leung, 2020).

Like Kahangamage and Leung (2020), Cao and Koretsky (2018) also discuss an engineering context. Even though Cao and Koretsky do not discuss a specific instructional design framework, they deal with elements that are often connected to instructional design. Cao and Koretsky (2018) developed what they refer to as "interactive virtual laboratories (IVLs)," (p. 656) and their goal was to use the sociocultural perspective to learn more about students' learning while engaging in thermodynamic work in IVLs. The authors also wanted to understand the elements that support students' idea development while using technology in these interactive environments (Cao & Koretsky, 2018). They use situated learning, or what is essentially learning in context, to ground their work, and they also focus on the human-technology interactions that are connected to that situated learning (Cao & Koretsky, 2018). In addition to the IVLs themselves, the authors also explore students and their environments, as noted in one of their emphasis areas (Cao & Koretsky, 2018). The IVLs were initially developed to help address the challenges students were having related to learning thermodynamics. There are several instructional design features included in IVLs to promote students' learning. For example, interactive virtual laboratories include, "inquiry-based scaffolding, a sequence of simulations and questions designed to guide students in building conceptual understanding, and multiple representations such as equations, graphs, and textual descriptions" (Cao & Koretsky, 2018, p. 664). In IVLs, students also conduct experiments and respond to prompts (Cao & Koretsky, 2018). Another instructional design component related to IVLs is the way in which students who are involved in Cao and Koretsky's (2018) study engage with these virtual labs. The number of students enrolled in a course impacts the numbers and types of sessions they must engage with (Cao & Koretsky, 2018). They found that students came up with helpful ideas that not only aided their understanding of the information, but also assisted them in overcoming challenges they had related to thermodynamic work.

Each of the frameworks and instructional design elements listed address the integration of technology. What this extant literature also shows is that many of the frameworks were developed or modified in response to the shifting of the overall technological environment. They were designed to help instructors of various subjects and topics better integrate technology into their classroom settings, whether formal or informal. Although these many works discuss everything from the integration of specific tools to general dispositions related to technology, there is yet another technological shift that necessitates the authors' development of instructional design interventions for mHealth—the influx of even more technology into higher education and the implications for data privacy. In addition to sharing frameworks, the extant literature provides a perspective on the technological context, primarily, of higher education. The various tools mentioned in some of the texts have changed what can happen in classrooms, and some of them also come with terms and conditions that impact users' data privacy. Even outside of situations related to health, the terms and policies of tools can seem somewhat invasive; this feeling may be greater when it comes to mHealth. The integration of technology has brought with it numerous policies related to how to use the tools and what companies can collect from those who use these tools, and that is why the authors' framework for mHealth interventions is so important. Just as those earlier frameworks assisted in showing the nuances of technology integration for instructional design, the authors' framework, too, will elucidate the perhaps less considered, but still important, areas of technology, data privacy, and mHealth.

Connection to Sociocultural Theory

Sociocultural theory (Vygotsky, 1978) recognizes the interactive components of learning, in addition to the focus on the various contexts and experiences students bring with them to classrooms, which includes adult learning classrooms (Wu & Wu, 2015), even though Vygotsky's theory initially started with a focus on children. For example, researchers have explored the use of sociocultural theory to incorporate student content for international courses in general (Kim, 2011), increased diversity in an international course (Snowball & McKenna, 2017), and similar studies have been done related to courses in the U.S. (Castillo-Montoya, 2017). These contexts are often discussed, as noted in the aforementioned literature, as instances that are unique to students' individual circumstances; however, there are areas of experience that, even when unique, are quite ubiquitous. An incredibly pervasive component of the general sociocultural context both for students and higher education broadly is technology. Although students' interactions with technology can be highly individualized and present an opportunity for learning based on both individual and social interactions, the larger technological milieu involves exchanges that are not always readily apparent to users. For example, some interactions, particularly those connected to software and app use, can often include more surreptitious engagements that could compromise users' privacy. User agreements and privacy policies for these various applications often disclose what they collect and how they use it, but these agreements are not always easy for users to access or decipher (Fowler et. al, 2020). Also, some apps may discuss how they can share information with partner organizations and fail to list those organizations in their terms and policies.

Furthermore, users sometimes assume that privacy measures such as Health Insurance Portability and Accountability Act (HIPAA) compliance are automatically associated with mHealth apps just because the apps are promoted, suggested, or used by certain companies or institutions, which may not be the case (Papandrea, 2019). These mHealth resources and their accompanying agreements are a part of the social context, and as the use of mHealth continues to grow in higher education, expanding the use of sociocultural theory to include attention to the implications of these various agreements and associations can assist designers and instructors in developing stronger learning interventions: interventions that acknowledge this overarching context and that support more transparency related to these critical privacy implications.

SOLUTIONS AND RECOMMENDATIONS

Application of Sociocultural Theory

Sociocultural theory is situated within constructivism, which says that "learning is the construction of meaning from experience," (Merriam & Bierema, 2014, p. 36). In Vygotsky's (1978) *Mind in Society*, he discusses the interconnectedness of learning and context. Again, although Vygotsky's work focuses on children, there are many uses for general and particular aspects of sociocultural theory in adult settings, as noted in the aforementioned extant literature. One area of sociocultural theory that could be especially helpful when developing mHealth interventions is a variation of the zone of proximal development (ZPD).

Vygotsky (1978) asserted that children who displayed knowledge at one grade level could add to that knowledge through interaction. He indicated that a child could come in with knowledge at grade level

6, and by interacting with the teacher and learning more through that interaction, the child could add to that knowledge. The space where that occurs is the zone of proximal development.

In the traditional sense, then, the zone of proximal development focuses on the learning that may not be accomplished individually occurring as a result of collaboration and interaction. Learners enhance their knowledge through engagement with other learners, with each bringing what they've gleaned from their own contexts. To apply ZPD to mHealth intervention development requires a wider view of both context and learners.

Technological Context

Because sociocultural theory often focuses on students' particularized contexts, and the authors' approach to mHealth using sociocultural theory involves recognizing a more expansive context, it is important to expound on that broader technological context, particularly as it relates to the zone of proximal development.

The massive volume of digital information college students regularly encounter fosters the need for levels of decision making related to technology engagement. For example, when browsing a website, students (or anyone interacting with websites) are faced with choices about whether or not to read a site's cookie policy before continuing with the site. Those particular messages are necessary for data transparency (Bauer et al., 2021; Meyers, 2019), but they are not the only policies users encounter, as the sites typically have terms and conditions and privacy policies in addition to those cookie policies. Users have to decide whether to invest the time it takes to read the numerous policies, which are sometimes quite lengthy, in order to engage with these sites. They may also make assumptions about the harmlessness of policies, figuring that they are much like the policies for other websites or that they will only be on the site for a short time and decide not to read them. Now, some users address the concern about websites' policies for tracking and privacy by clearing cookies and other web data or making adjustments to the types of browsers they use. However, these approaches require a relationship with technology that is not often fostered or necessarily encouraged.

The technological context is further broadened when considering the use of third-party technological tools in the classroom, particularly ones that are not affiliated with students' colleges or universities. The authors have previously noted that applications (apps) are a growing aspect of higher education broadly, and college and university classrooms are included in that growth (Ranga, 2018). Apps can be helpful supplemental tools for learning and course engagement, but they often come with a series of policies that may or may not be clear to users. If the app is available from a particular store, students have to understand the terms, conditions, and privacy policy for the app store, which usually tells them that the app they are trying to access will probably have its own set of terms, conditions, and privacy guidelines. If the instructor for a course decides to use multiple apps, then students save time if they have already read the policies for the app store, but for each app they have to use, there will likely be different policies.

These examples are not designed to critique the presence of policies because, again, transparency regarding how companies handle user data from websites, apps, and other tools is paramount; people have a right to know why and how their data is collected, used, and shared. These exemplars, instead, point to the widespread technological context that is present both within and outside the classroom. When considering mHealth specifically, the importance of recognizing this context is heightened because of the sensitive nature of the data that can be shared through mHealth.

The area of app use and development within this broader technological context is challenging, but there are efforts underway to improve aspects of data privacy that could be helpful to mHealth intervention design. For example, the authors just completed a project that involved both data collection and app development. The work explored the experiences people in the disability community have with trust and Internet-connected devices. The interdisciplinary team included faculty and student researchers, both graduate and undergraduate, from the areas of education, public health, philosophy, and computer science/computer engineering. The app, designed as a privacy-enhancing tool for Internet-of-things (IoT) devices, was developed based on feedback from study participants. The participatory design approach allows for more inclusion and greater transparency related to terms, conditions, and policies. The app is still in its early stages, but the support that it and other privacy-enhancing tools provide is growing and can be beneficial to the overall improvement of data privacy in mHealth. These types of tools can be deployed alongside mHealth interventions to ensure an added layer of transparency, protection, and agency for users. There are more developed privacy applications available from popular brands; however, some of the tools already on the market invade users' privacy as they attempt to protect it. Furthermore, the collecting and sharing of data is quite lucrative for many businesses, which can function as a disincentive for the much-needed data privacy protections for mHealth and other IoT interactions. Until apps like the one the authors helped create are more readily available, designers will need to consider other strategies for incorporating mHealth in a way that privileges users' privacy.

Therefore, employing sociocultural theory with the broader technological context in mind can assist instructional designers in developing mHealth interventions that consider these critical areas of data privacy and help others to use mHealth in a way that both acknowledges and addresses data privacy.

Higher Education Community as Learners

In addition to the focus on context, sociocultural theory generally, and ZPD specifically, also emphasize the knowledge that learners have already acquired; the goal is to grow that knowledge through social, interactive, collaborative endeavors. Obviously, colleges and universities are already communities of learners, as they are responsible for educating the millions of students who engage in some form of higher education. However, in order to develop mHealth interventions that address the ever-shifting information privacy landscape, the higher education community of learners must be framed in a slightly different way. Prior to the widespread introduction of apps and mobile devices, there may have been less interaction between various areas of higher education. These areas may have been more siloed. For example, what students were experiencing on online spaces such as social media may have been considered an issue for student affairs and not necessarily an issue for the classroom. However, now that these tools are also included in some classrooms (Blackmon, 2018; Abella-García et al., 2019; Rahman et al., 2019) there is less distance between areas that were once considered further apart.

A more helpful strategy, then, would be to understand the various areas across higher education as unique learning communities that are connected to each other and the larger technological context.

Putting It All Together

There are a few strategies that can help with applying the zone of proximal development from sociocultural theory to advance the development of mHealth interventions that consider data privacy. It is important to note that even though the connection to sociocultural theory and ZPD is highlighted, these strategies can maintain that connection and simultaneously layer in other theories instructional designers may use such as the many frameworks mentioned in the earlier sections of this work.

Understand Learner Groups

In recognizing each higher education unit as a different learner group, it allows for understanding their place on the technological context continuum. For example, upon preparing mHealth interventions, designers can examine how a particular unit uses mHealth as well as the privacy implications for how they use mHealth in their offices, knowing that this can vary from office to office. Designers who already use ADDIE could include this step as a part of their initial analysis (Salas, 2018; Stefaniak & Xu, 2020; Campbell, 2014). Counseling offices may use mHealth in ways that are very different from a student activities office, and the expectation for privacy may be very different as well, even if the data privacy guidelines may be the same depending on the technological tool. The broader technological context for a counseling office involves protected health information that would likely not be involved in a student activities unit, and because of that, students may assume that a level of privacy exists for mHealth use in counseling that may not be accurate. Extant literature indicates that even when insurance companies implement mHealth through third party tools, the responsibilities of the insurance company remain in place because of HIPAA, but the terms of mHealth use are guided by the terms of the particular app, especially if the app use is voluntary (Papandrea, 2019). Understanding these expectations as they relate to various units is valuable for developing more privacy-conscious mHealth interventions.

Establish Connections Between Learner Groups

Once an understanding of the various learner groups is established, recognizing the knowledge and information these groups bring with them—just as one would for higher education students in a classroom-will be crucial to establish the connections between these unique units, thereby leveraging ZPD. Although the various units' functions may be specialized, in order to enhance data privacy-protection measures, it will be vital to show how units can learn from each other. There is also the matter of establishing clear, efficient, and sustainable interventions. Understanding the particulars of various areas of higher education communities is necessary; however,designing an intervention for each department when integrating mHealth may be untenable. Also, it would miss an opportunity for departments to learn from each other. Determining the connections between units allows for a broader approach to data privacy considerations with mHealth interventions, and as with the traditional implementation of ZPD, attention to these connections can enhance knowledge about data privacy and mHealth.

Leverage Collaborative Knowledge

After understanding the learner groups and establishing connections between those groups to enhance data-privacy considerations in mHealth, those collaborative gains should be shared for sustained focus on data privacy. The goal of integrating ZPD into mHealth interventions is to grow the acknowledgement of and attention to data privacy, so helping users understand where these gains have been made and how the interactions with other learner groups helps to achieve those gains will be paramount to sustained focus on this important topic. As alluded to when discussing the overarching technological context, the way users engage with technology is constantly shifting, so mHealth interventions must also be designed to account for these shifts. By outlining the goals and objectives, as well as the tasks designed to help users accomplish them, the lessons from those collaborative interactions are clear, as are the steps learners can take when it is necessary to adjust or amend those lessons.

CONCLUSION

The growth of mHealth in the higher education community is evident. What must accompany this growth, however, is a focus on the privacy implications of mHealth use. By using sociocultural theory in mHealth intervention design, specifically with a focus on the zone of proximal development, units within colleges and universities can understand the larger technological context that influences how users may understand and experience interactions with their mHealth efforts. Furthermore, they can learn from other units about their experiences with mHealth use and collaboratively engage to enhance conversations and practices around data privacy considerations in mHealth.

ACKNOWLEDGMENT

Special thanks to William & Mary School of Education doctoral student and graduate assistant Daqian Yu for his assistance with citation support for this research.

REFERENCES

Abella-García, V., Delgado-Benito, V., Ausín-Villaverde, V., & Hortigüela-Alacalá, D. (2019). To tweet or not to tweet: Student perceptions of the use of Twitter on an undergraduate degree course. *Innovations in Education and Teaching International*, *56*(4), 402–411. doi:10.1080/14703297.2018.1444503

Alharbi, Y., Al-Mansour, M., Al-Saffar, R., Garman, A., & Alraddadi, A. (2020). Three-dimensional virtual reality as an innovative teaching and learning tool for human anatomy courses in medical education: A Mixed Methods Study. *Cureus*, *12*(2), e7085. doi:10.7759/cureus.7085 PMID:32226686

Barak, M. (2017). Cloud pedagogy: Utilizing web-based technologies for the promotion of social constructivist learning in science teaching preparation courses. *Journal of Science Education and Technology*, *26*(5), 459–469. doi:10.100710956-017-9691-3

Bauer, J. M., Bergstrøm, R., & Foss-Madsen, R. (2021). Are you sure, you want a cookie?—The effects of choice architecture on users' decisions about sharing private online data. *Computers in Human Behavior*, *120*, 106729. Advance online publication. doi:10.1016/j.chb.2021.106729

Blackmon, S. J. (2018). Beyond cybernation: Technology & teaching in doctoral educational leadership. In L. Hyatt & S. Allen (Eds.), *Advancing doctoral leadership education through technology* (pp. 56–74). Edward Elgar. doi:10.4337/9781786437020.00015

Blackmon, S. J., & Moore, R. L. (2020). A framework to support interdisciplinary engagement with learning analytics. In D. Ifenthaler & D. Gibson (Eds.), *Adoption of data analytics in higher education learning and teaching* (pp. 39–52). Springer. doi:10.1007/978-3-030-47392-1_3

Bruehlman-Senecal, E., Hook, C. J., Pfeifer, J. H., FitzGerald, C., Davis, B., Delucchi, K. L., Haritatos, J., & Ramo, D. E. (2020). Smartphone app to address loneliness among college students: Pilot randomized controlled trial. *JMIR Mental Health*, *7*(10), e21496. doi:10.2196/21496 PMID:33079071

Campbell, P. C. (2014). Modifying ADDIE: Incorporating new technologies in library instruction. *Public Services Quarterly*, *10*(2), 138–149. doi:10.1080/15228959.2014.904214

Cao, Y., & Koretsky, M. D. (2018). Shared resources: Engineering students' emerging group understanding of thermodynamic work. *Journal of Engineering Education*, *107*(4), 656–689. doi:10.1002/jee.20237

Castillo-Montoya, M. (2017). Deepening understanding of prior knowledge: What diverse first-generation college students in the U.S. can teach us. *Teaching in Higher Education*, *22*(5), 587–603. doi:10.1080/13562517.2016.1273208

Chen, J., Zhou, J., Wang, Y., Qi, G., Xia, C., Mo, G., & Zhang, Z. (2020). Blended learning in basic medical laboratory courses improves medical students' abilities in self-learning, understanding, and problem solving. *Advances in Physiology Education*, *44*(1), 9–14. doi:10.1152/advan.00076.2019 PMID:31821032

Czerkawski, B. C., & Lyman, E. W. III. (2016). An instructional design framework for fostering student engagement in online learning environments. *TechTrends*, *60*(6), 532–539. doi:10.100711528-016-0110-z

De Ponti, R., Marazzato, J., Maresca, A. M., Rovera, F., Carcano, G., & Ferrario, M. M. (2020). Pre-graduation medical training including virtual reality during COVID-19 pandemic: A report on students' perception. *BMC Medical Education*, *20*(1), 1–7. doi:10.118612909-020-02245-8 PMID:32977781

Fish, M. T., & Saul, A. D. (2019). The gamification of meditation: A randomized-controlled study of a prescribed mobile mindfulness meditation application in reducing college students' depression. *Simulation & Gaming*, *50*(4), 419–435. doi:10.1177/1046878119851821

Fowler, L. R., Gillard, C., & Morain, S. R. (2020). Readability and accessibility of terms of service and privacy policies for menstruation-tracking smartphone applications. *Health Promotion Practice*, *21*(5), 679–683. doi:10.1177/1524839919899924 PMID:32037887

France, D., Powell, V., Mauchline, A. L., Welsh, K., Park, J., Whalley, W. B., & Rewhorn, S. (2016). Ability of students to recognize the relationship between using mobile apps for learning during fieldwork and the development of graduate attributes. *Journal of Geography in Higher Education*, *40*(2), 182–192. doi:10.1080/03098265.2016.1154931

Goodman, B. E., Barker, M. K., & Cooke, J. E. (2018). Best practices in active and student-centered learning in physiology classes. *Advances in Physiology Education*, *42*(3), 417–423. doi:10.1152/advan.00064.2018 PMID:29972063

Hess, A. N. (2016). A case study of job-embedded learning. *portal. Portal (Baltimore, Md.)*, *16*(2), 327–347. doi:10.18438/eblip29526

Huberty, J., Green, J., Glissmann, C., Larkey, L., Puzia, M., & Lee, C. (2019). Efficacy of the mindfulness meditation mobile app "Calm" to reduce stress among college students: Randomized controlled trial. *JMIR mHealth and uHealth*, *7*(6), e14273. doi:10.2196/14273 PMID:31237569

Hyman, J. A., Moser, M. T., & Segala, L. N. (2014). Electronic reading and digital library technologies: Understanding learner expectation and usage intent for mobile learning. *Educational Technology Research and Development*, *62*(1), 35–52. doi:10.100711423-013-9330-5

Ibacache, K. (2019). Use of language-learning apps as a tool for foreign language acquisition by academic libraries employees. *Information Technology and Libraries*, *38*(3), 22–33. doi:10.6017/ital.v38i3.11077

Isaza-Restrepo, A., Gómez, M. T., Cifuentes, G., & Argüello, A. (2018). The virtual patient as a learning tool: A mixed quantitative qualitative study. *BMC Medical Education*, *18*(1), 297. doi:10.118612909-018-1395-8 PMID:30522478

Kahangamage, U., & Leung, R. C. K. (2020). Remodelling and engineering design subject to enhance students' learning outcomes. *International Journal of Technology and Design Education*, *30*(4), 799–814. doi:10.100710798-019-09519-3

Kazanidis, I., Pellas, N., Fotaris, P., & Tsinakos, A. (2018). Facebook and Moodle integration into instructional media design courses: A comparative analysis of students' learning experiences using the Community of Inquiry (CoI) model. *International Journal of Human-Computer Interaction*, *34*(10), 932–942. doi:10.1080/10447318.2018.1471574

Kazemi, D. M., Borsari, B., Levine, M. J., Shehab, M., Nelson, M., Dooley, B., Stinson, B., Fang, F., & Li, S. (2019). Real-time demonstration of a mHealth app designed to reduce college students hazardous drinking. *Psychological Services*, *16*(2), 255–259. doi:10.1037er0000310 PMID:30407059

Keifenheim, K. E., Teufel, M., Ip, J., Speiser, N., Leehr, E. J., Zipfel, S., & Herrmann-Werner, A. (2015). Teaching history taking to medical students: A systematic review. *BMC Medical Education*, *15*(1), 159. doi:10.118612909-015-0443-x PMID:26415941

Kim, H. Y. (2011). International graduate students' difficulties: Graduate classes as a community of practices. *Teaching in Higher Education*, *16*(3), 281–292. doi:10.1080/13562517.2010.524922

Kononowicz, A. A., Woodham, L. A., Edelbring, S., Stathakarou, N., Davies, D., Saxena, N., Tudor Car, L., Carlstedt-Duke, J., Car, J., & Zary, N. (2019). Virtual patient simulations in health professions education: Systematic review and meta-analysis by the digital health education collaboration. *Journal of Medical Internet Research*, *21*(7), e14676. doi:10.2196/14676 PMID:31267981

Lattie, E. G., Adkins, E. C., Winquist, N., Stiles-Shields, C., Wafford, Q. E., & Graham, A. K. (2019). Digital mental health interventions for depression, anxiety, and enhancement of psychological well-being among college students: Systematic review. *Journal of Medical Internet Research*, *21*(7), e12869. doi:10.2196/12869 PMID:31333198

Lee, J., & Jang, S. (2014). A methodological framework for instructional design model development: Critical dimensions and synthesized procedures. *Educational Technology Research and Development*, *62*(6), 743–765. doi:10.100711423-014-9352-7

Linn, M. C. (1995). Designing computer learning environments for engineering and computer science: The scaffolded knowledge integration framework. *Journal of Science Education and Technology*, *4*(2), 103–126. doi:10.1007/BF02214052

McLaughlin, J. E., Wolcott, M., Hubbard, D., Umstead, K., & Rider, T. R. (2019). A qualitative review of the design thinking framework in health professions education. *BMC Medical Education*, *19*(1), 98. doi:10.118612909-019-1528-8 PMID:30947748

Merriam, S. B., & Bierema, L. L. (2014). *Adult learning: Linking theory and practice*. Jossey-Bass.

Meyers, W. A. (2019). C if for cookie: Is the EU's new 'cookie law' good enough to protect my data? *International Lawyer*, *52*(3), 491–514.

National Council on Disability. (2017). *Mental health on college campuses: investments, accommodations needed to address student needs*. ncd.gov/sites/default/files/NCD_Mental_Health_Report_508.pdf

Papandrea, P. (2019). Addressing the HIPAA-potamus sized gap in wearable technology regulation. *Minnesota Law Review*. https://minnesotalawreview.org/wp-content/uploads/2019/12/Papandrea_FINAL_MLR104-Updated.pdf

Rahman, S., Ramakrishnan, T., & Ngamassi, L. (2019). Impact of social media use on student satisfaction in higher education. *Higher Education Quarterly*, *74*(3), 304–319. doi:10.1111/hequ.12228

Ranga, J. (2018). Multipurpose use of explain everything iPad app for teaching chemistry courses. *Journal of Chemical Education*, *95*(5), 895–898. doi:10.1021/acs.jchemed.7b00676

Reynolds, R. (2016). Defining, designing for, and measuring "social constructivist digital literacy" development in learners: A proposed framework. *Educational Technology Research and Development*, *64*(4), 735–762. doi:10.100711423-015-9423-4

Reynolds, R., & Harel Caperton, I. (2009, April). *Development of high school and community college students' contemporary learning abilities in Globaloria-West Virginia in the first pilot year*. Paper presented at the annual convention of the American Education Research Association, San Diego, CA.

Rhim, H. C., & Han, H. (2020). Teaching online: Foundational concepts of online learning and practical guidelines. *Korean Journal of Medical Education*, *32*(3), 175–183. doi:10.3946/kjme.2020.171 PMID:32894921

Ritz, L. T., & Buss, A. R. (2016). A framework for aligning instructional design strategies with affordances of CAVE immersive virtual reality systems. *TechTrends*, *60*(6), 549–566. doi:10.100711528-016-0085-9

Rouleau, G., Gagnon, M. P., Côté, J., Payne-Gagnon, J., Hudson, E., Dubois, C. A., & Bouix-Picasso, J. (2019). Effects of e-Learning in a continuing education context on nursing care: Systematic review of systematic qualitative, quantitative, and mixed-studies reviews. *Journal of Medical Internet Research*, *21*(10), e15118. doi:10.2196/15118 PMID:31579016

Seymour-Walsh, A. E., Bell, A., Weber, A., & Smith, T. (2020). Adapting to a new reality: COVID-19 coronavirus and online education in the health professions. *Rural and Remote Health*, *20*(2), 6000. doi:10.22605/RRH6000 PMID:32456441

Shum, S. B. (2012). *Learning analytics.* https://iite.unesco.org/pics/publications/en/files/3214711.pdf

Snowball, J. D., & McKenna, S. (2017). Student-generated content: An approach to harnessing the power of diversity in higher education. *Teaching in Higher Education, 22*(5), 604–618. doi:10.1080/13562517.2016.1273205

Stefaniak, J., & Xu, M. (2020). An examination of the systemic reach of instructional design models: A systematic review. *TechTrends, 64*(5), 710–719. doi:10.100711528-020-00539-8

van Merriënboer, J. J., Clark, R. E., & De Croock, M. B. (2002). Blueprints for complex learning: The 4C/ID-model. *Educational Technology Research and Development, 50*(2), 39–61.

Vygotsky (1978). *Mind in society: The development of higher psychological processes.* Harvard University Press.

Watkins, J. B., & Eisenberg, D. (2012). Increased demand for mental health services on college campuses: Perspectives from administrators. *Qualitative Social Work, 11*(3), 319–337. doi:10.1177/1473325011401468

Wu, Y. L., & Wu, H. C. (2015). Higher education learning experiences among Vietnamese immigrant women in Taiwan. *Adult Education Quarterly, 65*(2), 133–151. doi:10.1177/0741713614566673

Zhou, D., Gomez, R., Wright, N., Rittenbruch, M., & Davis, J. (2020). A design-led conceptual framework for developing school integrated STEM programs: The Australian context. *International Journal of Technology and Design Education.* doi:10.100710798-020-09619-5

ADDITIONAL READING

Fowler, L. R., Gillard, C., & Morain, S. R. (2020). Readability and accessibility of terms of service and privacy policies for menstruation-tracking smartphone applications. *Health Promotion Practice, 21*(5), 679–683. doi:10.1177/1524839919899924 PMID:32037887

Kazemi, D. M., Borsari, B., Levine, M. J., Shehab, M., Nelson, M., Dooley, B., Stinson, B., Fang, F., & Li, S. (2019). Real-time demonstration of a mHealth app designed to reduce college students hazardous drinking. *Psychological Services, 16*(2), 255–259. doi:10.1037er0000310 PMID:30407059

Merriam, S. B., & Bierema, L. L. (2014). *Adult learning: Linking theory and practice.* Jossey-Bass.

Meyers, W. A. (2019). C if for cookie: Is the EU's new 'cookie law' good enough to protect my data? *International Lawyer, 52*(3), 491–514.

KEY TERMS AND DEFINITIONS

Application (App): Software for a computer or mobile device.

Collaborative Knowledge: Information and/or skills acquired through working with and learning from others, especially as it relates to communities of learners.

Data Privacy: The protection of data that includes sensitive and confidential information, as well as information that users would otherwise not want shared without their knowledge or permission.

Family Education Rights and Privacy Act (FERPA): A United States (U.S.) federal law that governs the rights of parents and others to access education records for children (K-12) and postsecondary students over age 18.

Higher Education Community: Includes colleges and universities as a whole with a focus on students, professors/instructors, staff/administrators both singly and collectively, particularly as it relates to addressing data privacy.

Internet of Things: The various objects connecting and exchanging data using the internet.

Technology Integration: The incorporation of technology—digital and non-digital—into personal and professional spaces. The current work has a particular emphasis on digital technology integration.

Chapter 10
Methadone Referrals Demystified:
A Client's Journey Into Methadone Treatment – Social Constructivism and the Use of Video-Based Content in Medical Provider Education

Katarzyna M. Sims
Yale School of Medicine, USA

Maximilian D. Wegener
Yale School of Medicine, USA

Ralph Brooks
Yale School of Medicine, USA

Merceditas S. Villanueva
Yale School of Medicine, USA

Lisa Nichols
Yale School of Medicine, USA

ABSTRACT

This chapter considers social constructivism as an educational theory for the development of multimedia content to assist primary-care providers, particularly those in HIV clinics and other clinicians, and support staff involved in the care of patients with substance use disorders in better understanding the intake processes at the Methadone clinics. Main aspects of social constructivism with its focus on the collaborative and generative learning and the importance of a cultural and social context are elaborated within the framework of the multimedia design. A series of four videos were developed that feature interviews with patients who describe their experience on Methadone. In addition, medical providers and medical staff describe the intake procedures for Methadone. Also discussed is the instructional design process and the Bergman and Moore instructional design model that informed the design.

DOI: 10.4018/978-1-7998-9490-2.ch010

INTRODUCTION

The COVID-19 pandemic resulted in increased drug use and overdose deaths, which escalated the demand for Methadone services (Holland et al., 2021). Most states witnessed large-scale increases, with the highest in West Virginia, Kentucky, and Tennessee (Friedman & Akre, 2021). The Connecticut Office of the Chief Medical Examiner reported 1,378 confirmed drug overdose deaths in 2020 in Connecticut, an increase of 14.3% compared to 2019. As of the second week of August, there were 878 confirmed drug overdose deaths in Connecticut in 2021 (Clinton, 2021).

Methadone is a full opioid agonist[1] and the oldest of the medications used to treat opioid use disorder. It has been in use since 1972 (Cooper et al., 2020). Methadone controls cravings and prevents opioid withdrawal. It has been effective in reducing opioid use as well as the harms associated with opiate use disorders (OUD) such as fatal overdose, acquisition of HIV, and hepatitis C (HCV) infection. Additionally, Methadone has been linked to a reduction of incarceration rates and improving employment (Cooper et al., 2020). Other medications approved by the Food and Drug Administration (FDA) for opioid use disorder include buprenorphine and naltrexone (Cooper et al., 2020; Seval et al., 2020).[2] All medications must be prescribed by licensed healthcare providers.

Given the opioid epidemic, the need to expand referrals to substance use disorder (SUD) clinics that are licensed to dispense Methadone for OUD prompted an examination of provider-identified gaps in knowledge. The synthesis of HIV, HCV, and opioid use disorders has raised questions surrounding improved collaboration between providers of HIV and OUD services. Specifically, providers of HIV clinical services were generally not co-located with providers of OUD services in Connecticut, leading to suboptimal bidirectional referrals.

As part of our grant-funded project to optimize the treatment of HCV for persons with HIV, improving communication between HIV and OUD providers who operated in siloed institutions became an important goal. During the project, it was identified that HIV providers and support personnel within HIV clinics lacked a full understanding of the processes surrounding Methadone treatment. Thus, the authors embarked on creating a series of videos to fill this gap.

The COVID-19 pandemic has had a major impact on traditional in-person teaching, assessment methods, student–teacher relationships, and student and teacher well-being leading the authors to choose video intervention as an instructional method (Smith & Boscak, 2021; Kaini & Motie, 2021; Wong, 2020). The pandemic accelerated the global use of online learning platforms (e-learning). Due to the disruption of health services and health education, many institutes that offer advanced degrees in medical education have shifted from in-person to virtual learning, using technologies such as artificial intelligence for adaptive learning, virtual reality, and e-learning (Dhawan, 2020; Peisachovich et al., 2020; Sandars et al., 2020). A recent call for a national, virtual, video-based curriculum for urology residents to design surgical skill training is a perfect illustration of those changes (Tabakin et al., 2021).

Health care conferences have also adapted quickly to the pandemic by shifting to e-learning. E-learning has redefined the standard presentation and poster formats, as organizers adapted to the needs of attendees who no longer could participate in person. Thus, multiple conference planning committees switched to virtual conference models or offered alternative formats such as pre-recorded sessions with live question forums. Currently, two years into the pandemic, hybrid sessions are still in place.

The video intervention discussed in this chapter allows for a multi-layered discourse among health care providers about the program linkage processes, Methadone assisted treatment stigma, and client access to medical care. Specifically, the videos explain what happens when a health care provider refers a client to a SUD program. They explore the processes around dose adjustment and take-home bottles, counseling options, screenings, potential side effects, myths, and stigma surrounding the treatment. Three Connecticut SUD programs participated in the creation of the videos: the Recovery Network of Programs, located in Bridgeport; the APT Foundation, located in New Haven; and the Root Center for Advanced Recovery, located in Hartford. All four videos are currently available on a major educational platform hosted by the Connecticut NEAETC (New England AIDS Education Training Center) Regional Partner's website (www.aetcct.org) as well as on the Target HIV website (www.targethiv.org) and AETC National Coordination Resource Center website (www.aidsct.org). These sites serve as a free resource for programs, clinicians, and clients.

Finally, it is important to mention that the use of online learning approaches has been well received by learners in the medical field over the years. A national survey conducted in August 2018 of U.S. physicians, nurse practitioners, and physician assistants, which examined what influences the choice of continuing medical education (CME) modalities, showed that online training was equally as appealing as live training. The activities that the respondents anticipated using in the future were live (mean 3.8 [1 = *not likely*, 5 = *very likely*]), online (mean 3.5), point-of-care (mean 3.5), and print-based (mean 3.5) activities. For online CME, clinicians valued time flexibility (mean 4.4), the self-directed pace (mean 4.2), and cost-efficiency (mean 4.2; O'Brien et al., 2020). Apart from the delivery method, major factors that influenced providers' choices of online CME training included topic (best–worst scaling net positivity 0.54), quality of the content (0.51), availability of CME credit (0.43), and clinical practice focus (0.41; O'Brien et al., 2020).

Despite increased use of video-based instruction for medical students, there remains a need to establish its role as an instructional method in more generalized provider training. To date, the video-based approach has proven effective in telehealth consultations, post-workshop reflections, and prerecorded lectures for continuing education (CE).

Video communications allow medical personnel to evaluate patients and diagnose illnesses in real-time without the need for either the patient or the practitioner to travel. Medical professionals also use video communications to access certification programs, for continuing medical education (CME), and to train others. (Williams, 2020, para. 2)

There have been successful attempts to create interactive online curricula that significantly reduce the time spent during in-person training and offer flexibility to complete the training from the comfort of home. One such example was the first video-based curriculum in surgical education, developed by the Pediatric Intensive Care Unit (PICU) in El Salvador in 2020. It taught local providers on pediatric advanced airway management and surgical approach to patients requiring airway reconstruction, and it demonstrated considerable improvement in those skills among surgeons, anesthesiologists, intensivists, and speech pathologists (Ghersin, 2020).

The main objectives of this chapter are:

1. Explain the relationship between the theory of social constructivism and video-based content in medical education.
2. Describe how the instructional design process informed the development of multimedia content.
3. List and describe the phases of the Bergman and Moore instructional design model that guided the design and development process.

THEORETICAL BASIS

The precise beginnings of constructivism are unknown, though the movement developed in the 1990s as a variation of the cognitive learning theory, bringing a shift in thinking about the learning processes (Molenda, 2020). Constructivists' main contribution to the learning sciences was emphasizing the social aspect of learning. This approach was different from the pure cognitive understanding, which was steeped in the retrieval and memorization practices. To constructivists, knowledge is a social and cultural construct, where individuals create meaning through their interactions with each other and with the environment they live in, hence, assimilating new information with their current abilities and state of knowledge (Ernest, 1999; Gredler, 1997; Kanselaar, 2002; Prawat & Floden, 1994).

Constructivism-based learning is frequently used in medical education to analyze clinical cases, evaluate clinical performance, and improve cognitive learning. Specifically, video interventions seem to be effective in breast self-examination, prostate cancer screening, sunscreen adherence, self-care in patients with heart failure, HIV testing, and treatment adherence (Tuong et al., 2014). A review of one of the endocrine and reproductive pathophysiology courses at Harvard Medical School revealed that a majority of students (59%) and tutors (78%) preferred video-based cases over text-based case studies (Basu Roy, 2012). In addition, video-based assessments offer numerous advantages over immediate observations of clinical performance in terms of objectivity, time-efficacy, and practicality (McQueen et al., 2019). They enhance quality assurance of examiner's grading and improved feedback practices (Yeates et al., 2020).

In an educational setting, the learner actively co-constructs, redefines, and renegotiates meaning within a given cultural and social context by setting their own goals and controlling the learning process. By interacting with others, the learner becomes aware of the different ways one acquires and interprets knowledge and is then able to select, explain and organize the information independently (Kanselaar, 2002). John Dewey (1859–1952) summarized this idea succinctly by saying that learners assume a role of an actor rather than a spectator (Dewey, 1938).

Social constructivism (or socio-cultural theory of learning) emerged as a variation of the cognitive learning theory in the 1990s and is characterized as a subset of constructivism (Molenda, 2020). The major difference is a greater emphasis on collaborative learning, which can take different forms such as joint teaching, peer collaboration, WebQuests (a form of blended learning where the information comes from the web), problem-based instruction, and other methods that involve learning with others (Shunk, 2000). Jerome S. Bruner (1915–2016) suggested that learners employ various thinking approaches, depending on their previous knowledge, situation, and type of learning materials used (Rannikmäe et al., 2020). Therefore, learning is more effective when it includes exposure to multiple ways of thinking and social negotiation of meanings. Students should then be given opportunities to reflect on their thinking and to discuss it with peers.

In cognitive sciences, learning is described in terms of information processing (see Figure 1). It means that our minds process, discard, or store the external data when they receive it. Information is processed at first in working memory. It is then retained and transferred to long-term memory. For the new information to be stored in long-term memory, it needs to be interpreted by prior knowledge and then connected to existing knowledge (Dennick, 2016). Consequently, our experiences are being constantly integrated and sorted through the pre-existing notions and beliefs.

Figure 1. Knowledge transfer diagram
(Adapted from Shank, 2018, p. 14).

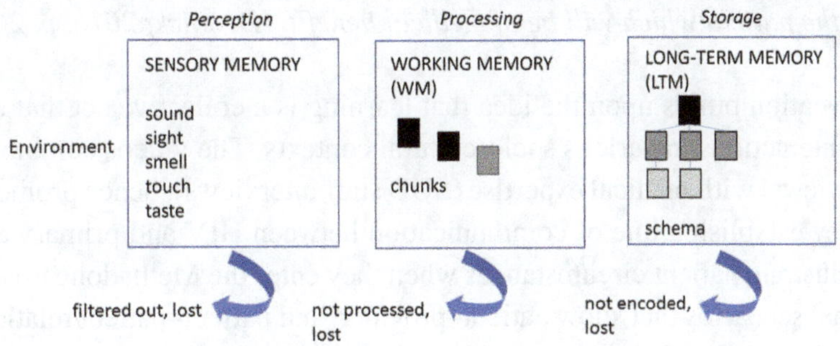

The model in Figure 1 explains how information processing works, including the selection, organization, and integration of new information. The role of instructional designers is thus to assist in this process by reducing the *cognitive load*, the term coined by John Sweller (1988) that presupposes that working memory is only able to hold a small amount of information at any time.

The most recognizable theory of social construction was offered by Lev Vygotsky (1896–1934), who contended that learner construction of knowledge is the result of social interaction, interpretation, and understanding (Vygotsky, 1962). Rogoff (1990) referred to this practice as *guided participation*, in which a learner acquires new culturally valuable skills through collaborative instruction with a more experienced facilitator, called the *more knowledgeable other* (MKO). In this way, the learner operates within the *zone of proximal development* (ZPD) that Vygotsky defines as a space between the present knowledge level and the potential levels of development under structured guidance (Vygotsky, 1978). Language and dialogue play a key role in this process; language plays a crucial role in shaping thought, and dialogue allows building connections between people from different cultures and backgrounds (Adams, 2006). Although Vygotsky originally investigated learning processes among children, his theory is now applied to adult learning as well. In Vygotsky's words:

Learning awakens a variety of internal developmental processes that are able to operate only when the child is interacting with people in his environment and with his peers . . . learning is not development; however, properly organized learning results in mental development and sets in motion a variety of developmental processes that would be impossible apart from learning. Thus, learning is a necessary and universal aspect of the process of developing culturally organized, specifically human, psychological functions. (Vygotsky, 1978, p. 90)

There is a direct link between the medical field and socio-constructivist theory. As in social constructivism, interpersonal communication is very important in the medical field. Red Dennick observed that communication skills such as the ability to listen and interpret what the patient is saying and to give them advice and proper information in the manner that the patient understands are evidence of good medical practice (Dennick, 2016). In this patient-centered approach, which is similar to the learner-centered approach in the social theory of learning, the patient generates the knowledge, and the provider assists and supports them in expanding their prior knowledge. Dennick explained:

If constructivist pedagogy is used to establish prior knowledge it is also used in helping the patient/providers to construct their understanding of their condition and to help the doctor to establish potentially new behaviours in the patient which will be of medical benefit. (Dennick, 2016, p. 203)

Our video intervention builds upon the idea that learning is a collective act that occurs through in-person and online interactions in various socio-cultural contexts. The videos combine personal experiences (patient interviews) with medical expertise (SUD staff interviews), hence promoting collaboration and discussion. They establish a line of communication between HIV and primary care providers and their patients and illustrate patient circumstances when they enter the Methadone treatment program. In addition, the fictional scenarios that show patient–provider, and patient–patient relationships encourage metacognition over formal instruction. Medical knowledge about Methadone is continuously redefined and renegotiated by exposing the learner to the facets of Methadone treatment from different perspectives.

The main premise of the videos is to improve providers' knowledge about Methadone treatment to provide better care and to illustrate complex patient–doctor interactions that would ultimately help patients in their treatment. In his review of the OUD treatment training offered for medical students and residents in the United States, Lyle Cooper stated the need for more training that would focus on the skillsets and emotional intelligence required to work with patients struggling with opioids and heroin addiction (Cooper et al., 2020). Similarly, Madison Ratycz has advocated for the incorporation of heroin and fentanyl education into medical school curricula. She observed that many physicians are not well prepared to address OUD regarding assessment and management. Ratycz noted potential in simulation-based medical education that would include training on harm reduction interventions and overdose reversal, including training about treating OUD and co-occurring chronic pain (Ratycz et al., 2018).

"METHADONE REFERRALS DEMYSTIFIED: A CLIENT'S JOURNEY INTO METHADONE TREATMENT"

Structure and Content

To support social constructivist learning around Methadone use, the authors chose video as the medium for an online delivery method. Using video as an online streaming medium contributes to the widespread consumption of educational content and thus builds on the ideas of constructivism. Video-based education supports deeper content processing and improves learner engagement (Heath et al., 2007; Hendricks et al., 2018). A recent study showed a slight improvement in student learning from prerecorded videos than live lecturers. A sample of 7,776 students was introduced to prerecorded videos instead of existing teaching methods, leading to small-scale improvements in their learning ($g = 0.28$). Adding video to existing teaching led to strong learning benefits ($g = 0.80$; Noetel et al., 2021).

As shown in Figure 2, the video intervention consists of four episodes, approximately nine-minutes long, that follow the five-step intake process into a Methadone clinic. One of the Methadone clinics in Connecticut provided a written explanation of this process. They reported that once a patient calls the clinic, they try to complete a prescreening over the phone (Step 1). Next, they schedule an appointment to complete the admission. During the admission process, the clinic would ask for a copy of the patient's photo ID and insurance card, and they would collect a urine sample (Step 2). The patient would then be scheduled with one of the medical providers for an admission physical (Step 3). Afterward, they meet

Figure 2. Patient journey into Methadone treatment

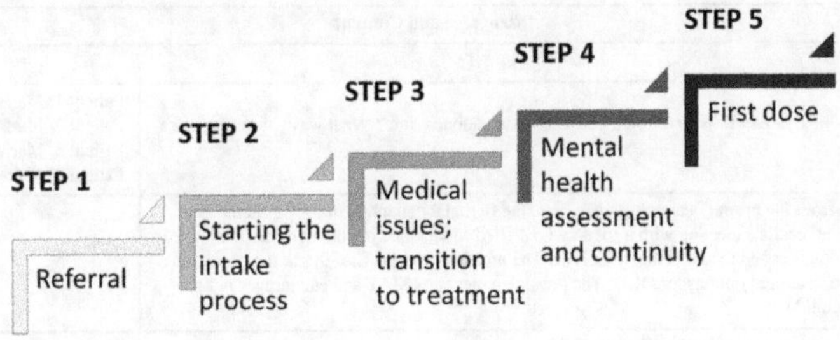

with one of the counselors for their intake assessment (Step 4). The entire intake process takes a few hours, but typically, everything is completed in one day, including the first dose of Methadone (Step 5).

The authors chose interviews as an inquiry method for the video intervention, rather than seeking to interpret and paraphrase statements by the medical staff and the patients. This allowed them to remain as objective and unbiased as possible. They interviewed four patients, one medical provider (who is both a primary care provider and SUD clinic provider), two counselors, and one clinical coordinator.

All interviewed patients were between the ages of 45 and 63 and were undergoing Methadone treatment. The patients were stable in recovery, receiving take-home bottles, and meeting with a counselor monthly. They were chosen by the SUD clinics based on the criteria provided by the development team. The criteria included: duration of the treatment, age, gender, and race. All patients signed a consent to participate in the project. The names of the patients have not been altered, but the authors did not list the Methadone program the patients were affiliated with. Thomas (Patient 4) had spent two years in treatment, which is the shortest time, whereas Maria (Patient 1) had been in treatment the longest, 15 years. Patient testimonials are embedded in the videos in a way that they provide a distinct perspective on the treatment practices discussed by the medical personnel. Patients describe how they have made decisions about their medication based on the assistance provided by the clinic, highlighting the challenges and the successes of the treatment. Based on the five-step process outlined in Figure 2, the authors developed four episodes, called *chapters*. Chapters 1–4 describe the patient's journey through the Methadone treatment according to the intake pathway (see Figure 3).

Figure 3. Four chapters corresponding to the five-step Methadone treatment process

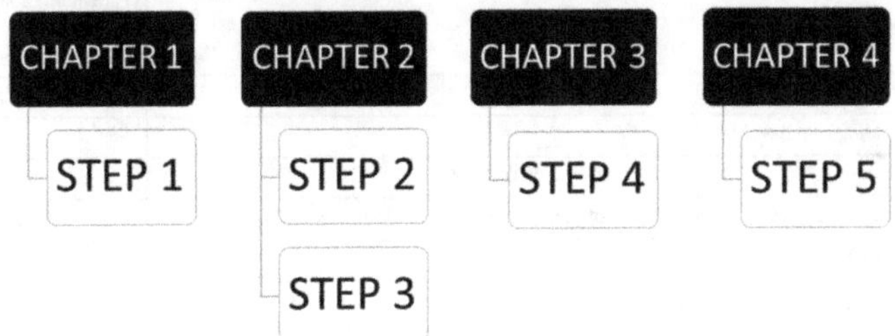

Chapters 1, 3, and 4 include short vignettes that showcase a fictional patient, Lisa, and her interactions inside and outside of the Methadone clinic setting before and during treatment. The goal was to show events that could unfold between a patient and individuals linked to the treatment and that could be

Table 1. Structure and interview questions corresponding to the intake procedures described in Figure 1

Structure and Content		
Chapter 1	*Getting Started*	**Interviewee**
Why did you decide to enter the Methadone treatment? Who referred you to the Methadone clinic? What was your experience entering the clinic?		Patient 1: Maria Patient 2: Mark Patient 3: Maria Patient 4: Thomas
Scenario 1	Referral from the primary care physician: Lisa, the fictional patient, is in the physician's office. She recalls a meeting with a friend who started Methadone treatment to battle his opioid addiction and recommends it for Lisa. The meeting prompts Lisa to ask the physician about the treatment options for OUD. The physician mentions MAT and encourages her to call the clinic.	
What are some of the reasons patient mentions when they enter the program?		Clinical coordinator
What did you want to achieve when you decided to start the treatment?		Patient 1: Maria Patient 3: Maria
What are the medical benefits of Methadone? What are the common misconceptions around Methadone?		Medical provider
What is the stigma surrounding Methadone treatment?		Clinical coordinator Patient 2: Mark
How can the primary care provider facilitate the referral process to a Methadone clinic? What do you want the primary care doctors to know when referring someone for Methadone treatment? Have you talked to your primary care doctor about Methadone treatment?		Patient 2: Mark Patient 4: Thomas Medical provider
What is the role of the primary care provider when speaking with the patient with OUD?		Medical provider
What are some of the benefits of staying on Methadone?		Patient 2: Mark
Chapter 2	***Transition To Treatment (Part 1)***	
What is the most difficult part of the treatment? How can a referral be made?		
What is the first step of the intake process? What does the intake process look like? How is the client admitted?		Medical provider
What questions do you ask when admitting a patient to a Methadone program?		Clinical coordinator
What is the screening process? When do you perform urine toxicology screening? What does it detect? What screenings do you offer during treatment?		Clinical coordinator Medical provider
What is Methadone, and how does it compare with other medications? What is the goal of the medical provider assessment? What topics are discussed during the assessment?		Medical provider Patient 4: Thomas
What are the side effects of MAT?		Medical provider
What do the clients struggle with in the first 90 days of the program? What are some of the challenges that patients encounter while on Methadone? How many clients continue after 90 days?		Clinical COORDINATOR
What does the first week on Methadone look like? What are some of the challenges you encountered when entering the treatment? What are the biggest challenges of being on Methadone?		Patient 2: Mark Patient 4: Thomas
Chapter 3	***Transition To Treatment (Part 2)***	
Scenario 2	Meeting with the intake counselor: Lisa meets with the intake counselor and learns about the intake process and the counseling.	
How does the intake counselor get assigned? What are the recurring topics during counseling sessions?		Clinical coordinator
When does the counseling start? What topics are discussed during the intake with the counselor? How often does the counseling happen? What are the types of sessions you offer?		Substance abuse counselor
How often does the counseling happen? What are the recurring topics during counseling sessions?		Patient 4: Thomas
What is the role of the counselor and the counseling?		Senior counselor
What is the role of counseling? What are the counseling options? How long are the sessions?		Substance abuse counselor
What have you learned through counseling?		Patient 4: Thomas Patient 1: Maria Patient 2: Maria
When does the counseling end?		Clinical coordinator
In what areas of their lives does the counseling help the clients?		Senior counselor
Chapter 4	***First Dose and Next Steps***	
Scenario 3	The first dose: Lisa receives her first dose of Methadone at the medicating window.	
Why are there different colors of Methadone?		Clinical coordinator
What are some positive changes that you have experienced when being on Methadone?		Patient 3: Mark Patient 2: Maria
What is the starting Methadone dose?		Medical provider
How do you adjust the dose?		Patient 2: Maria Patient 3: Mark
How long do clients stay on Methadone? How do you adjust the dose? What is the process for dose adjustments?		Clinical coordinator
How do you earn take-home bottles? What screenings do you undergo during treatment?		Patient 4: Thomas

continued on following page

Table 1. Continued

Structure and Content		
Chapter 1	*Getting Started*	**Interviewee**
How do you monitor client progress? What is the process regarding take-home bottles?		Clinical coordinator
Scenario 4	Lisa's journey—next steps: Lisa stumbles upon her friend and describes her experience when in MAT	
How long does a patient stay on Methadone? How does counseling help with dose adjustments?		Clinical coordinator Substance abuse counselor
How long do you plan to stay in MAT? What did you learn from being in the treatment program? How did the treatment help you move on with your life?		Patient 2: Maria Patient 1: Maria Patient 3: Mark Patient 4: Thomas

challenging to film due to the Health Insurance Portability and Accountability Act (HIPAA) regulations. The authors created a sequence of four scenarios around the fictional patient, Lisa, which show a referral through a friend (Scenario 1)—which is usually the most common way that a patient is referred, that is, by a friend or a family member, a meeting with the primary care doctor (Scenario 1) and the intake counselor (Scenario 2), the administration of the first Methadone dose (Scenario 3), and what happens when the patient is stable in treatment (Scenario 4). The videos assist the viewer in constructing their understanding of patient experiences in the Methadone clinic through the testimonials of actual patients intertwined with medical expertise (see Table 1). Videos offer a common space in which the viewer is exposed to multiple perspectives concerning the treatment. As such, they promote collaboration and knowledge sharing—one of the main principles of social constructivism.

THE DESIGN PROCESS

The design for this project was broken up into three distinct phases, as shown in Figure 4.

Figure 4. Design process

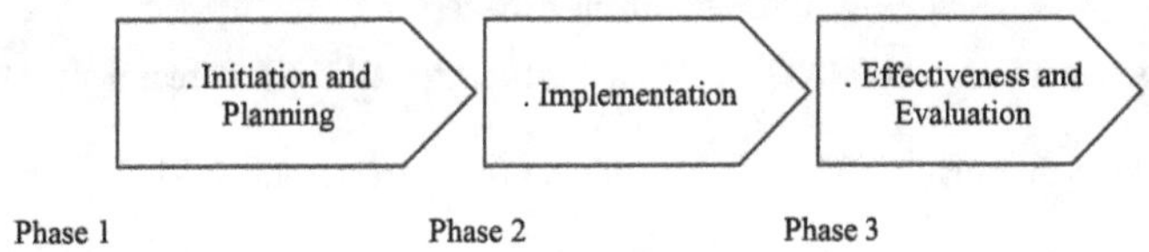

Phase 1: Initiation and Planning

In Phase 1, the core team, consisting of a training development specialist, data manager, and AIDS education and training center (AETC) coordinator, set the goals and the timeline of the project to span through twelve months, including the pre-production, recording, and post-production. The team performed needs analysis using qualitative methods, including medical provider surveys that were distributed among the faculty in the AIDS Program at Yale School of Medicine and focus groups with the SUD clinics. As a result of the provider survey, additional interview questions about Methadone adjustment were identified that included interactions with other medications a patient may be prescribed elsewhere, such as benzos or prescription opioids.

Through focus groups with SUD clinics, the team verified the interview questions and the interview process. The team distributed the script to SUD clinics and the stakeholders for review and adjusted the questions based on their feedback. Since the recording took place on SUD clinic sets, the team also explained the precautions that need to take place when filming during the COVID-19 pandemic. Finally, the team produced storyboards for stakeholders to review and performed casting for the scenarios. To complete Phase 1, the team confirmed the product format, scheduled tasks, and approved the spending plan.

Phase 2: Implementation

In Phase 2, our core team completed all tasks determined earlier in Phase 1. The team then monitored project progress through formative feedback collected from SUD clinics and the AIDS Program at Yale School of Medicine faculty by reviewing sections of edited footage during Zoom meetings. The team adjusted project deliverables based on the feedback. After one of the review phases with medical providers, the authors included the language primer in the videos (see Figure 5). The proposed terminology destigmatizes the patient experience and the Methadone treatment.

Figure 5. Language primer
Source: Tetrault et al. (n.d.)

Avoid these terms...	Use these instead...
Addict, user, drug abuser, junkie, alcoholic	Person with *substance* use or patient with *substance use disorder*
Addicted baby	Baby born with neonatal abstinence syndrome
Substance abuse or dependence	Substance use disorder
Problem	Disease
Habit	Drug addiction
Clean or dirty urine test	Negative (appropriate) or positive (inappropriate) urine drug test
Medication Assisted Treatment (MAT)	Medications for Addiction Treatment (MAT)
Opioid substitution therapy	Opioid agonist treatment
Relapse	Return to use
Treatment failure	Treatment attempt
Being clean	Being in remission or recovery

YALE PROGRAM IN ADDICTION MEDICINE

Phase 3: Effectiveness and Evaluation

In Phase 3, the authors used focus groups to evaluate the videos. SUD partners found the videos to be useful during their new staff orientations. The authors also organized focus groups with the staff members from the Service Syringe Programs (SSPs) in Connecticut (Advancing CT Together and the Yale Healthcare Van), which provided recommendations to improve the videos, and, overall, found the videos useful for the linkage processes between the clinics and their patients.

The development team continues promoting the videos on the New England Connecticut AETC Partner website, where videos are housed currently, and it encourages the completion of a brief feedback survey on the website.

The data on the effectiveness of the videos is primarily based on the results available through Google Analytics that has been installed on the New England Connecticut AETC Partner website at the end of September 2021. The videos have been watched by 40 users from the United States from September 1, 2021, to January 2, 2022. The average session lasted 2 minutes 57 seconds, where a single session is the time a user is actively engaged with the page.

INSTRUCTIONAL DESIGN APPROACH

Instructional Design Models Based on a Socio-Constructivist Approach

Instructional design models serve as theoretical, management, and communication tools for analyzing, designing, developing, implementing, and evaluating (ADDIE) guided instruction (Cheung, 2016). They help ensure that the learning objectives align with the learning outcomes, the designed activities support the learning objectives, the learner's backgrounds and educational needs are properly analyzed, and the assessments measure proficiency effectively (West, 2018). Currently, there exist over 30 instructional design models that are used for the design and development of learning experiences (West, 2018). The ADDIE framework constitutes the foundation of instructional design regardless of which model is used (Gustafson & Branch, 1997).

Instructional design models based on the social constructivist view highlight the need for collaboration among learners. Lave and Wenger (1991) asserted that organizations promoting social collaborations, such as communities of practice, are bearers of society's practical knowledge (Lave & Wenger, 1991). Fardanesh (2006) elaborated that the models based on the constructivist approach enable students to learn through the creation of meaning in their minds. There is no need to frame the learning process defined by the input, activities, and output. Instead, various learning experiences are applied, such as learning in an authentic context through the process of knowledge construction, in which the preconceptions, beliefs, and concepts are tested and redefined or the exposure to different perspectives (Fardanesh, 2006). The teaching and learning approaches include problem-based learning, project method, discovery learning, anchored instruction, and generative learning, among others (Fardanesh, 2006).

Generative Learning and the Constructivist Approach

Generative learning involves actively engaging in cognitive processes during learning–including the selection of relevant material, organizing it into a coherent structure, and integrating it into prior knowledge

(Fiorella & Mayer, 2015). These processes have been concisely illustrated earlier in this study in Figure 1. In the title of their study, Bonn and Grabowski (2001) called generative learning theory the "practical cousin of constructivism." In other words, generative learning offers practical implementation of the constructivist approach. It is also intended for learners with high prior knowledge, who benefit most from using imagining as a learning method that involves the creation of mental images of the presented content. Equally suitable are the strategies of self-testing, self-explaining, and enacting (Fiorella & Mayer, 2015). Medical providers belong to a group of learners who possess such a high degree of prior knowledge.

Merlin Wittrock (1931–2007), the founder of the generative model of comprehension, elucidated in "Generative Learning Processes of the Brain" that the learning processes "include and extend beyond the relations among individual words to sentences, large blocks of text, images, and procedures that characterize meaningful learning from instruction and teaching" (Wittrock, 1992, p. 552). According to Wittrock, understanding happens through relationship building rather than just storing and retrieving the information, as is the case in the cognitive approach.

Of course, learning also depends on what is presented. The content needs to be structured in such a way that allows the learner to generate the relationships mentioned by Wittrock. The instructor's role is then to "know how and when to facilitate the learner's construction of relations[hips]" (Wittrock, 1990, p. 352). Hence, Wittrock identified two types of generative learning strategies that lead to the creation of meaning: first, among the various elements of instruction and the memory components such as "demonstrations, metaphors, analogies, examples, pictures, applications, interpretations, paraphrases, and inferences" (as information being perceived) and second, between that information and the learner's prior knowledge (Wittrock, 1992, p. 354).

The emphasis of the videos is on the generation of deep meaning through constructing relations between new and existing knowledge. The resource allows for such generative learning, where patient interviews interlace with scenarios and medical expertise. Also, the content is divided into four chapters, which allows for better information processing. Other elements that facilitate information processing are graphics such as Figure 2 (patient's journey into Methadone treatment) and Figure 5 (language primer), as well as statistics that provide data on the opioid overdose epidemic in the United States.

The Bergman and Moore Instructional Design Model

The authors created an online resource that is available to providers to access at any time, considering the time constraints that medical providers often face. Although they envisioned that the user would interact with the content independently, at their own pace, and without a facilitator, the videos can also be used in a group setting, where screenings with subsequent discussions take place and involve a moderator—very much in line with social constructivism approach. The resource is free, easily accessible, and widely available.

An instructional design model such as that of Bergman and Moore (1990) reflects the conceptual approach behind our videos. The video intervention meets all four key criteria for the Bergman and Moore model as described in Gustafson and Branch's "Revisioning Models of Instructional Development" (1997):

a. The instructional product is needed.

b. Something needs to be produced rather than selected from existing materials.

c. There will be a considerable emphasis on tryout and revision.

d. The product must be usable by learners with facilitators available, not teachers (Gustafson and Branch, 1997, p. 48)

The Bergman and Moore model is a product-oriented model that encourages self-paced instruction and mindful reflection. It focuses on the delivery of high-quality instructional materials such as interactive, online multimedia content that users can use immediately, without the instructor's guidance (Gustafson & Branch, 1997). It is one of the innumerous models that do not require an extensive needs assessment since the main emphasis is on product quality and product development. The time spent on trial and revisions during the development phase is also high in comparison to the classroom orientated models like, for example, ASSURE (analyze, state, select, utilize, require, and evaluate), in which there is no need for revisions until the product is complete (Brinkerhoff, 2001).

The Bergman and Moore model recognizes six distinct phases: analysis, design, development, production, authoring, and validation. Each of those phases includes three subphases: input, deliverables (output), and evaluation, as shown in Figure 6. The output of each phase provides input for the subsequent phase

Figure 6. The Bergman and Moore instructional design model
(© 2015, Association for Educational Communications and Technology, p. 62. Used with permission.)

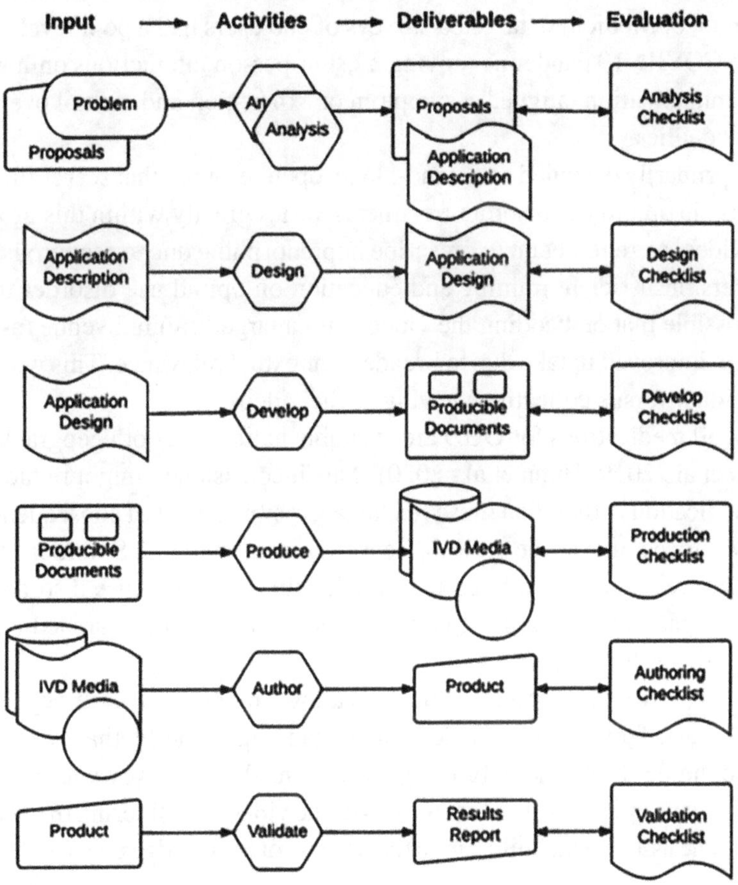

(Branch & Dousay, 2015). In the analysis phase, the instructional need is specified: Learning objectives are established, evaluated, and revised by the development team and the stakeholders, who, in our case, consisted of the faculty of the AIDS Program at Yale School of Medicine.

The design phase started with the review of the project description and the project goals. Based on this evaluation, the development team outlined a plan for the development of the media. By the end of this phase, a detailed design plan included the specification of media, necessary equipment, and the discussion of design principles, timelines, and interaction strategies, and the assessment methodology was formulated and evaluated again by the stakeholders.

During the development phase, the core team designed storyboards that showed the scene sequencing and sample graphics of the lower third and the opening. The authors created the audio script with shot descriptions and interview questions. They then delivered the concept in the production phase and provided a close to the final product in the authoring phase, which also included formative assessments by the stakeholders and the SUD partners. Internal final reviews and target audience reviews were facilitated as part of the validation phase. Subtitles were added to the final video to ensure accessibility.

CHALLENGES AND RECOMMENDATIONS

The evaluation of the effectiveness of the videos posed a major challenge. As opposed to the regular, organized focus groups (with our SUD and later SSP partners, as well as with the faculty of the AIDS Program at Yale School of Medicine), targeted surveys of end users had a poor level of uptake. This may have been due to the COVID-19 pandemic moving most in-person interactions online. Many employees reported "virtual communication fatigue," a symptom of exhaustion and mental overload caused by the overuse of online modalities.

Our videos were primarily designed as a stand-alone, open resource that serves the medical providers community. Expertise in opioid use disorder treatments varies greatly within this group. A 2018 survey mentioned that providers were reluctant to prescribe buprenorphine due to numerous personnel barriers such as, among others, insufficient training and education on opioid use disorder treatment (Haffajee et al., 2018). It is possible that embedding the videos into a larger training venue (as opposed to stand-alone) would result in improved uptake due to broader contextual relevance. This would allow exploring the process of individual versus collective viewing of the videos.

Additionally, not all medications for OUD are available nationally, both geographically and through Medicaid (Andrews et al., 2019; Huhn et al., 2020). This inconsistency might reduce the motivation to learn about OUD medications other than those readily accessible and, as a consequence, affect the value of the educational resources such as the videos discussed in this study. As Solomon et al. (2022) pointed out, the connection between greater availability of medication for opioid use disorder (MOUD) and the use of MOUD among patients in treatment facilities needs to be still researched as access to MOUD continues to be a public health challenge.

Varying levels of expertise discouraged us from creating a more specific survey in which the authors could assess both the basic familiarity and a deep understanding of the Methadone intake processes and the difficulties surrounding it. Instead, a brief, open-form feedback survey was created on the website (www.aetcct.org). The survey assessed the usefulness of the videos considering the goals, objectives, and abilities of the users. The assessment builds upon the process of knowledge construction, which is distinct for each user, who continually refines and reshapes their view of reality based on their newly acquired knowledge. The common evaluation methods involved self- and peer-assessment (Laskaris et al., 2017).

Several recommendations were made after reviewing the videos with our senior program management, as well as with our Connecticut SSP and SUD stakeholder partners. The recommendations include:

1. The need to produce a video about client background stories.
2. The need to create an online training program about the biology and psychology of addiction.
3. The need to create a Q&A section on the Connecticut NEAETC Regional Partner's website (www.aetcct.org) that would address the following questions that the clinics posed:
    a. What kinds of drugs could be detected in the urine testing? Can Methadone be detected in the urine testing?
    b. What are the main differences between the clinics in their intake and monitoring criteria?

Finally, more curricular changes in medical education to include awareness of the opioid epidemic are needed. Both in-person and online OUD training programs have been reported nationwide in recent years as a response to the growing opioid use epidemic—numerous training programs aimed at health professionals and health care centers. Between July 2019 and June 2020, a hybrid training to reduce provider stigma toward harm reduction and pharmacotherapy for OUDs (Methadone, buprenorphine, and naltrexone) was delivered to 147 health professionals in Utah, including 40 SUD treatment professionals. The training significantly reduced the total stigma score toward harm reduction (Sulzer et al., 2021). Another example of an educational program was the extension for community healthcare outcomes (ECHO) to expand access to medications for the treatment of opioid use disorder among rural primary care clinics in New Mexico (Salvador et al., 2020). The training was delivered as a 12-week online course, with 67 primary care staff across 27 rural clinics in New Mexico participating, including 32 prescribers and 35 clinic support staff. The efforts made by the Idaho State University Physician Assistant (PA) program to incorporate medication for assisted treatment (MAT) training for future health care providers into its curriculum are also worth mentioning (Phelps et al., 2021). The course content was redesigned from the already existing free online materials available through the American Academy of Physician Assistants and the American Society of Addiction Medicine. Two online modules were created: the eight-hour module was modified to fit PA and NP needs, with the second module of 16 hours of additional training.

CONCLUSION

Drawing upon socio-constructivist learning theory, the authors created four educational videos to illustrate the five-step admission process into Methadone clinics in Connecticut. The main goal of the videos is to assist the primary care providers, particularly those in HIV clinics and other clinicians and support staff involved in the care of patients with SUDs, in better understanding the intake procedures to the Methadone treatment programs in Connecticut.

The videos feature interviews with patients undertaking Methadone treatment and with medical providers and SUD personnel. The video intervention builds upon the idea that learning is a collective act that occurs during in-person and online interactions in various socio-cultural contexts involving exploration and experimentation. The socio-constructivist theory assumes that personal experience cannot be separated from knowledge. It presupposes that the individuals interact with the world to extract meaning from it to construct a logical and consistent cognitive model based on outside stimuli like images, texts, words, and sounds. The learners examine these constructs by interacting with each other and are ultimately responsible for their learning.

The video as an online modality provides the opportunity to capture the complexity of the intake process, where patients experience the treatment on a personal level. At the same time, it allows for clarification of this process from the perspective of the medical staff. The video intervention has been effective in revealing a range of phenomena and complexities surrounding Methadone treatment, including stigma, myths, and misconceptions around its efficacy, the process around take-home bottles and dose adjustments, the potential side effects, or the counseling options.

ACKNOWLEDGMENT

This research was supported by the Health Resources and Services Administration (HRSA) of the U.S. Department of Health and Human Services (HHS) [HRSA 017-047 Curing Hepatitis C Among People of Color Living with HIV].

This research was also supported by:

1. APT Foundation, New Haven, Connecticut
2. Recovery Network of Programs, Inc., Bridgeport, Connecticut
3. Root Center for Advanced Recovery, Hartford, Connecticut

REFERENCES

Adams, P. (2006). Exploring social constructivism: Theories and practicalities. *Education, 34*(3), 243–257.

Andrews, C. M., Abraham, A. J., Grogan, C. M., Westlake, M. A., Pollack, H. A., & Friedmann, P. D. (2019). Impact of Medicaid restrictions on availability of buprenorphine in addiction treatment programs. *American Journal of Public Health, 109*(3), 434–436. doi:10.2105/AJPH.2018.304856 PMID:30676789

Basu Roy, R., & McMahon, G. T. (2012). Video-based cases disrupt deep critical thinking in problem-based learning. *Medical Education, 46*(4), 426–435. doi:10.1111/j.1365-2923.2011.04197.x PMID:22429179

Bonn, K. L., & Grabowski, B. L. (2001). *Generative learning theory: A practical cousin to constructivism* [Paper presentation]. Joint Mathematics Meetings, New Orleans, LA.

Branch, R. M., & Dousay, T. A. (2015). *Survey of instructional development models* (5th ed.). Association for Educational Communications and Technology.

Brinkerhoff, D. A. (2001). Survey of instructional development models. *TechTrends, 45*(1), 48–50. doi:10.1007/BF02763388

Cheung, L. (2016). Using an instructional design model to teach medical procedures. *Medical Science Educator, 26*(1), 175–180. doi:10.100740670-016-0228-9 PMID:27182457

Clinton, H. (2021). *Connecticut Department of Public Health drug overdose monthly report.* https://public.tableau.com/app/profile/heather.clinton/viz/SUDORS_Dashboard_final2/OverdoseDashboard

Cooper, R. L., Ramesh, A., Juarez, P. D., Edgerton, R., Paul, M., Tabatabai, M., Brown, I. K., & Matthews-Juarez, P. (2020). Systematic review of opioid use disorder treatment training for medical students and residents. *Journal of Health Care for the Poor and Underserved, 31*(5), 26–42. doi:10.1353/hpu.2020.0136 PMID:35061607

Dennick, R. (2016). Constructivism: Reflections on twenty-five years teaching the constructivist approach in medical education. *International Journal of Medical Education, 7*, 200–205. doi:10.5116/ijme.5763.de11 PMID:27344115

Dewey, J. (1938). *Logic: The theory of inquiry*. Holt.

Dhawan, S. (2020). Online learning: A panacea in the time of COVID-19 crisis. *Journal of Educational Technology Systems, 49*(1), 5–22. doi:10.1177/0047239520934018

Ernest, P. (1999). *Social constructivism as a philosophy of mathematics: Radical constructivism rehabilitated. A 'historical paper'*. Available at www. people. ex.ac.uk/PErnest

Fardanesh, H. (2006). *A classification of constructivist instructional design models based on learning and teaching approaches*. https://files.eric.ed.gov/fulltext/ED491713.pdf

Fiorella, L., & Mayer, R. E. (2015). *Learning as a generative activity*. Cambridge University Press. doi:10.1017/CBO9781107707085

Friedman, J., & Akre, S. (2021). COVID-19 and the drug overdose crisis: Uncovering the deadliest months in the United States, January–July 2020. *American Journal of Public Health, 111*(7), 1284–1291. doi:10.2105/AJPH.2021.306256 PMID:33856885

Ghersin, Z. J., Yager, P., Cummings, B. M., Hersh, C., Cayer, M., Callans, K. M., Zablah, J. E., Gallagher, T., Abrego, S., Bonilla, J., Sanchez Vela, O., Guzman, L., Aguilar, A., & Hartnick, C. J. (2020). A multidisciplinary, video-based, curriculum for management of the intubated and surgical airway patient for a pediatric hospital in El Salvador. *International Journal of Pediatric Otorhinolaryngology, 128*, 109732. doi:10.1016/j.ijporl.2019.109732 PMID:31644996

Gredler, M. E. (1997). Learning and instruction. *Theory into Practice*.

Gustafson, K., & Branch, R. (1997). Revisioning models of instructional development. *Educational Technology Research and Development, 45*(3), 73–89. doi:10.1007/BF02299731

Haffajee, R. L., Bohnert, A. S., & Lagisetty, P. A. (2018). Policy pathways to address provider workforce barriers to buprenorphine treatment. *American Journal of Preventive Medicine, 54*(6), S230–S242. doi:10.1016/j.amepre.2017.12.022 PMID:29779547

Heath, C., Luff, P., & Sanchez Svensson, M. (2007). Video and qualitative research: Analysing medical practice and interaction. *Medical Education, 41*(1), 109–116. doi:10.1111/j.1365-2929.2006.02641.x PMID:17209899

Hendricks, M., Nair, G., Staunton, C., Pather, M., Garrett, N., Baadjies, D., Kidd, M., & Moodley, K. (2018). *Impact of an educational video as a consent tool on knowledge about cure research among patients and caregivers at HIV clinics in South Africa*. Academic Press.

Holland, K. M., Jones, C., Vivolo-Kantor, A. M., Idaikkadar, N., Zwald, M., Hoots, B., Yard, E., D'Inverno, A., Swedo, E., Chen, M. S., Petrosky, E., Board, A., Martinez, P., Stone, D. M., Law, R., Coletta, M. A., Adjemian, J., Thomas, C., Puddy, R. W., ... Houry, D. (2021). Trends in U.S. emergency department visits for mental health, overdose, and violence outcomes before and during the COVID-19 pandemic. *JAMA Psychiatry*, *78*(4), 372–379. doi:10.1001/jamapsychiatry.2020.4402 PMID:33533876

Huhn, A. S., Hobelmann, J. G., Strickland, J. C., Oyler, G. A., Bergeria, C. L., Umbricht, A., & Dunn, K. E. (2020). Differences in availability and use of medications for opioid use disorder in residential treatment settings in the United States. *JAMA Network Open*, *3*(2), e1920843–e1920843. doi:10.1001/jamanetworkopen.2019.20843 PMID:32031650

Kaini, S., & Motie, L. Z. (2021). Virtual vs Online: Insight from Medical Students. Comment on "Effectiveness of virtual medical teaching during the COVID-19 crisis: Systematic review.". *JMIR Medical Education*, *7*(2), e27020. doi:10.2196/27020 PMID:33988518

Kanselaar, G. (2002). Constructivism and socio-constructivism. *Constructivism and Socio-Constructivism*, 1–7.

Laskaris, D., Kalogiannakis, M., & Heretakis, E. (2017). "Interactive evaluation" of an e-learning course within the context of blended education. *International Journal of Technology Enhanced Learning*, *9*(4), 339–353. doi:10.1504/IJTEL.2017.087793

Lave, J., & Wenger, E. (1991). Legitimate peripheral participation. *Situated Learning: Legitimate Peripheral Participation, 1*, 29-43.

Madden, E. F. (2019). Intervention stigma: How medication-assisted treatment marginalizes patients and providers. *Social Science & Medicine*, *232*, 324–331. doi:10.1016/j.socscimed.2019.05.027 PMID:31125801

McQueen, S., McKinnon, V., VanderBeek, L., McCarthy, C., & Sonnadara, R. (2019). Video-based assessment in surgical education: A scoping review. *Journal of Surgical Education*, *76*(6), 1645–1654. doi:10.1016/j.jsurg.2019.05.013 PMID:31175065

Molenda, M. H. (2020). *The elements of instruction: A framework for the age of emerging technologies*. Routledge. doi:10.4324/9781315194721

Noetel, M., Griffith, S., Delaney, O., Sanders, T., Parker, P., del Pozo Cruz, B., & Lonsdale, C. (2021). Video improves learning in higher education: A systematic review. *Review of Educational Research*, *91*(2), 204–236. doi:10.3102/0034654321990713

O'Brien Pott, M., Blanshan, A. S., Huneke, K. M., Baasch Thomas, B. L., & Cook, D. A. (2020). What influences choice of continuing medical education modalities and providers? A National Survey of U.S. physicians, nurse practitioners, and physician assistants. *Academic Medicine*, *96*(1), 93–100. doi:10.1097/ACM.0000000000003758 PMID:32969838

Peisachovich, E., Da Silva, C., Penhearow, N. J., Sombilon, E. V., & Koh, M. (2020). Implementing virtual simulated person methodology to support the shift to online learning: Technical report. *Cureus*, *12*(6). Advance online publication. doi:10.7759/cureus.8864 PMID:32754403

Phelps, P., Rodríguez, M. M. D., de la Caridad Alvarez, M., & Johnson, J. L. (2021). Shifts in attitudes and intentions to practice following medication-assisted treatment training. *The Journal of Physician Assistant Education: the Official Journal of the Physician Assistant Education Association*, *32*(3), 182–184. doi:10.1097/JPA.0000000000000368 PMID:34224540

Prawat, R. S., & Floden, R. E. (1994). Philosophical perspectives on constructivist views of learning. *Educational Psychologist*, *29*(1), 37–48. doi:10.120715326985ep2901_4

Rannikmäe, M., Holbrook, J., & Soobard, R. (2020). Social Constructivism—Jerome Bruner. In B. Akpan & T. J. Kennedy (Eds.), *Science Education in Theory and Practice. Springer Texts in Education*. Springer. doi:10.1007/978-3-030-43620-9_18

Ratycz, M. C., Papadimos, T. J., & Vanderbilt, A. A. (2018). Addressing the growing opioid and heroin abuse epidemic: A call for medical school curricula. *Medical Education Online*, *23*(1), 1466574. doi:10.1080/10872981.2018.1466574 PMID:29708863

Rogoff, B. (1990). *Apprenticeship in thinking*. Oxford University Press.

Salvador, J. G., Bhatt, S. R., Jacobsohn, V. C., Maley, L. A., Alkhafaji, R. S., Rishel Brakey, H., Myers, O. B., & Sussman, A. L. (2020). Feasibility and acceptability of an online ECHO intervention to expand access to medications for treatment of opioid use disorder, psychosocial treatments and supports. *Substance Abuse*, *42*(4), 1–8. PMID:32814005

Sandars, J., Correia, R., Dankbaar, M., de Jong, P., Goh, P. S., Hege, I., Masters, K., Oh, S., Patel, R., Premkumar, K., Webb, A., & Pusic, M. (2020). Twelve tips for rapidly migrating to online learning during the COVID-19 pandemic. *MedEdPublish*, *9*(1), 3068.

Seval, N., Eaton, E., & Springer, S. A. (2020, January). Beyond antibiotics: A practical guide for the infectious disease physician to treat opioid use disorder in the setting of associated infectious diseases. *Open Forum Infectious Diseases*, *7*(1), ofz539. doi:10.1093/ofid/ofz539 PMID:31993454

Shank, P. (2018). *Manage memory for deeper learning: 21 evidence-based and easy-to-apply tactics that support memory while learning and beyond*. Learning Peaks LLC.

Shunk, D. H. (2000). Learning: introduction, issues, and historical perspectives. In *Learning theories: An educational perspective* (pp. 1–29). Upper Saddle River, NJ: Pearson Education.

Smith, E., & Boscak, A. (2021). A virtual emergency: Learning lessons from remote medical student education during the COVID-19 pandemic. *Emergency Radiology*, *28*(3), 445–452. doi:10.100710140-020-01874-2 PMID:33420528

Solomon, K. T., Bandara, S., Reynolds, I. S., Krawczyk, N., Saloner, B., Stuart, E., & Connolly, E. (2022). Association between availability of medications for opioid use disorder in specialty treatment and use of medications among patients: A state-level trends analysis. *Journal of Substance Abuse Treatment*, *132*, 108424. doi:10.1016/j.jsat.2021.108424 PMID:34144299

Sulzer, S. H., Prevedel, S., Barrett, T., Voss, M. W., Manning, C., & Madden, E. F. (2021). Professional education to reduce provider stigma toward harm reduction and pharmacotherapy. *Drugs Education Prevention & Policy*, *28*(2), 1–11. doi:10.1080/09687637.2021.1936457

Tabakin, A. L., Patel, H. V., & Singer, E. A. (2021). Lessons learned from the COVID-19 pandemic: A call for a national video-based curriculum for urology residents. *Journal of Surgical Education, 78*(1), 324–326. doi:10.1016/j.jsurg.2020.07.013 PMID:32741691

Tetrault, J. M., Krause, R., Roessler, E., Heimer, R., Powell, M. L., Drew, S., & Edens, E. (n.d.). *Addiction treatment: Clinical skills for healthcare providers*. https://www.coursera.org/lecture/addiction-treatment/how-do-you-talk-about-addiction-YVN5U

Tuong, W., Larsen, E. R., & Armstrong, A. W. (2014). Videos to influence: A systematic review of effectiveness of video-based education in modifying health behaviors. *Journal of Behavioral Medicine, 37*(2), 218–233. doi:10.100710865-012-9480-7 PMID:23188480

Vygotsky, L. S. (1962). *Thought and language*. MIT Press. doi:10.1037/11193-000

Vygotsky, L. S. (1978). *Mind in society: The development of higher psychological processes*. Harvard University Press.

Waters, E., & Sroufe, L. A. (1983). Social competence as a developmental construct. *Developmental Review, 3*, 79–97.

West, R. E. (2018). *Foundations of learning and instructional design technology* (1st ed.). EdTech Books.

Williams, T. (2020). The benefits of using video in healthcare. *Health Tech Digital*. https://www.healthtechdigital.com/the-benefits-of-using-video-in-healthcare/

Wittrock, M. C. (1992). Generative learning processes of the brain. *Educational Psychologist, 27*(4), 531–541. doi:10.120715326985ep2704_8

Wong, R. Y. (2020). Medical education during COVID-19: Lessons from a pandemic. *BCMJ, 62*(5), 170–171.

Yeates, P., Moult, A., Lefroy, J., Walsh-House, J., Clews, L., McKinley, R., & Fuller, R. (2020). Understanding and developing procedures for video-based assessment in medical education. *Medical Teacher, 42*(11), 1250–1260. doi:10.1080/0142159X.2020.1801997 PMID:32749915

ADDITIONAL READING

Broadhead, R. S., Heckathorn, D. D., Altice, F. L., Van Hulst, Y., Carbone, M., Friedland, G. H., O'Connor, P. G., & Selwyn, P. A. (2002). Increasing drug users' adherence to HIV treatment: Results of a peer-driven intervention feasibility study. *Social Science & Medicine, 55*(2), 235–246. doi:10.1016/S0277-9536(01)00167-8 PMID:12144138

Grabowski, B. L. (2013). Generative learning contributions to the design of instruction and learning. In D. Jonassen & M. Driscoll (Eds.), *Handbook of research on educational communications and technology* (pp. 713–737). Routledge.

Johnston, L., Williams, S. B., & Ades, A. (2018, March). Education for ECMO providers: Using education science to bridge the gap between clinical and educational expertise. *Seminars in Perinatology*, *42*(2), 138–146. doi:10.1053/j.semperi.2017.12.010 PMID:29336833

Kodjo, C. M., & Klein, J. D. (2002). Prevention and risk of adolescent substance abuse. The role of adolescents, families, and communities. *Pediatric Clinics of North America*, *49*(2), 257–268. doi:10.1016/S0031-3955(01)00003-7 PMID:11993282

Moemennasab, M., Rahemi, S., Ayatollahi, A., & Aeen, M. (2002). The effect of video-based instruction on students' cognitive learning. *Journal of Medical Education*, *1*(3).

Myrick, K., & Del Vecchio, P. (2016). Peer support services in the behavioral healthcare workforce: State of the field. *Psychiatric Rehabilitation Journal*, *39*(3), 197–203. doi:10.1037/prj0000188 PMID:27183186

KEY TERMS AND DEFINITIONS

Harm Reduction: A public health approach to regulate and minimalize drug use.

MAT: Medications for assisted treatment is a method to treat substance use disorder that involves a combination of medication treatment with counseling and behavioral therapy.

Methadone: A synthetic opioid agonist that prevents opioid withdrawal symptoms.

OUD: Opioid use disorder, a chronic disorder that involves dependence and addiction to opioids used to produce subjective feelings of euphoria in the brain.

Social Constructivism: A learning theory developed by Russian psychologist Lev Vygotsky, which presupposes that students learn through social interactions and are active participants in the creation of their knowledge.

SSP: Syringe services programs are community-based prevention organizations that prevent the spread of infectious disease through injection drug use by facilitating the safe disposal of used needles and syringes.

SUD: Substance use disorder is a mental disorder that happens through misuse of alcohol and/or another substance (drugs or medications), which leads to health issues and/or problems at work, school, or home.

ENDNOTES

1 Methadone is a synthetic opioid agonist, which means that it prevents opioid withdrawal symptoms, and does not produce feelings of euphoria or heavy sedation (Madden, 2019). It is taken daily in form of a pill or liquid.

2 Buprenorphine, similarly, to Methadone, alleviates acute withdrawal symptoms and can be administered daily as a tablet, every six months as a subdermal implant, or as a monthly injection (Seval et al., 2020). Instead of controlling withdrawal and cravings, naltrexone is an opioid antagonist, and, unlike Methadone and Buprenorphine, it blocks the euphoric effects of opioids (Seval et al., 2020).

Chapter 11
Leveraging Instructional Technology to Design Diverse Learning Experiences Through Collaborative Stakeholder Engagement

Jessica Andrea Giraldo
Herbert Wertheim College of Medicine, USA & Florida International University, USA

Samantha Marina Lemus-Martinez
Herbert Wertheim College of Medicine, Florida International University, USA

Garamis E. Campusano
Center for the Advancement of Teaching, Florida International University, USA

ABSTRACT

Medical educators often receive minimal formal pedagogical and technological training. The COVID-19 pandemic made this gap even more apparent, necessitating the development of a multidisciplinary team approach to design and implement quality online learning interactions. The team is composed of faculty development and instructional design personnel, who are positioned to provide the pedagogical, technological, and theoretical expertise and guidance on how to design and develop diverse digital learning experiences. This team works within an iterative, development process that encourages collaboration by assisting faculty in shifting from lecture-based instruction to active learning, providing medical educators a form of reverse faculty development by engaging medical students as co-curriculum constructors, informing faculty regarding the implications of cognitive load and the science of learning, and cultivating positive experiences for faculty when working with the multidisciplinary team that encourages future repeated engagement.

DOI: 10.4018/978-1-7998-9490-2.ch011

INTRODUCTION

This chapter describes a multidisciplinary approach to designing and implementing quality online learning interactions. This approach utilizes well-supported theory and an iterative development process that encourages collaboration among key stakeholders as its central tenets. Faculty were consistently exposed to this approach when a multidisciplinary team assisted them in redesigning their passive, lecture-based online sessions to active e-learning experiences. Faculty were provided with two methods of support: (a) a reverse faculty development approach that engaged students as co-curriculum constructors and (b) a multidisciplinary team consisting of faculty development and instructional design personnel who support medical educators through their pedagogical, technological, and theoretical expertise on how to develop exemplar diverse digital learning experiences.

BACKGROUND

Most of today's students enter medical school accustomed to using technology (Guze, 2015) to engage with the content in their courses and to quickly access a wealth of information (Sheehy, 2019). The evolution of the medical profession is constantly making advancements in how healthcare is provided, such that it is necessary to build the digital literacy skills for all students in this increasingly technology-supported practice, regardless of whether they are versed in technology or not (Aungst & Patel, 2020). Additionally, medical students continuously engage more with online educational tools (Hughes, 2018) to supplement their in- and out-of-classroom learning experiences (Bauzon, 2021). According to Graff et al. (2021) "students' enjoyment and comprehension of material is enhanced by interactive, multimedia education that incorporates multiple learning modalities. The integration of faculty-made technological resources…has been described as highly favored by medical students" (pp. 8-9). Thus, medical educators must answer the call to become early adopters of technology (Simpson et al., 2018) as well as assist in closing the professional gap between themselves and students (Sheehy, 2019). However, medical educators often receive minimal formal, pedagogical (Alpert et. al, 2019; Haber et al., 2006) and technological training (Torda, 2020). Their professional degree programs focus mainly on the practice of medicine. Additionally, upon graduating, their careers evolve at a fast pace, often leaving limited time to learn (Alpert et al, 2019; Bing-You & Sproul, 1992; Dandavino et al., 2007; Haber et al, 2006) and adopt the skills necessary to enhance student learning.

While the medical education community has been discussing the need for further faculty competency in digital fluency and next steps (Simpson et al., 2018; Torda, 2020), the rapid shift to remote instruction during the COVID-19 pandemic ultimately forced educators to reflect on and analyze on their current use of educational technology and its implications on student learning (Torda, 2020). Through this reflection, it became apparent that while instructional sessions were able to be moved online, faculty's current minimal use of education technology tools and overuse of traditional, passive, lecture-based methods resulted in a critical missing piece: engagement and interactions that stimulated student learning.

At Florida International University's Herbert Wertheim College of Medicine (HWCOM), this realization guided the development of new online sessions that placed active learning at the forefront and emphasized the need to shift away from traditional, lecture-based methods. Faculty at the college were not only asked to challenge their pedagogical paradigms, but a multidisciplinary support team also encouraged and assisted them in the selection, use, and assessment of appropriate technology tools

(Simpson et al, 2018). during the development process of the new sessions. The multidisciplinary support team, composed of faculty development and instructional design personnel at HWCOM, worked alongside faculty and medical students to develop engaging online experiences that were grounded in instructional theory.

Theoretical Framework for Intervention Goals and Design

The Technological Pedagogical Content Knowledge (TPACK) framework developed in 2006 by Matthew J. Koehler and Punya Mishra is most relevant to supporting and informing the identified needs of medical education faculty discussed in this chapter. Koehler and Mishra's original work enhanced that of Lee Shulman's teacher knowledge construct, formally known as pedagogical content knowledge (PCK), by integrating technological knowledge as necessary to effective instruction. TPACK is a model that identifies teacher knowledge as a complex interplay of three primary forms: Content Knowledge (CK), Pedagogy (PK), and Technology (TK). According to Youm and Corral (2019), the TPACK framework has been validated in K-12 and higher education, with one validation study in medical education. In their validation study, faculty from two medical schools demonstrated they were confident in their content knowledge, but required further training in pedagogy, technology, and the intersection between technological and pedagogical knowledge. Instructional designers and faculty development programming were identified as bridges to closing the gap in faculty's pedagogical, and especially technological knowledge, which is "the greatest perceived deficit of medical educators" (p. S72).

While additional studies are necessary to further support the generalizability of Youm and Corral's research findings in medical education, a clear need for faculty development in each type of knowledge domain must be addressed equally and no one domain should be overlooked over another. Therefore, to address the levels of knowledge in the TPACK framework's domains of pedagogy and technology, a grassroots intervention at HWCOM was essential to the development of our medical educators. This intervention utilizes a multidisciplinary team approach for the design and development of instructional sessions. The team, models for faculty how pedagogical and technological knowledge intersect, which is critical to the effective design and delivery of diverse learning experiences.

Intervention Goals

To achieve the aims of this multidisciplinary intervention, HWCOM's faculty development and instructional design personnel focused on the following four goals: (a) assisting faculty in shifting from lecture-based instruction to active learning methods, including a flipped classroom approach; (b) providing medical educators a form of reverse faculty development by engaging medical students as co-curriculum constructors; (c) informing faculty regarding the implications of cognitive load and the science of learning; and, (d) cultivating positive experiences for faculty when working with the multidisciplinary team that encourages future repeated engagement.

Lecture-Based to Active Learning

Medical education is not exempt from the higher education practice of passive teaching methods, or death by PowerPoint, despite the call for change (Zakrajsek, 2018). There is a long-standing tradition of rote memorization in higher education (Irby, et al. 2010; Prober & Norden, 2021) and the belief that the only way an educator can ensure students are learning the content is through verbal delivery. There is also a misconception that once taught, the concepts will be retained long-term by the student (Ahmed, et al. 2021). In medical school, this is exacerbated by the pressure on the faculty to provide *all* the information necessary to prepare students to be competent, future physicians. The resistance from faculty to move away from lecture-based teaching has "critically slowed the adoption of more contemporary evidence-based teaching strategies that would likely have advanced student learning" (Zakrajsek, 2018, p. 1). These beliefs prevent the development of self-directed learners as well as students being able to apply newly acquired knowledge in diverse ways.

It is, however, important to acknowledge that some faculty have made the attempts to implement more active learning methods as opposed to running courses that are strictly lecture-based. For example, Schwartzstein and Roberts (2017) state that "lecture-based teaching has increasingly been replaced by team-based learning, interprofessional education, and exercises integrating clinical medicine and basic science" (p. 606). This is in part due to the Liaison Committee on Medical Education (LCME)'s accreditation requirement to increase self-directed and active learning in classrooms, causing medical schools to emphasize active learning and team-based activities. According to Ginzburg (2018), self-directed learning is "integral to the … shift towards basic, clinical and social sciences content integration and outcomes-based medical education" (p. 1). This helps students "develop the capacity for self-reflection and lifelong learning," and is considered an "essential skill for the development of a successful professional career" (p. 1). Approaches delineated by Ginzburg (2018) to integrate self-directed learning are small and large group sessions, such as problem-based learning. These sessions provide students with opportunities to examine, explore and consolidate knowledge while also increasing student engagement (Fong, 2016).

Faculty in higher education have made best efforts to adopt and implement new pedagogical methods, such as team-based learning or a flipped classroom approach. As a result, they have felt "liberated from the tyranny of the requirement to 'cover' everything since acquisition of the information is accomplished by the student" (Schwartzstein & Roberts, 2017, pp. 606-607). However, there is still much to be learned from the intentionality of selecting and implementing active learning methods. While Zakrajsek (2018) promotes the idea that a means to facilitate acceptance and adoption of evidence-based strategies is to recognize that there is a place for well-delivered and thought-provoking lectures, he also warns against "poorly executed continuous exposition lectures" in which learning is impacted (p. 2).

Reverse Faculty Development

The allocation of human capital and funding resources that develop and train faculty is typically limited (Servey, et al. 2020), resulting in a lack of necessary support. An additional barrier to faculty participating in development opportunities is their lack of institutionally protected time, which would allow for them to engage in their own development. One way in which to address faculty development needs in resource-deprived settings and institutions where faculty time is not protected, is to engage medical students who are interested in teaching. This approach can focus on building the (TK) and Pedagogy (PK) knowledge of medical education faculty through an inverted method whereby students support faculty in developing new digital learning experiences that are interactive and leverage educational technology. This will also enable students to support the medical school curriculum while also becoming better future educators that are knowledgeable about teaching practices and educational technology tools.

There are currently two models available to students interested in teaching at the Herbert Wertheim College of Medicine: (1) the academic medicine pipeline program is a rigorous four-year longitudinal program that scaffolds the teaching of critical teaching and learning skills, and (2) the teaching skills elective is a two or four-week course offered to fourth-year medical students. The fourth-year elective is generally taken by students who either later realized their interest in teaching or did not want to engage in the longitudinal program with a rigorous teaching concentration. The medical students engaged in these initiatives receive training in the areas of curriculum and instruction and support through the college's multidisciplinary team of faculty development and instructional design personnel. A benefit of the initiatives is the opportunity for faculty and students to engage in a partnership where faculty can remain content experts while students model effective curriculum design and instructional teaching methods, similar to a "train the trainer" approach or reverse mentorship model (Leh, 2005).

Cognitive Load and the Science of Learning

Medical education faculty often approach the design and delivery of content as experts and may lose sight of how a novice learner experiences the intake of knowledge for the first time (Persky & Robinson, 2017). This experience is often exacerbated in a medical school setting where overloading is the norm as a result of the sheer amount of medical information that students are expected to learn. Lectures within the medical school curriculum have been likened to "drinking from a 'firehose of information'" (Ahmed, et al., 2021). For example, Ahmed et al. (2021) stated that "a preclinical curriculum of25,000 slides had to be covered in just a year and a half" (p. 718). This overload of information thus increases the cognitive load on the learner and impacts their long-term retention of information (Lewis, 2016).

Lewis (2016) states that cognitive load is defined as the "stress put on our brain when we learn new data and skills" (p. 877). Our brain's working memory can only hold "7 ± 2 pieces of information at one time," which must be "either moved to long-term memory very fast or it is lost" (p. 877). Cognitive load is affected by the complexity of information, the amount of information and how it is presented as well as the audience (e.g., novice learners) (Lewis, 2016) and is an important factor for enhancing student learning outcomes (Mayer and Chandler, 2001)). Lectures filled with overloaded PowerPoint slides misrepresent the act of teaching and assume that a student has learned what was presented (Schwartzstein & Roberts, 2017. While it may seem efficient to load students with as much information as possible, it is "unlikely to be an effective way to learn" (p. 605) due to our brain's limited processing capacity. By reducing cognitive load, we can maximize learning and aid in the long-term retention of information (Lewis, 2016). Therefore, understanding the science of learning, specifically cognitive load, and its implications for teaching and curriculum design is important in the development and implementation of specific strategies and evidence-based approaches that improve students' learning and success (Gooding et al., 2016).

The multidisciplinary team at HWCOM has employed a variety of strategies to assist in changing the culture that has normalized the overuse of PowerPoints and the information overload in instructional sessions. For example, faculty engage in lecture rehearsals where they receive feedback on their slide design and content organization, and they discuss opportunities to further synthesize or distill the content into manageable chunks to reduce extraneous load. These sessions may also involve suggesting to faculty where passive methods can be substituted by active learning strategies when optimal. Following the consultation, faculty may choose to meet independently with an instructional designer to work on the implementation of the active learning strategies that involve the design of digital learning experiences, which are created in alignment with evidence-based techniques.

Continuous Engagement With a Multidisciplinary Team

According to Hirumi (2021), medical faculty development and instructional design personnel are positioned to provide expert advice and guidance on the "how and why people learn, how to design training and educational systems, and how to work with [subject matter experts] SMEs to mold content into effective, efficient, and engaging coursework" (p. S9). However, channeling this message to faculty must be done in a methodical manner, ensuring that faculty buy-in to the curricular, instructional, and technological changes that medical education demands. This process entails a respectful, collaborative approach that acknowledges faculty as key stakeholders and autonomous in their teaching practice. Approaching faculty development in this way cultivates positive experiences, which, in turn, encourages future repeated engagement with a multidisciplinary team.

Systematic Instructional Design Approach

Instructional design and technology professionals leverage systematic processes to design intentional learning experiences (Dick et al. 2015). Systematic means that there is a "orderly, logical, method of identifying, developing, and evaluating" instructional strategies to meet learning outcomes (Rose, 2004, p. 5). This systematic approach is composed of interdependent inputs and outputs, i.e., the learners, instructor, objectives, learning activities, and the environment (Dick et al., 2015).

This systemic approach to instructional design can be traced to World War II, where psychologists and educators developed training materials (Reiser, 2001) and combined their research with instructional media to create instructional design (Rose, 2004). The field continued to develop following the war, influenced by the work of Robert Gagné and Leslie Briggs, B.F. Skinner as well as Ralph Tyler, Benjamin Bloom and Robert Glaser (Rose, 2002). During the 1970s, their independent efforts combined to develop the body of knowledge on a systematic approach to instructional design (Rose, 2002). The 1980s brought forth the merging of instructional design with technology (with the advent of personal computers), which continues to be an instrumental component of instructional design today (Rose, 2002).

These historical events led to the development of a systems approach model to instructional design, commonly known as "ADDIE" (Molenda, 2003; Reiser, 2001). From this generic model, numerous others were developed that are either more or less complex, but the major components they all have in common are the "analysis of instructional problems and the design, development, implementation, and evaluation of…materials" (Reiser, 2001, pp. 6-7). Broadly speaking, (a) analyze involves defining the instructional problem and identifying a solution, (b) design involves drafting the instructional strategy, (c) development entails creating and assembling the assets, (d) implementation is how the instruction is delivered and how learners use the solution, and (e) evaluation measures the impact of the instruction. ADDIE and its derivatives are collectively known as instructional systems development or ISD (Dick et al., 2015; Molenda, 2003).

This systematic approach helps to standardize the design and development of instruction, thereby minimizing "reliance on intuition or trial-and-error" (Rose, 2004, p. 6). There is ultimately a flexibility built-in to the process that allows instructional designers and faculty developers to apply the practices and learning theory that make the most sense in their context and with their learners. For example, the authors of this chapter who comprise the multidisciplinary team at HWCOM used Bloom's taxonomy (Bloom, 1956) to create learning objectives that clarify what the learner is expected to do, which falls under the analysis component of the ADDIE paradigm. In the design phase, backwards design—beginning with the end in mind—was used when crafting instruction (Wiggins & McTighe, 1998), while also leveraging Mayer's 10 multimedia principles (Mayer, 2008) in the development phase, Gagné's nine events of instruction (Gagne, 1965) during implementation, and Kirkpatrick's four levels of evaluation in the final phase (Kirkpatrick & Kirkpatrick, 2016). In other words, learning theories are tools in a toolbox that instructional designers and faculty developers can pull from to help meet the objectives of the intervention.

In addition to the systematic approach to design, it is important to note the attitudes, skills, and collaborative approaches necessary to analyze, design, develop, implement, and evaluate instruction while paying attention to the limitations in time and resources that can affect ISD. Instructional designers and faculty developers often rely on faculty as the subject-matter experts; therefore, they must work collaboratively with their SMEs to design effective instruction. This partnership also requires critical thinking and problem-solving skills, including staying open-minded and listening to opposing views as well as the ability to ask good questions that help verify instructional goals and identify solutions (Dick et al., 2015). Faculty and support personnel can work together to create shared meaning at the intersection of curricular development and instructional systematic design processes. Further, how and whether instruction is designed is influenced by the amount of time for development and delivery. Other considerations include the experience of the instructional designer or faculty developer and any political or budget considerations (Dick et al., 2015).

Integration of Instructional Technology

The COVID-19 pandemic has only helped to exacerbate the process of integrating educational technology in the classroom. For the past decade, educational research has been focused on analyzing the effectiveness of faculty transitioning from a more passive approach (e.g., using only PowerPoints to relay information to students) in their teaching to a more active approach using technology. Still, the literature is clear on how challenging it can be to transition faculty from using this passive method of teaching to a more engaging one, and there are several factors to consider when implementing such a strategy in the medical classroom. For one, we must acknowledge that faculty may not be comfortable or familiar with technology, that they may, in fact, according to Youm & Corral (2019), lack pedagogical and more specifically technological knowledge. This is especially important when we consider that there is a consistent need/demand for faculty to be more familiar with technology integration on account of the rise of digital natives in the classroom. In addition to this, we must also consider well-supported pedagogical principles like addressing cognitive load when designing and delivering instruction in an online or blended setting. Bridging these challenges can be especially daunting for medical faculty, considering the sheer amount of information that they must disseminate to their own students. The multidisciplinary approach we developed intentionally is set to inspire prolonged adoption of instructional technology grounded in learning theory by faculty. In giving faculty the opportunity to learn more about the instructional design and integration process through several tiers of support, faculty can use their expertise (CK) to help begin and continue the integration process while meeting the increasing needs for teaching with technology and creating more engaging and effective learning experiences for their students. What faculty lack in (PK) and (TK), they can obtain by working in partnership with faculty development and instructional design personnel and student co-curriculum constructors. Of course, the benefits of such a multidisciplinary instructional integration approach are many, including: (a) supplementing traditional teaching, (b) enhancing student motivation and engagement, and (c) promoting higher thinking (Chen, 2019; Eady, 2013).

However, our end goal was never simply to integrate technology successfully in the classroom as a one-off but rather to continue to help faculty move towards transitioning into being able to employ more active and engaging methods of teaching through the use of technology into the foreseeable future and to continue to help them develop the pedagogical and technology skills necessary to do so.

Exemplar Learning Experiences

By using the multidisciplinary team approach, undergraduate medical education faculty have the opportunity to leverage the pedagogical and technological expertise of HWCOM's faculty development and instructional design personnel. Initial meetings consist of determining the scope of the project, such as whether the topic has been covered in previous years through traditional teaching methods or if it is an entirely new session. Other elements of discussion include identifying the desired student learning outcomes and allowing the faculty member to fully articulate their vision for the proposed instructional session. These conversations that integrate the ADDIE model help to facilitate the multidisciplinary team's ability to offer the faculty a variety of suggestions of evidence-based strategies and complementary instructional technology tools that would best align with what faculty are ultimately trying to achieve.

Examples of learning experiences that were developed by using ADDIE include:

- Self-paced modules
- Online, synchronous modules to facilitate collaborative learning
- Gamification activities
- Instructor-led training

Self-Paced Modules

Self-paced modules typically allow for learners to explore content at their own pace in a scaffolded manner. The learner may be provided with flexibility in terms of where and when they engage with the material. These modules can be utilized to flip the classroom, facilitating more time for in-class engagement between the faculty and students.

Self-paced modules were created by fourth-year medical students in the teaching skills elective course, whereby they partnered with faculty advisors, who are content experts, to develop the materials for the modules. Students were trained and coached by the elective course director on the principles of teaching and learning as well as assisted in navigating the collaborative relationship between the members of the multidisciplinary team. The students consulted with the multidisciplinary team's instructional designer for the visual design principles and usage of the educational technology. All key stakeholders were engaged in the review of module content and its development and implementation.

Examples that were developed through this initiative include: (a) an interventional radiology module to promote awareness of the specialty among first and second year medical students, (b) a nutrition module that assisted in educating medical students on proper nutrition counseling and resources available to provide future patients with proper nutrition education, (c) an eye disease module for medical students in the clinical skills course intended to prepare them to identify common presentations of eye disease in a primary care setting and, (d) a research module to support the learning of students interested in medical education research. The research module provided information regarding annotated bibliographies and included videos and self-assessments, as well as interactive activities that tested the students' ability to analyze the components of a journal article.

Online, Synchronous Modules to Facilitate Collaborative Learning

Online, synchronous modules were developed to facilitate collaborative learning in the absence of a physical space. Two examples of interactive modules designed in the authoring tool Articulate Rise, which were developed for small group learning, include: (a) a series of problem-based learning cases and (b) a dermatology case. For the problem-based learning cases, modules were developed to integrate Google documents as an alternative white board that could update live as the case unfolded in small group breakout rooms. The Google documents allowed for students in their respective groups to collaborate on various aspects of the case and facilitated in eliminating the need for faculty and students to toggle between multiple screens. For the dermatology case, a group of medical students interested in dermatology developed content with their faculty advisor for a clinical skills remote session on identifying racial and ethnic variations in the clinical presentation of common skin conditions. The module was delivered to an entire cohort of second year medical students as a primer to the patient encounter that would take place in small groups.

Gamification Activities

Through the teaching elective offered to fourth year medical students interested in gaining experience in teaching and curriculum design, one student collaborated with the Internal Medicine Co-Clerkship Director, the elective course director, and one of the instructional designers (from the multidisciplinary team) to design the framework for a virtual escape room on patient safety issues. The Internal Medicine Co-Clerkship Director was consulted for their expertise on patient safety, while the instructional designer was engaged on developing a 360 virtual image of a room with activities that medical students interacted with to earn clues to escape the room. The teaching skills elective course director partnered with the faculty member to assist in the development of learning objectives and assessments that were implemented to measure the impact of the learning experience. The delivery of the activity is ongoing and early results from three of the six instructional sessions have demonstrated improvement in patient safety knowledge.

An additional example of a gamified learning experience led by a fourth-year teaching elective student was a pharmacology "Jeopardy" styled game. The faculty member, faculty developer and elective student worked collaboratively to identify the appropriate category titles and corresponding content. An instructional designer was engaged to recreate the gamification components of the "Jeopardy" styled game show while ensuring that no copyright laws were infringed upon. The elective student worked with the faculty member and course director to create the rules for the game and the logistics of the event for 120 students in an auditorium setting.

Instructor-Led Training

The medical students in the college's advanced medicine pipeline program for future medical educators work alongside faculty to assist in enhancing the visual design of PowerPoint presentations. Students are involved in the co-construction of the presentations and model good design principles when working with faculty on the refinement and development of PowerPoint presentations. Additionally, the Director of Teaching and Learning (the college's faculty developer) engaged one of the college's instructional designers to deliver a workshop to these medical students that targeted how to approach powerful presentation design and good design principles. The central focus for this initiative is the early intervention of pedagogical training for future medical educators while modeling the benefits of a multidisciplinary team approach.

APPROACH FOR SELECTION AND IMPLEMENTATION OF INSTRUCTIONAL TECHNOLOGY TOOLS

When considering the integration of instructional technology, it is critical to clearly identify the instructional goal and desired student learning outcomes prior to selecting a tool. As part of our multidisciplinary team approach, the instructional design personnel provided guidance and expertise on the educational technology tools that are best aligned with the purpose of the instruction. When engaging the team, the faculty developer and instructional designer ask clarifying questions that determine the goal, learning environment, timing and assessment needs of the instruction. These components are necessary as any one element can affect the selection of the tools. For example, having a couple of weeks versus several months for development can make the difference between using an application that is free, low-cost and with a low-skill entry (e.g., Google documents) versus using an advanced, customizable authoring tool (e.g., Articulate Storyline) that requires specialized training and knowledge.

Once it is clear what the parameters of the intended instruction are, our multidisciplinary team showcased solutions or prior examples of interventions that met a similar need. This aided in faculty understanding the capacity of the educational technology, its ease of use and helped them visualize its implementation in the classroom. When proposing an instructional technology tool, the instructional designer helped faculty members understand its limitations. For example, Articulate Rise is a web-based authoring tool that has the capacity to embed quizzes that report a grade to a learning management system (e.g., Canvas). However, the quiz settings that are built-in cannot be customized to meet every learning need. Sometimes, a previous intervention can be replicated to meet the same need, but depending on the goal, other solutions may require further investigation. For example, another faculty member desiring to implement an escape room activity; however, what was previously created was designed for a virtual setting, while the faculty member needs to implement it in person, requiring a different approach to implementation. Our multidisciplinary team approach involves consulting one another, colleagues and/or searching the learning and development community (e.g., eLearning Heroes, Canvas Community, ATD, etc.) for potential options. Following this exploration, our team proposes three options, the selection of which depends upon how much time and resources the key stakeholders (i.e., faculty member, medical student or other content creator) may have to provide feedback and develop content: (a) a low-level option that may satisfy critical needs for the instruction; (b) a mid-level option that may satisfy some, but not all needs, but provides some customization, which requires a little more time; and (c) a high-level, completely customizable option that will require significant more time investment from all stakeholders.

The next phase of this process involves the rapid prototyping of the potential solution. For example, the instructional designer may use PowerPoint or Word to create a storyboard, which gives a sense for the flow of the information and possible visual and interactive elements. Regardless of the format of the draft, its evaluation requires timely and specific feedback from the subject matter experts to begin or continue development. This iterative process also requires testing of the functionality, ease of use and flow, preferably from the key stakeholders as well as colleagues that would be experiencing it for the first time. This can aid in identifying any functional, aesthetic or content issues and help in creating a better learning experience. Then, our multidisciplinary team coaches and guide the faculty in the implementation of the intervention, including testing of the technology in a simulated learning environment (e.g., testing integration with the setting of the intended space for delivery) as well as offering further technology support as part of the instructional session.

Throughout this process, it is the goal of our multidisciplinary team to address any barriers to the implementation of new pedagogical and technological approaches to designing instruction. By demonstrating the possibilities of instructional technology, providing the support necessary to effectively implement them, and creating a collaborative approach that respects the autonomy of the faculty, the authors aim to build the capacity of medical faculty to leverage instructional technology in the future.

CHALLENGES AND RECOMMENDATIONS FOR IMPROVING PRACTICE

The challenges in developing diverse digital learning experiences involve three main areas: (1) finance, (2) continuity and (3) time. Licenses for authoring tools and educational technology can be cost-prohibitive and unexpected. For example, Articulate Storyline and Rise were used to develop self-paced learning modules that supplemented the curriculum. Articulate licenses cost from $700 to $3,000 per user, per year, while stock image subscriptions can average $1,000 per year. Proactively budgeting for these tools can assist departments in ensuring that they can support the development of online instruction effectively. Alternatively, one can consult with instructional design and faculty development personnel to explore free and low-cost options and leverage departmental or unit resources. The instructional designers often have subscriptions to various educational technology tools, and the college's IT department can vet and source the purchase of new tools. Continuity can be challenged when a key stakeholder leaves the organization, such as a faculty or staff member or even when a student graduates and the implementation of the module remains in the development phase. Detailed project documentation and open lines of communication and cohesion among support personnel may serve to minimize interruptions. Lastly, the design of learning experiences requires time to develop and should be refined with sufficient feedback to make changes that improve future outcomes. A clear understanding of timelines is necessary to manage expectations and create a learning experience that meets the needs of all users.

FUTURE RESEARCH DIRECTIONS

With the professionalization of medical education and the practice of teaching, future research is needed on the impact of a reverse faculty development approach that utilizes undergraduate medical education students as agents of change. Longitudinal studies are necessary to measure the success of such an initiative and whether there is also an impact on the future generation of medical educators. While the authors of this chapter would want to measure the influence of the initiative immediately, students engaged in the program must first complete their residency and potentially fellowship programs, which would therefore delay their entrance into academia.

An additional area for future research is whether faculty are more confident in designing, developing, and implementing diverse learning experiences that incorporate the evidence-based practices that have been modeled through the multidisciplinary team approach. With the trend of neuroscience, cognitive and behavioral psychology informing educators on the way students learn, more research is needed on whether medical faculty are implementing the principles grounded in those fields into their everyday teaching or if they continue to primarily rely on traditional teaching methods that do not place the student and their learning at the center.

CONCLUSION

The COVID-19 pandemic has disrupted medical education in such a way that it has forced medical educators to innovate their pedagogical and technological practices in light of the shift to remote instruction. At HWCOM, a multidisciplinary team approach was developed to bridge the gaps in pedagogical and technological practices by engaging in a collaboration among key stakeholders to design digital learning experiences that were grounded in instructional theory. The faculty development and instructional design personnel partnered with medical students as co-curriculum constructors and faculty as subject matter experts. By modeling evidence-based teaching and learning practices, our multidisciplinary team built the faculty and students' capacity to impact the existing curriculum and, we hope, the future of medical education. The approach outlined in this chapter also leveraged instructional technology to meet the needs of a medical curriculum that transitioned to online formats during the COVID-19 pandemic. The multidisciplinary team assisted faculty in the selection, use and implementation of educational technology tools that were aligned with the faculty member's vision for the instruction. Taking this multidisciplinary approach to the next level involves incorporating instructional design personnel into other faculty development programming available, such as teaching squares, creating an opportunity to follow through with educational ideas that come out of this type of programming.

Lastly, there is an opportunity to develop a center for innovation focused on medical education at individualized institutions that serves as a platform to bring together faculty members, support personnel and future medical educators for the experimentation of new ideas, including the development of workshops to learn new skills, hack-a-thons to deep dive into solving a specific problem with educational technology, presentations, a book club to engage in meaningful discussions, poster presentations and gaming simulations to explore innovative technologies, and the development of a micro-credential to encourage the use of best practices in teaching and learning.

This research received no specific grant from any funding agency in the public, commercial, or not-for-profit sectors.

REFERENCES

Ahmed, O. M., Juthani, P. V., Green, M. L., & Moeller, J. J. (2021). Optimizing preclinical learning with retrieval practice: A call to action. *Medical Teacher*, *43*(6), 718–720. doi:10.1080/0142159X.2020.1788212 PMID:32643504

Alpert, C., Sinha, S., & Cullen, M. (2019). Teaching tomorrow's teachers: An innovative model of clinician-educator development for fellows-in-training. *Journal of the American College of Cardiology*, *73*, 22.

Aungst, T. D., & Patel, R. (2020). Integrating Digital Health into the Curriculum-Considerations on the Current Landscape and Future Developments. *Journal of Medical Education and Curricular Development*, *7*. doi:10.1177/2382120519901275 PMID:32010795

Bauzon, J., Alver, A., Ravikumar, V., Devera, A., Mikhael, T., Nauman, R., & Simanton, E. (2021). The Impact of Educational Resources and Perceived Preparedness on Medical Education Performance. *Medical Science Educator*, *31*(4), 1–8. doi:10.100740670-021-01306-x PMID:34457974

Bing You, R. G., & Sproul, M. S. (1992). Medical students' perceptions of themselves and residents as teachers. *Medical Teacher*, *14*(2-3), 133–138. doi:10.3109/01421599209079479 PMID:1406122

Bloom, B. (1956). Taxonomy of Educational Objectives: The Classification of Educational Goals. Handbook 1 Cognitive Domain.

Chen, H. J., Liao, L. L., Chang, Y. C., Hung, C. C., & Chang, L. C. (2019). Factors influencing technology integration in the curriculum for Taiwanese health profession educators: A mixed-methods study. *International Journal of Environmental Research and Public Health*, *16*(14), 2602. doi:10.3390/ijerph16142602 PMID:31336610

Dandavino, M., Snell, L., & Wiseman, J. (2007). Why medical students should learn how to teach. *Medical Teacher*, *29*(6), 558–565. doi:10.1080/01421590701477449 PMID:17922358

Dick, W., Carey, L., & Carey, J. O. (2015). *The systematic design of instruction*. Pearson.

Eady, M., & Lockyer, L. (2013). Tools for learning: Technology and teaching. *Learning to Teach in the Primary School, 71*.

Fong, S. F., Sakai, D. H., Kasuya, R. T., Kramer, K., Wong, V. S., Haning, W., Asano, I., Uyehara-Lock, J. H., Thompson, K., Omori, J. S., Hirose-Wong, S. M., & Horio, D. T. (2016). Medical School Hotline: Liaison Committee on Medical Education Accreditation, Part IV: Pre-clerkship Education. *Hawai'i Journal of Medicine & Public Health: a Journal of Asia Pacific Medicine & Public Health*, *75*(2), 48–51. PMID:26918209

Gagné, R. M., Biggs, L. J., & Wager, W. W. (1992). *Principles of instructional design* (4th ed.). Harcourt Brace Jovanovich, Publishers.

Ginzburg, S. (2018). Curriculum Inventory in Context: Use of Self-Directed Learning in U.S. and Canadian Medical Schools. *AAMC, 5*(5).

Graff, C. J., Kaljo, K., Treat, R. W., & Dielentheis, K. (2021). The Adaptive Learner: How Faculty and Medical Students' Perceptions of Learning Needs and Desires Differ. *WMJ: Official Publication of the State Medical Society of Wisconsin*, *120*(1), 8–16. PMID:33974759

Guze, P. A. (2015). Using Technology to Meet the Challenges of Medical Education. *Transactions of the American Clinical and Climatological Association*, *126*, 260–270. PMID:26330687

Haber, R. J., Bardach, N. S., Vedanthan, R., Gillum, L. A., Haber, L. A., & Dhaliwal, G. (2006). Preparing fourth-year medical students to teach during internship. *Journal of General Internal Medicine, 21*(5), 518–520. doi:10.1111/j.1525-1497.2006.00441.x PMID:16704402

Hirumi, A. (2021). IAMSE 2021—Plenary Session: Top 10 Ways an Instructional Designer Can Help You Define the New Normal. *Medical Science Educator, 31*(S1), 1–8. doi:10.100740670-021-01400-0 PMID:34567833

Hughes, J. (n.d.). *Communicating with Generation Z: Everything You Need to Know*. Keystone Academic. https://www.keystoneacademic.com/news/communicating-with-generation-z-everything-you-need-to-know

Irby, D. M., Cooke, M., & O'Brien, B. C. (2010). Calls for reform of medical education by the Carnegie Foundation for the Advancement of Teaching: 1910 and 2010. *Academic Medicine, 85*(2), 220–227. doi:10.1097/ACM.0b013e3181c88449 PMID:20107346

Kirkpatrick, J. D., & Kirkpatrick, W. K. (2016). *Kirkpatrick's four levels of training evaluation*. Association for Talent Development.

Knowles, M. S., Holton, E. F., & Swanson, R. A. (1998). *The Adult Learner: the Definitive Classic in Adult Education and Human Resource Development*. Gulf Publishing Company.

Koehler, M. J., & Mishra, P. (2009). What is technological pedagogical content knowledge? *Contemporary Issues in Technology & Teacher Education, 9*, 60–70.

Leh, A. S. (2005). Lessons learned from service learning and reverse mentoring in faculty development: A case study in technology training. *Journal of Technology and Teacher Education, 13*(1), 25–41.

Lewis, P. J. (2016). Brain Friendly teaching – Reducing Learners' Cognitive Load. *Academic Radiology, 23*(7), 877-880.

Mayer, R. E. (2008). Applying the science of learning: Evidence-based principles for the design of multimedia instruction. *The American Psychologist, 63*(8), 760–769. doi:10.1037/0003-066X.63.8.760 PMID:19014238

Mayer, R. E., & Chandler, P. (2001). When learning is just a click away: Does simple user interaction foster deeper understanding of multimedia messages? *Journal of Educational Psychology, 93*(2), 390–397. doi:10.1037/0022-0663.93.2.390

McMillan, C., Loads, D., & McQueen, H. A. (2018). From students to scientists: The impact of interactive engagement in lectures. *New Directions in the Teaching of Physical Sciences*, (13).

Molenda, M. (2003). In search of the elusive ADDIE model. *Performance Improvement, 42*(5), 34–37. doi:10.1002/pfi.4930420508

Oyedotun, T. D. (2020). Sudden change of pedagogy in education driven by COVID-19: Perspectives and evaluation from a developing country. *Research in Globalization, 2*(100029), 100029. Advance online publication. doi:10.1016/j.resglo.2020.100029

Pan, Scott, & Phillips. (2021). Using Learning Experience Design to Optimize Digital Instruction During COVID-19 and Beyond. *Academic Medicine, 96*(5). doi:10.1097/ACM.0000000000003889

Persky, A. M., & Robinson, J. D. (2017). Moving from novice to expertise and its implications for instruction. *American Journal of Pharmaceutical Education, 81*(9), 6065. doi:10.5688/ajpe6065 PMID:29302087

Prober, C. G., & Norden, J. G. (2021). Learning Alone or Learning Together: Is It Time to Reevaluate Teacher and Learner Responsibilities? *Academic Medicine*, *96*(2), 170–172. doi:10.1097/ACM.0000000000003741 PMID:32910002

Rose, E. (2004). Instructional Design and Curriculum Development: Deconstructing the Difference. *Educational Technology*, *44*(2), 3–12. https://www.jstor.org/stable/44428883

Schartzstein, R., & Roberts, D. (2017). Saying Goodbye to Lectures in Medical School – Paradigm Shift or Passing Fad? *The New England Journal of Medicine*, *377*(7), 605–607. doi:10.1056/NEJMp1706474 PMID:28813217

Servey, J. T., Hartzell, J. D., & McFate, T. (2020). A faculty development model for academic leadership education across a health care organization. *Journal of Medical Education and Curricular Development*, *7*. Advance online publication. doi:10.1177/2382120520948878 PMID:32851193

Sheehy, R. (2019). This is Not Your Grandfather's Medical School: Novel Tools to Enhance Medical Education. *Missouri Medicine*, *116*(5), 371–375. PMID:31645786

Simpson, D., Marcdante, K., Souza, K. H., Anderson, A., & Holmboe, E. (2018). Job Roles of the 2025 Medical Educator. *Journal of Graduate Medical Education*, *10*(3), 243–246. doi:10.4300/JGME-D-18-00253.1 PMID:29946376

Youm, J., & Corral, J. (2019). Technological Pedagogical Content Knowledge Among Medical Educators: What Is Our Readiness to Teach With Technology? *Academic Medicine*, *94*(11S), S69–S72. doi:10.1097/ACM.0000000000002912 PMID:31365390

Zakrajsek, T. (2018). Reframing the lecture versus active learning debate: Suggestions for a new way forward. *Educ Health Prof*, *1*(1), 1–3. doi:10.4103/EHP.EHP_14_18

ADDITIONAL READING

Kalynych, C., Edwards, L., West, D., Snodgrass, C., & Zenni, E. (2021). Tuesdays Are Great for Teaching Tips: A Spaced Education Strategy for Faculty Development. *Journal of Graduate Medical Education*, *13*(3), 434–435. doi:10.4300/JGME-D-20-01249.1 PMID:34178279

Parmelee, D., Roman, B., Overman, I., & Alizadeh, M. (2020). The lecture-free curriculum: setting the stage for life-long learning: AMEE Guide No. 135. *Medical Teacher*, *42*(9), 962–969. doi:10.1080/0142159X.2020.1789083 PMID:32644866

Reis, S. (2018). Curriculum reform: Why? What? How? and how will we know it works? *Israel Journal of Health Policy Research*, *7*(1), 1–4. doi:10.118613584-018-0221-4 PMID:29880061

Sağin, F. G. (2020). How to use educational technology to make education better-Not just different or entertaining! *Biologia Serbica, 41*(2).

Sewell, J. L., Bowen, J. L., Cate, O. T., O'Sullivan, P. S., Shah, B., & Boscardin, C. K. (2020). Learning challenges, teaching strategies, and cognitive load: Insights from the experience of seasoned endoscopy teachers. *Academic Medicine, 95*(5), 794–802. doi:10.1097/ACM.0000000000002946 PMID:31425188

Skochelak, S. E., & Stack, S. J. (2017). Creating the medical schools of the future. *Academic Medicine, 92*(1), 16–19. doi:10.1097/ACM.0000000000001160 PMID:27008357

Song, H. S., Pusic, M., Nick, M. W., Sarpel, U., Plass, J. L., & Kalet, A. L. (2014). The cognitive impact of interactive design features for learning complex materials in medical education. *Computers & Education, 71*, 198–205. doi:10.1016/j.compedu.2013.09.017 PMID:27274609

Ward, R. A., Ting, A. S. J., & Peyton, E. M. (2020). A medical student's perspective on' students as catalysts for curricular innovation: A change management framework'. *Medical Teacher, 42*(12), 1427–1428. doi:10.1080/0142159X.2020.1739256 PMID:32174223

KEY TERMS AND DEFINITIONS

Educational Technology: Any program, application or the use of any program or application in the design and delivery of learning experiences.

Faculty Developer: A dedicated instructional support personnel that directs and supports college-wide educational effectiveness through the development and training of faculty, including delivering workshops, onboarding, faculty observations and evaluations, support for small group teaching, instructor assessments, and student teacher development.

Instructional Designer: A dedicated instructional support personnel that develops and designs resources and workshops, contributes to curriculum enhancement projects, and provides leadership and guidance on the effective use of technology to support learning.

Instructional Systems Development: A systemic approach to instructional design that involves the analysis design, development, implementation, and evaluation of instruction.

Multidisciplinary Team Approach: A collaborative team comprising of instructional support personnel who work closely with faculty to facilitate changes in their instructional practice.

Reverse Faculty Development: The use of specially trained medical students to model evidenced-based teaching and learning strategies to faculty, similar to a train the trainer approach.

Self-Directed Learning: The ability to direct one's own learning without the guidance of an instructor.

Undergraduate Medical Education: A four-year medical education leading up to residency.

Chapter 12
Telehealth Use in Interdisciplinary Health Professions Student Groups to Support Improved Outcomes

LuAnn Etcher
Sacred Heart University, USA

Donna Faye McHaney
Sacred Heart University, USA

ABSTRACT

The intervention is presented within an academic setting. Clinical site shortages for all health professions students has been compounded by the recent pandemic, with a logical desire to leverage and expand the use of telehealth in this regard. The overarching purpose was to provide clinical encounters for a blend of interdisciplinary health professions students via telehealth care, while improving healthcare access and outcomes in underserved populations. A systematic instructional design approach was utilized. The approach included a needs analysis for gathering background information, followed by the design phase will commence where the project model can be initially designed and reviewed prior to launch. In the development phase, the project is finalized, implemented, and then evaluated for necessary changes to improve outcomes and foster sustainability. A discussion of challenges and recommendations for improved practice is included.

INTRODUCTION

The advent of the COVID-19 pandemic has created significant waves of disruption within university educational delivery, including undergraduate and graduate level health professions programs since it began, with issues occurring on many levels (Diaz, et al., 2021; Hoofman, et al., 2019). In graduate level health professions programs, meeting programmatic requirements (such as testing and monitoring

DOI: 10.4018/978-1-7998-9490-2.ch012

of student symptom status) during the initial early days of the outbreak was followed by the issue of assuring current COVID-19 initial 'jab' and booster vaccination status (Drenkard, et al., 2022). Among the most problematic of issues was that many graduate level health professions students were left wanting in terms of clinical placements due to scarcity of preceptors and organizational hesitancy to take on students during the pandemic.

All graduate level health professions programs require that a student spend a specified number of hours in the clinical setting, where they learn from experiences in working alongside licensed health care providers in their field of practice or specialty. While the number and type of clinical hours required for graduation varies by program specialty, in the United States each graduate level health professions student must meet their program specifications in terms of number of clinical hours (as well as any other programmatic requirements) in order to successfully complete their health professions program. In the United States, students must show proof of successful program completion through official academic program transcripts in order to qualify to take the national professional board examination for their specialty, which they must then pass in order to begin the process of becoming licensed in their home state of residence.

Securing clinical placements for graduate level health professions students has become increasingly competitive over time. The paucity of preceptors and clinical sites is due to multiple factors such as the expanding volume of graduate level health professions programs, increasing numbers of students desiring to enter the health professions, retirement of many providers from the Baby Boomer' generation, and reduced willingness of seasoned providers to precept students. Many preceptors today are also requiring students pay the preceptor for each preceptorship they engage in.

While most graduate level health professions programs place the primary burden to locate preceptors and clinical placement locales on their students, if the students are unable to secure a preceptor and site then the responsibility falls on program faculty to support students in their search. The lack of available clinical placements and the requirement that faculty step up and support students in securing clinical sites and preceptors when students fail to do so has added significantly to the already full workload of faculty in graduate level health professions programs. On top of the issues that had naturally resulted in increasing competitiveness for preceptors and clinical sites (e.g., retiring preceptors, increasing numbers of graduate level health professions programs and therefore students) is the fact that the pandemic caused many health care organizations and hospital systems to place moratoriums or severe limits on student access to their facilities for the purpose of academic clinical site placement.

In response to the clinical placement constraints imposed by the pandemic, creative solutions were sought which could potentially help to fill the gap and support students to successfully complete both didactic (Hao, et al., 2021) and clinical course hour programmatic requirements (Triemstra, et al., 2021). The issue of how to deal with loss of the standard classroom and clinical environments impacted students from university educational programs across many health professions domains, including dental programs, nursing programs (Huang, 2021), pharmacy programs (Etando, et al., 2021), physical therapy programs (Ng, et al., 2021), as well as physician and other medical school based specialty programs (Martinelli, et al., 2021; Song, et al., 2021); Su et al., 2021; Al-Balas, et al., 2020). This problem of being able to secure clinical site placements and preceptors for the purposes of fulfilling academic health professions program requirements has not been limited to the United States. The peer-reviewed literature contains papers describing the issues encountered in securing clinical placements due to the COVID-19 pandemic by health professions students and faculty in many nations across the globe, including Africa

(Etando, et al., 2021), China (Su, et al. 2021), Europe, (Hempel, et al., 2021), Jordan (Al-Balas, et al., 2020), among others.

The use of telehealth has already been identified as an acceptable way for students in many graduate level health professions programs to meet a small portion of the clinical hours they are required to complete. One opportunity that may hold potential promise as a way for students to complete clinical hours and to work alongside other graduate level health professions students is through leveraging of telehealth using one site for a group of students. The potential to combine students from across health care professional domains within a single setting where a cadre of providers works using telehealth to see patients is attractive on multiple levels which will be expounded upon later in this chapter.

The driving motives for developing the project include both the need for student clinical sites and to find a way to meet needs to provide quality care in underserved populations due to COVID-19. The overarching purpose is to provide clinical preceptors and sites for a blend of interdisciplinary graduate level health professions students via telehealth care, while improving health care access and outcomes in underserved populations using a program developed to be decidedly feasible and acceptable to all involved.

In this chapter, the content will address the following objectives:

- Introduce and discuss remotely delivered health care, what it consists of and its potential as a clinical learning source for graduate level health professions program students.
- Explicate the systematic instructional design process in developing out the proposed project.
- Define and describe the theoretic underpinnings that inform the program design and approach.
- Describe the interdisciplinary graduate level health professions student telehealth program.
- Discuss program evaluation methods.
- Discuss program challenges and recommendations for next steps.

BACKGROUND

Clinical site shortages for all graduate level health professions students have been compounded by the recent COVID-19 pandemic, with a logical desire to leverage and expand the use of telehealth in this regard. The proposed intervention is based on identified needs within academic graduate level health professions programs, and in light of considerations imposed by the recent COVID-19 pandemic.

While hospitals were overflowing with patients suffering the catastrophic effects of COVID-19, the ability of patients to see their health care providers face to face in the office was reduced to emergencies only, or was halted altogether (Atchley, et al., 2021). Within the outpatient healthcare system, the transition to using remote and virtual alternatives for health care encounters began escalating over time and remained high even with the ebbs and flows of the COVID-19 pandemic. With the change in health care delivery to remote and virtual means, patients who normally filled provider offices suddenly found themselves outside the purview of the healthcare system. An example is that of older adults with knowledge deficits and challenges around technology, who suffered physical and psychological impacts during the pandemic through reduced activity levels, increased isolation, and loss of social connections, and lapses in routine medical care (Kroll, et al., 2021).

Because of the laborious processes required to ensure universal precautions and personal protection from infection, effort was put into defining best practices for managing outpatient visits in terms of reducing wait times while improving outcomes, satisfaction, quality, and continuity of care even with the constraints imposed by pandemic precautions (Atchley, et, al., 2021). With this increased focus on patient flow, the ability for health care settings and providers to accommodate taking on students for clinical rotations waned.

Academe is a traditionally slow-moving system. Faculty overseeing graduate level health professions programs and their students were blind-sided when clinical sites and preceptors began routinely turning down requests for placement during the COVID-19 pandemic.

THEORETICAL UNDERPINNINGS

Deciding on a theoretical framework for an intervention is vitally important because it sets the tone for the work. Selecting an appropriate theoretical framework can support and serve to brace up the work as a whole and provide consistency across the project as it is threaded through. Most importantly, a well-fitting theoretical framework can purposefully inform the development of an intervention as well as how the work will subsequently be approached, conducted, and then finally evaluated. Several theories were selected and are discussed in terms of suitability to serve in supporting and informing the project work in terms of design and approach in the following sections of this chapter.

The Quality-Caring Model (QCM)

To begin, the Quality-Caring Model (QCM) by Duffy (2003) is an appropriate selection to frame the locus and serve as a theoretical compass for the project. The findings from a study by Salinas et al. (2020) demonstrated that employing the elements of the QCM resulted in participant reports of "feeling cared for". The authors state that such feelings have potential to be generated as a result of 'multiple caring behaviors enacted simultaneously by clinicians" (Salinas et al, 2020). In an additional study employing the QCM, narrative findings from key stake holders enrolled in the study demonstrated positive themes around care quality (Haex, et al., 2021). Given the above, threading use of the QCM approach through the project is anticipated to support students from varying disciplines who are engaged in the project to learn through the collaborative caring delivery of services while improving access to care and quality outcomes for the patients being seen for visits during the project time period.

The Community of Inquiry Framework (CoI)

Next the Community of Inquiry Framework, or CoI, developed by Garrison and colleagues (2001), is selected to serve as the theoretical framework for the teaching-learning "classroom". The CoI was selected for its potential in supporting students to engage in Purposeful Interpersonal Interaction, or PII. Purposeful Interpersonal Interaction (PII) is high quality interpersonal interaction that occurs in the classroom, and which has been demonstrated in the literature to lead to better student outcomes (Mehall, 2021). In addition, Purposeful Interpersonal Interaction has been found to have potential to enhance meaningful collaboration among the student disciplines as well with the patients being seen during care encounters (Mehall, 2021).

Trauma Informed Approach to Education (TIE)

Because pandemic-related trauma has been known to flow into the classroom from outside sources (Black, 2022) and has been shown to impede student learning and progress (Black, 2022), a trauma informed approach to education (TIE) will be employed by program faculty (Goddard, et al., in review; Hess, et al., 2022). Adopting a trauma-informed educational approach is a way in which faculty can act proactively (Goddard, et al., in review) in considering and addressing in their students the trauma encountered universally across the global population during the COVID-19 pandemic (Shah, et al., 2020). Using a trauma informed approach to education can support the construction of a milieu conducive to student learning and has demonstrated such during the pandemic in both clinical (Goddard, et al., in review) and non-clinical classroom settings (Hess, et al., 2022).

USING A SYSTEMATIC INSTRUCTIONAL DESIGN APPROACH

The systematic instructional design approach utilized in this project consists of three phases. Phase One consists of planning for the work in terms of assessment and innovation. Phase Two consists of undertaking the work in terms of design development and implementation. Phase Three consists of evaluation.

Phase One - Assessment

The needs analysis for the project takes place in the first phase, and should consist of assessing needs of the students, faculty involved, and the graduate level health professions program requirements that need to be met through the course where the project is being launched. A variety of methods can be used to carry out the needs assessment. A common method is to use a Strengths – Weaknesses – Opportunities – Threats, or SWOT analysis (Morrison, 2016). The SWOT analysis process was developed at Stanford University in the decade of the 1970s and has been widely used over time as a way to easily assess the four areas important in identifying needs versus assets (Morrison, 2016). SWOT stands for strengths, weaknesses, opportunities, and threats to the project. Project lead faculty and instructional designers can use a SWOT analysis to collect data on the strengths, weaknesses, opportunities, and threats for specified areas, then come back together to discuss the findings. There are many types of needs assessments that can be selected for use in assessing the strengths, weaknesses, opportunities, and threats to the project, so select and utilize an assessment that works for the program and situation (Sava, 2012). Once the needs assessment is completed, and the project design and development can commence.

Phase One - Innovation During Design and Development

During the first phase of design and development, innovative ideas on design and development should align with the project goals and the objectives and be fitting in terms of feasibility and acceptability for the students, faculty, patients served during the clinical practicum. Threading theories through the project such as the QCM and CoI will provide support and PII in both the didactic and clinical course. Supporting students though the collaborative caring delivery of services and PII enhances meaningful collaboration among students and patients as well. The project should have provisions for the inclusion of both didactic and clinical course content to be housed within the learning management system utilized by the institution. This will provide for a central location which is familiar to students and faculty where course materials can be housed and accessed over the semester.

Phase One – Resource Planning

As Phase One should include resource planning and should take place after your needs assessment. Gathering background information which can inform the developer regarding the resources at hand for use, as well as any resource gaps that could send the project going awry should be included. Examples of the types of information that the project leaders should gather should include: information on the types of graduate academic programs to be involved, academic level of students to be included (e.g., first year, second year, and so on.), how many academic faculty will be available and working to teach both the clinical course and didactic course sections during the project, the types of software and hardware equipment needed to carry out the project successfully (versus what is available), the types and volume of clinical equipment needed to carry out the project successfully, and the number of instructional design staff assigned to work on the project.

Within Phase One, faculty and instructional designers heading up the project should also plan for identifying faculty education and training needs. Because the faculty are the student guides throughout the project and essential to the success of the project, assuring they are competent in the areas of telehealth care is vital. If there are gaps in competencies, education to meet the needs and bring the faculty up to the level of expectation for the project should be initiated and completed before the course portion of the project begins.

The largest resource that will need to be planned for is the clinical sites for where students will attend clinical through engaging in telehealth care. The innovative part of this project is not the use of telehealth care, it is the collaboration between programs in an interdisciplinary way where students can learn from one another, and facullty have potential to expand their clinical site resources though the project work,

The expansion of clinical sites is important and should be carefully reflected on in order to make sure your programs are maximizing use of each site without overburdening the preceptor or clinical site. The clinical preceptors and clinical sites should be treated in a way that conveys that you understand how precious a resource they are. In examining and evaluating the programs use of clinical preceptors and clinical sites, faculty should:

- Know the rules and regulations:
  - What is the maximum student:preceptor ratio? How many students can attend clinical with a single preecptor on any given day?
  - How many telehealth hours does the certifying body allow a program to count?
  - Do other types of activities count toward the required number of clinical hours (e.g., simulation, professional activities, observation hours, and so on.)?
- If it is allowable to have a preceptor take more than one student per day:
  - Make sure the precpetor and clinical site agree it is feasible and acceptable. If yes, consider sending more than one student to the clinical site with that preceptor each week.
  - First semester clinical students are less experienced and can be more difficult to find clinical placements for. If a preceptor and site can comfortably accept more than one student on a day, consider placing a first semester student (one doing a larger amount of observation) and a more advsanced student together with the one preceptor on the same day. The more

novice student can take advantage of observation of gthe preceptor, while the more advanced student is being overseen by the precpetor in patient visits.
    - If not, consider asking whether a precptor can accept students more than one day per week.
- Does the clinical site conduct telehealth visits?
    - If yes, find out the depth of visits they conduct and whether they use any remote physical examination tools and what they are.
        - Know the rules and regulations on how many and what type of telehealth clinical hours can be counted toward clinical practice hour completion.
        - Know the precpetor to student ratio for telehealth clinical visits.
    - If the clinical site and/or preceptor does not conduct telehealth visits, consider working with the clinical site to offer education to support them to begin conducting telehealth care visits with their patients.

In working on expanding the number of clinical placement site and preceptors you have to work with, consider also:

- Partnering with the other health professions programs in your colloege or university.
- Partnering with local hospitals and health care agencies who might be willing to work with you on developing a project such as the one desctibed in this chapter in order to be a part of any publications that might come of the work.
- Give back to the preceptors and clinical sites thst you work with:
    - It should go without saying that sending a Letter of Verification on the hours each preceptor spent precepting for the semester should always be provided for preceptors.
    - If your college ot university has capacity to provide free continuing education course offerings, that is a very nice way to say thank you.
    - Consider whether library access can be offered to your precptors.
    - Consider whether adjunct status can be offered to your preceptors.

Phase Two – Project Design, Development, and Implementation

The project should align in terms of course and content with the usual course offering for all student disciplines. It is assumed that all graduate level health programs would be on the same academic calendar. If not, that would require consideration before moving forward.

The course faculty would manage developing the course content and the instructional design staff would be responsible to manage and facilitate set up of the learning management system. The project can be designed to take several forms. Table 1 contains several versions for consideration when setting up the project. In reviewing the content in Table 1, it is observed all students across disciplines are able to take part in clinical case conferences together on Monday mornings between 8 A.M. to 12 P.M., where patients and/or their family members engage with each specialty during the meeting at this hypothetical clinical site. The nature of the clinical site lends itself to such collaborative experiences among the three disciplines. A similar type of care conferencing may also be conducted in sub-acute rehab and skilled nursing facilities. These facilities also routinely have nurse practitioners, social workers, and physical therapists on site.

Table 1. Possible design versions for use with the project

Version	Health Professions Programs (Students Assigned to the Project)	Clinical Site / Central Visiting Nurse Association and Hospice	Preceptor Schedule Telehealth (E) Onsite (O) Home Visits (H) Day: M, T, W, Th, F	Student Clinical Assignments Site 1 - 8 Hours / Week Central Visiting Nurse Association and Hospice
Version One	Nursing (2 / 2) Family Nurse Practitioner (2), Adult Gerontology Primary Care Nurse Practitioner (2)	Smith, RN Adams, RN	Smith (E) T, Th (O) M WF Adams (E) T, Th (O) M W F	Family Nurse Practitioner (2) Monday (O) Care Conferences 8 AM – 12 N with Smith 1-5 PM office with Smith Adult Gerontology Primary Care Nurse Practitioner (2) Monday (O) Care Conferences 8 AM – 12 N with Adams 1-5 PM office with Adams
Version Two	Nursing (2 /2) Family Nurse Practitioner (2), Adult Gerontolgy Primary Care Nurse Practitioner (2) Social Work (2)	Smith, RN Adams, RN Jones, SW	Smith (E) T, Th (O) M W F Adams (E) T, Th (O) M W F Jones (E) M, T, Th (O) W F (H) M 1 – 5 PM	Family Nurse Practitioner students - 2 Monday (O) Care Conferences 8 AM – 12 N with Smith; 1-5 PM office with Smith Adult Gerontology Primary Care Nurse Practitioner Students - 2 Monday (O) Care Conferences 8 AM – 12 N with Adams 1-5 PM office with Adams Jones (E) 2 social work students Monday care conferences 8 AM to 12 N (E); SW student #1: M 1-5 PM Jones – home visits; SW student #2: Tuesday 8 AM – 5 PM Jones
Version Three	Nursing (2 / 2) Family Nurse Practitioner (2), Adult Gerontology Primary Care Nurse Practitioner (2) Social Work (2) Physical Therapy (2)	Smith, RN Adams, RN Jones, SW Jackson, PT	Smith (E) T, Th (O) M W F Adams (E) T, Th (O) M W F Jones (E) M, T, Th (O) W F (H) M 1 – 5 PM Jackson (E) M, T, Th (O) W F (H) M 1 – 5 PM	Family Nurse Practitioner students - 2 Monday (O) Care Conferences 8 AM – 12 N with Smith 1-5 PM office with Smith Adult Gerontology Primary Care Nurse Practitioner students - 2 Monday (O) Care Conferences 8 AM – 12 N with Adams 1-5 PM office with Adams Jones (E) 2 social work students SW Student #1: Monday care conferences 8 AM to 12 N (E) SW student #1: M 1-5 PM Jones –home Visits; Jones (E) SW student #2: Tuesday 8 AM – 5 PM Jackson (E) 2 physical therapy students PT Student #1: Monday care conferences 8 AM to 12 N (E) PT student #1: M 1-5 PM Jackson –home visits 1-5 PM; Jackson (E) PT student #2: Tuesday 8AM – 5 PM

Phase Three – Evaluation

The final phase of the process in evaluation. It is anticipated that students who take part in the project will be enrolled in a clinical course with paired didactic elements housed within a learning management system, or LMS. Because the project is designed for pilot during an active course with interdisciplinary student cohorts, it is important to have the ability to make improvements quickly and while the course is in motion.

Therefore, the project will leverage the "Plan – Do – Study – Act", or PDSA model during project implementation (Byrk, et al., 2015). The Plan – Do – Study - Act is a highly utilized means of evaluation where nimble analyses regarding 'what works and what does not work' can be conducted and changes made in real time to address issues and support the success of the project and all involved (Byrk, et al., 2015).

Post-course evaluations should be delivered as usual for the course in order to collect all of the normative metrics that are required by the program and department for end of semester faculty and course evaluation. In addition to the usual course evaluations, the program faculty and course design staff should develop evaluation metrics based on the course content and delivery. This additive program-based evaluation should include information important to assuring the project is feasible and acceptable to all involved. Depending on the level of interface, evaluations designed to query the faculty, instructional designers, students, preceptors, and clinical site staff would all be important. Evaluation data should be reviewed with the course faculty that were involved during the project piloting. In addition, data can be shared with others from the above group of involved individuals, depending on the type and nature of the data. Reporting back to involved key players is important in projects such as this (Wong & Hendrick, 2020).

CHALLENGES, SOLUTIONS, AND RECOMMENDATIONS

Challenges for the project include obtaining buy-in at all levels of the theoretical frameworks (e.g., The Quality-Caring Model, The CoI, and TIE) for program start up, support, and sustainability.

Not touched on in this chapter is the issue of whether such a project would need to go through the organizational Institutional Review Board for approval before it could be launched. Because the work is toward improvements in quality of education, it would seem that many institutions and organizations would not require an institutional board review and approval to commence, but because this is questionable it behooves faculty to check with the institutional review boards at the university and clinical sites to be sure. If the institutional review board review is required, be sure to allow at least 3 to 6 months for the reviews to be completed in successive order depending on the institutions and organizations involved.

FUTURE DIRECTIONS FOR TELEHEALTH RESEARCH AND PRACTICE

More work needs to be accomplished in terms of research as well as in policy initiatives to expand the appropriate use of telehealth. Research aimed at examining the adequacy with which such projects can meet student learning needs, and how the project performs to support faculty in terms of pedagogical objectives and programmatic requirements are needed. In addition, future applications of projects such as this one in which data are collected on program efficacy, feasibility, acceptability are warranted in order to define next steps and future directions in the use of telehealth settings for graduate health professions clinical requirements. Recommendations for practice improvement that stem from carrying out such a project will emerge from the data collected and from comparative review and analysis with existing literature on the topic at hand. Telehealth should be viewed as an accepted modality for clinical experiences across graduate level health professions programs, and the number of hours allowed to be used in programs should continue to be evaluated as the availability of equipment for remote monitoring becomes more widely available for use by students engaging in the clinical setting with their preceptors. New directions for telehealth practice will emerge as organizations begin to acquire higher levels of technology coupled with the education to apply the modalities remotely in patient care. Because the cost of equipment designed for remote assessment is prohibitive, few to date have been able to afford much of the variety of equipment available for use. Until then providers will continue to employ the use of electronic connect applications, virtual connection platforms and phone to provide telehealth care.

CONCLUSION

In this chapter, remotely delivered health care was discussed in terms of what it consists of as well as its potential as a substantive clinical learning environment for graduate level health professions students. The systematic instructional design for such a project was discussed and described including table-based versions which can be modeled in real life settings. The advent of the COVID-19 pandemic has created significant waves of disruption within university educational delivery, including undergraduate and graduate level health professions programs since it began, with issues occurring on many levels (Diaz, et al., 2021; Hoofman, et al., 2019).

All graduate level health professions programs require that a student spend a specified number of hours in the clinical setting, where they learn from experiences in working alongside licensed health care providers in their field of practice or specialty. In response to the clinical placement constraints imposed by the pandemic, creative solutions were sought which could potentially help to fill the gap and support students to successfully complete both didactic (Hao, et al., 2021) and clinical course hour programmatic requirements (Triemstra, et al., 2021). The driving motives for developing the project include both the need for student clinical sites and to find a way to meet needs to provide quality care in underserved populations due to COVID-19.

More work needs to be accomplished in terms of research as well as in policy initiatives to expand the appropriate use of telehealth. Telehealth should be viewed as an accepted modality for clinical experiences across graduate level health professions programs, and the number of hours allowed to be used in programs should continue to be evaluated as the availability of equipment for remote monitoring becomes more widely available for use by students engaging in the clinical setting with their preceptors.

Projects such as the one presented here are important: initiatives where the goal is to expand the use of telehealth care as a means to increase clinical practice sites for graduate level health professions students are vitally needed. In addition, using telehealth appropriately can provide care modalities and an able venue through which traditionally difficult to reach populations who may not be able to travel to clinic settings for provider visits.

ACKNOWLEDGMENT

This work received no specific grant from any funding agency in the public, commercial, or not-for-profit sectors.

REFERENCES

Al-Balas, M., Al-Balas, H. I., Jaber, H. M., Obeidat, K., Al-Balas, H., Aborajooh, E. A., Al-Taher, R., & Al-Balas, B. (2020). Distance learning in clinical medical education amid COVID-19 pandemic in Jordan: Current situation, challenges, and perspectives. *BMC Medical Education*, *20*(1), 341. doi:10.118612909-020-02257-4 PMID:33008392

Atchley, M. D., Kroll, N. P., & Etcher, L. A. (2021). Reducing the wait: When time is priceless. *The Nurse Practitioner*, *46*(2), 50–55. doi:10.1097/01.NPR.0000731576.93905.48 PMID:33475331

Black Thomas, L. M. (2022). Stress and depression in undergraduate students during the COVID-19 pandemic: Nursing students compared to undergraduate students in non-nursing majors. *Journal of Professional Nursing*, *38*, 89–96. doi:10.1016/j.profnurs.2021.11.013 PMID:35042595

Bryk, A. S., Gomez, L. M., Grunow, A., & LeMahieu, P. G. (2015). *Learning to improve: How schools can get better at getting better.* Harvard Education Press.

Diaz, K., Staffileno, B. A., & Hamilton, R. (2021). Nursing student experiences in turmoil: A year of the pandemic and social strife during final clinical rotations. *Journal of Professional Nursing, 37*(5), 978–984. doi:10.1016/j.profnurs.2021.07.019

Drenkard, K., Sakallaris, B., Deyo, P., Abdillahi, S., & Hahn, H. (2021). University COVID -19 Surveillance Testing Center: Challenges and Opportunities for Schools of Nursing. *Journal of Professional Nursing, 37*(5), 948–953. doi:10.1016/j.profnurs.2021.07.004

Duffy, J., & Hoskins, L. (2003). The Quality-Caring Model©: Blending dual paradigms. *Advances in Nursing Science*, *26*(1), 79–90. doi:10.1097/00012272-200301000-00010 PMID:12611432

Etando, A., Amu, A. A., Haque, M., Schellack, N., Kurdi, A., Alrasheedy, A. A., Timoney, A., Mwita, J. C., Rwegerera, G. M., Patrick, O., Niba, L. L., Boahen-Boaten, B. B., Tabi, F. B., Amu, O. Y., Acolatse, J., Incoom, R., Sefah, I. A., Guantai, A. N., Opanga, S., ... Godman, B. (1722). Challenges and Innovations Brought about by the COVID-19 Pandemic Regarding Medical and Pharmacy Education Especially in Africa and Implications for the Future. *Healthcare (Basel, Switzerland)*, *9*(12), 1722. Advance online publication. doi:10.3390/healthcare9121722

Gagné, R. M., Briggs, L. J., & Wager, W. W. (1992). *Principles of instructional design* (4th ed.). Harcourt Brace Jovanovich College Publishers.

Garrison, D. R., Anderson, T., & Archer, W. (2000). Critical inquiry in a text-based environment: Computer conferencing in higher education. *The Internet and Higher Education*, *2*(2-3), 87–105. doi:10.1016/S1096-7516(00)00016-6

Gergen, K. J. (1999). *An invitation to social construction.* Sage Publications.

Haex, R., Thoma-Lürken, T., Zwakhalen, S., & Beurskens, A. (2020). The needs of key-stakeholders for evaluating client's experienced quality of home care: A qualitative approach. *Journal of Patient-Reported Outcomes, 4*(1), 96. doi:10.118641687-020-00260-3 PMID:33169288

Hallberg, D., & Salimi, N. (2020). Qualitative and Quantitative Analysis of Definitions of e-Health and m-Health. *Healthcare Informatics Research, 26*(2), 119–128. doi:10.4258/hir.2020.26.2.119 PMID:32547809

Hao, X., Peng, X., Ding, X., Qin, Y., Lv, M., Li, J., & Li, K. (2022). Application of digital education in undergraduate nursing and medical interns during the COVID-19 pandemic: A systematic review. *Nurse Education Today, 108*, 105183. doi:10.1016/j.nedt.2021.105183 PMID:34741918

Hempel, G., Weissenbacher, A., & Stehr, S. N. (2021). COVID-19: eine Chance zur Digitalisierung der Lehre?: Erfahrungsbericht und Ergebnisse einer Umfrage zur digitalen Lehre im Bereich Anästhesiologie, Intensiv-, Notfall-, Schmerz- und Palliativmedizin an der Universität Leipzig [COVID-19: a chance for digitalization of teaching?: Report of experiences and results of a survey on digitalized teaching in the fields of anesthesiology, intensive care, emergency, pain, and palliative medicine at the University of Leipzig]. *Der Anaesthesist*, 1–9. Advance online publication. doi:10.100700101-021-01016-4 PMID:34338817

Hess, K., McAuliffe, E. L., Gleckman-Krut, M., & Shapiro, S. (2022). Learning from 2020: How the Challenges of Remote Teaching Reinforce the Need for Care-Informed Pedagogy. *Teaching Sociology, 50*(1), 3–16. https://doi org.sacredheart.idm.oclc.org/10.1177/0092055X211060344

Hoofman, J., & Secord, E. (2021). The Effect of COVID-19 on Education. *Pediatric Clinics of North America, 68*(5), 1071–1079. doi:10.1016/j.pcl.2021.05.009 PMID:34538299

Huang, C. L. (2021). Article. *Hu Li Za Zhi, 68*(5), 4–6. doi:10.6224/JN.202110_68(5).01 PMID:34549401

Interactions, A. (2021). *E-Learning development with SAM*. Allen Interactions. Retrieved from: https://www.alleninteractions.com/services/custom-learning/sam/elearning-development

Kroll, N. L., Sanchez-Jones, T., Atchley, M. D., & Etcher, L. A. (2021). COVID-19 and the golden years. *The Nurse Practitioner, 46*(6), 37–42. doi:10.1097/01.NPR.0000743320.82081.6a PMID:34004640

Martinelli, S. M., Chen, F., Isaak, R. S., Huffmyer, J. L., Neves, S. E., & Mitchell, J. D. (2021). Educating Anesthesiologists During the Coronavirus Disease 2019 Pandemic and Beyond. *Anesthesia and Analgesia, 132*(3), 585–593. doi:10.1213/ANE.0000000000005333 PMID:33201006

Mehall, S. (2021). Purposeful interpersonal interaction and the point of diminishing returns for graduate learners. *The Internet and Higher Education, 48*, 100774. Advance online publication. doi:10.1016/j.iheduc.2020.100774

Morrison, M. (2006). *SWOT Analysis*. https://www.rapidbi.com/history-of-the-swot-analysis/

Ng, L., Seow, K. C., MacDonald, L., Correia, C., Reubenson, A., Gardner, P., Spence, A. L., Bunzli, S., & De Oliveira, B. (2021). eLearning in Physical Therapy: Lessons Learned From Transitioning a Professional Education Program to Full eLearning During the COVID-19 Pandemic. *Physical Therapy, 101*(4), pzab082. doi:10.1093/ptj/pzab082

Salinas, M., Salinas, N., Duffy, J. R., & Davidson, J. (2020). Do caring behaviors in the quality caring model promote the human emotion of feeling cared for in hospitalized stroke patients and their families? *Applied Nursing Research, 55*, 151299. doi:10.1016/j.apnr.2020.151299 PMID:32518006

Sava, S. (2012). Methods of Needs Analysis in Educational Context. In *Needs Analysis and Programme Planning in Adult Education* (1st ed., pp. 59–119). Verlag Barbara Budrich. doi:10.2307/j.ctvbkjvs2.8

Shah, S. M. A., Mohammad, D., Qureshi, M. F. H., Abbas, M. Z., & Aleem, S. (2021). Prevalence, Psychological Responses and Associated Correlates of Depression, Anxiety and Stress in a Global Population, During the Coronavirus Disease (COVID-19) Pandemic. *Community Mental Health Journal, 57*(1), 101–110. doi:10.100710597-020-00728-y PMID:33108569

Song, Y., Ding, Y., Ren, X., Liu, B., & Ma, H. (2021). Experience in online teaching and examining of histological experiments based on digital slices, Rain Class and QQ group class. *Chin J Histochem Cytochem., 1*, 102–106. doi:10.16705/j.cnki.1004-1850.2021.01.017

Su, B., Zhang, T., Yan, L., Huang, C., Cheng, X., Cai, C., & Cui, D. (2021). Online Medical Teaching in China During the COVID-19 Pandemic: Tools, Modalities, and Challenges. *Frontiers in Public Health, 9*, 797694. doi:10.3389/fpubh.2021.797694 PMID:34988057

Transforming and Scaling Up Health Professionals' Education and Training: World Health Organization Guidelines. (n.d.). *World Health Organization*. https://www.ncbi.nlm.nih.gov/books/NBK298950/

Triemstra, J. D., Haas, M., Bhavsar-Burke, I., Gottlieb-Smith, R., Wolff, M., Shelgikar, A. V., Samala, R. V., Ruff, A. L., Kuo, K., Tam, M., Gupta, A., Stojan, J., Gruppen, L., & Ellinas, H. (2021). Impact of the COVID-19 Pandemic on the Clinical Learning Environment: Addressing Identified Gaps and Seizing Opportunities. *Academic Medicine, 96*(9), 1276–1281. doi:10.1097/ACM.0000000000004013 PMID:34432665

Wong, B. M., & Headrick, L. A. (2020). Application of continuous quality improvement to medical education. *Medical Education, 55*(1), 72–81. doi:10.1111/medu.14351 PMID:32790930

World Health Organization. (2013). *Annex 1, Definition and list of health professionals*. From.

ADDITIONAL READING

Al-Mamun, M. A., Lawrie, G., & Wright, T. (2020). Instructional design of scaffolded online learning modules for self-directed and inquiry-based learning environments. *Computers & Education, 144*, 103695. doi:10.1016/j.compedu.2019.103695

Chang, J. E., Lai, A. Y., Gupta, A., Nguyen, A. M., Berry, C. A., & Shelley, D. R. (2021). Rapid Transition to Telehealth and the Digital Divide: Implications for Primary Care Access and Equity in a Post-COVID Era. *The Milbank Quarterly, 99*(2), 340–368. doi:10.1111/1468-0009.12509 PMID:34075622

Coleman, E., & O'Connor, E. (2019). The role of WhatsApp® in medical education; a scoping review and instructional design model. *BMC Medical Education, 19*(1), 1–13. doi:10.118612909-019-1706-8 PMID:31345202

Iancu, A. M., Kemp, M. T., & Alam, H. B. (2020). Unmuting Medical Students' Education: Utilizing Telemedicine During the COVID-19 Pandemic and Beyond. *Journal of Medical Internet Research*, *22*(7), e19667. doi:10.2196/19667 PMID:32614776

Jackson, D. N., Trivedi, N., & Baur, C. (2021). Re-Prioritizing Digital Health and Health Literacy in *Healthy People 2030* to Affect Health Equity. *Health Communication*, *36*(10), 1155–1162. doi:10.1080/10410236.2020.1748828 PMID:32354233

Kruse, C., & Heinemann, K. (2022). Facilitators and Barriers to the Adoption of Telemedicine During the First Year of COVID-19: Systematic Review. *Journal of Medical Internet Research*, *24*(1), e31752. doi:10.2196/31752 PMID:34854815

Melrose, S., Park, C. L., & Perry, B. (2013). *Teaching Health Professionals Online : Frameworks and Strategies*. AU Press. doi:10.15215/aupress/9781927356654.01

Office of Disease Prevention and Health Promotion. (n.d.). *Healthy People 2030*. U.S. Department of Health and Human Services. https://health.gov/healthypeople/about

Scott Kruse, C., Karem, P., Shifflett, K., Vegi, L., Ravi, K., & Brooks, M. (2018). Evaluating barriers to adopting telemedicine worldwide: A systematic review. *Journal of Telemedicine and Telecare*, *24*(1), 4–12. doi:10.1177/1357633X16674087 PMID:29320966

World Health Organization. (2013). *Transforming and Scaling Up Health Professionals' Education and Training: World Health Organization Guidelines*. World Health Organization. https://www.ncbi.nlm.nih.gov/books/NBK298953/

KEY TERMS AND DEFINITIONS

eHealth (or eMedicine): Electronic health (i.e., eHealth) or electronic medicine (i.e., eMedicine) refers to services that are electronically based that are used in healthcare or healthcare delivery.

Health Professional: Health professionals are ethically principled providers educated to care for people, their families and/or their communities utilizing evidence-based professional practice in accordance with the training they received, and within the limits of their licenses and certifications.

Instructional Design Theory: A theory that informs and aims to support the systematic or process-based development of instructional material.

mHealth: Mobile health (i.e., mHealth) refers to services electronic health care services that are used or delivered using mobile and wireless modalities.

Systematic Instructional Design: The process involved with creating and delivering instructional materials in a way that is systematic and proven to be effective for the learner population.

Telecare: Personal electronic and/or digital applications that support individuals to independently self-monitor designated biopsychosocial parameters for the purpose of safety, health maintenance or wellness.

Telehealth: Healthcare services beyond the doctor-patient relationship delivered via telecommunication technology. Telehealth care can refer to education, support, or care services provided by health care professionals other than physicians.

Telemedicine: Medical care delivered via telecommunication technology. This can include diagnostic and treatment-related elements of medical care.

Trauma Informed Education: Education delivery from the perspective and understanding that that trauma is a universal construct and has been experienced by all to some degree since the onset of COVID-19.

Underserved Population: The Department of Health and Human Services (n.d.) characterizes as underserved, vulnerable, and special needs populations as those that include minority members or individuals who have experienced health disparities.

Compilation of References

Aamir, J., Ali, S. M., Boulos, M. N. K., Anjum, N., & Ishaq, M. (2018). Enablers and inhibitors: A review of the situation regarding mHealth adoption in low-and middle-income countries. *Health Policy and Technology*, *7*(1), 88–97. doi:10.1016/j.hlpt.2017.11.005

Abella-García, V., Delgado-Benito, V., Ausín-Villaverde, V., & Hortigüela-Alacalá, D. (2019). To tweet or not to tweet: Student perceptions of the use of Twitter on an undergraduate degree course. *Innovations in Education and Teaching International*, *56*(4), 402–411. doi:10.1080/14703297.2018.1444503

Adams, P. (2006). Exploring social constructivism: Theories and practicalities. *Education*, *34*(3), 243–257.

Agarwal, R., Bills, J. E., Hecht, T. J., & Light, R. P. (2011). Role of home blood pressure monitoring in overcoming therapeutic inertia and improving hypertension control: A systematic review and meta-analysis. *Hypertension*, *57*(1), 29–38. doi:10.1161/HYPERTENSIONAHA.110.160911 PMID:21115879

Ahern, D. K., Kreslake, J. M., Phalen, J. M., & Bock, B. (2006). What is ehealth (6): Perspectives on the evolution of ehealth research. *Journal of Medical Internet Research*, *8*(1), e4. doi:10.2196/jmir.8.1.e4 PMID:16585029

Ahmed, O. M., Juthani, P. V., Green, M. L., & Moeller, J. J. (2021). Optimizing preclinical learning with retrieval practice: A call to action. *Medical Teacher*, *43*(6), 718–720. doi:10.1080/0142159X.2020.1788212 PMID:32643504

Akeel, A. U., & Mundy, D. (2019). Re-thinking technology and its growing role in enabling patient empowerment. *Health Informatics Journal*, *25*(4), 1278–1289. doi:10.1177/1460458217751013 PMID:29366367

Alaiad, A., Alsharo, M., & Alnsour, Y. (2019). The determinants of m-health adoption in developing countries: An empirical investigation. *Applied Clinical Informatics*, *10*(05), 820–840. doi:10.1055-0039-1697906 PMID:31667819

Alam, M. Z., Hoque, M. R., Hu, W., & Barua, Z. (2020). Factors influencing the adoption of mHealth services in a developing country: A patient-centric study. *International Journal of Information Management*, *50*, 128–143. doi:10.1016/j.ijinfomgt.2019.04.016

Al-Balas, M., Al-Balas, H. I., Jaber, H. M., Obeidat, K., Al-Balas, H., Aborajooh, E. A., Al-Taher, R., & Al-Balas, B. (2020). Distance learning in clinical medical education amid COVID-19 pandemic in Jordan: Current situation, challenges, and perspectives. *BMC Medical Education*, *20*(1), 341. doi:10.118612909-020-02257-4 PMID:33008392

Alessi, S. M., & Trollip, S. R. (2001). *Multimedia for learning: methods and development* (3rd ed.). Allyn and Bacon.

Alharbi, Y., Al-Mansour, M., Al-Saffar, R., Garman, A., & Alraddadi, A. (2020). Three-dimensional virtual reality as an innovative teaching and learning tool for human anatomy courses in medical education: A Mixed Methods Study. *Cureus*, *12*(2), e7085. doi:10.7759/cureus.7085 PMID:32226686

Aljunid, S. M. (2021). Obesity, a costly epidemic. In S. Al-Sabah., A. Aminian, L. Angrisani, E. Al Haddad, & L. Kow (Eds.), Laparoscopic Sleeve Gastrectomy. Springer. https://doi.org/ doi:10. 1007/978-3-030-57373-7_2

Alpert, C., Sinha, S., & Cullen, M. (2019). Teaching tomorrow's teachers: An innovative model of clinician-educator development for fellows-in-training. *Journal of the American College of Cardiology*, *73*, 22.

Altschuld, J. W., & Kumar, D. D. (2010). Needs assessment: An overview. *Sage (Atlanta, Ga.)*.

Altschuld, J. W., & Witkin, B. R. (2000). From needs assessment to action: Transforming needs into solution strategies. *Sage (Atlanta, Ga.)*.

American Heart Association. (2021). *Center for Health Technology and Innovation*. Retrieved from: https://www.ahahealthtech.org

American Hospital Association (AHA). (2019, Feb). *Factsheet: Telehealth*. https://www.aha.org/system/files/2019-02/fact-sheet-telehealth-2-4-19.pdf

Anderson, E. S., Wojcik, J. R., Winett, R. A., & Williams, D. M. (2006). Social-cognitive determinants of physical activity: The influence of social support, self-efficacy, outcome expectations, and self-regulation among participants in a church-based health promotion study. *Health Psychology*, *25*(4), 510–520. doi:10.1037/0278-6133.25.4.510

Andrews, C. M., Abraham, A. J., Grogan, C. M., Westlake, M. A., Pollack, H. A., & Friedmann, P. D. (2019). Impact of Medicaid restrictions on availability of buprenorphine in addiction treatment programs. *American Journal of Public Health*, *109*(3), 434–436. doi:10.2105/AJPH.2018.304856 PMID:30676789

Angell, S. Y., McConnell, M. V., Anderson, C. A., Bibbins-Domingo, K., Boyle, D. S., Capewell, S., Ezzati, M., De Ferranti, S., Gaskin, D. J., Goetzel, R. Z., Huffman, M. D., Jones, M., Khan, Y. M., Kim, S., Kumanyika, S. K., McCray, A. T., Merritt, R. K., Milstein, B., Mozaffarian, D., ... Warner, J. J. (2020). The American Heart Association 2030 impact goal: A presidential advisory from the American Heart Association. *Circulation*, *141*(9), e120–e138. doi:10.1161/CIR.0000000000000758 PMID:31992057

Antunes, C., Azadfard, M., Hoilat, G. J., & Gupta, M. (2020). Fatty Liver. StatPearls Publishing.

Arigo, D., Jake-Schoffman, D. E., Wolin, K., Beckjord, E., Hekler, E. B., & Pagoto, S. L. (2019). The history and future of digital health in the field of behavioral medicine. *Journal of Behavioral Medicine*, *42*, 67–83. doi:10.100710865-018-9966-z

Arnold School of Public Health. (n.d.a). *About the center.* https://sc.edu/study/colleges_schools/ public_health/research/research_centers/techealth/about/index.php

Arnold School of Public Health. (n.d.b). *Health promotion, education, & behavior.* https://sc.e du//study/colleges_schools/public_health/study/areas_of_study/health_promotion_education_and behavior/index.php

Arnold School of Public Health. (n.d.c). *Mission, vision and values*. https://sc.edu/study/college s_schools/public_health/about/mission_vision_values/index.php

Arnold School of Public Health. (n.d.d). *Web development and communications core.* https://sc. edu/study/colleges_schools/public_health/internal/faculty_staff/administrative_departments/ope rations_and_accreditation/web_development_and_communciations/index.php

Artinian, N. T., Fletcher, G. F., Mozaffarian, D., Kris-Etherton, P., Van Horn, L., Lichtenstein, A. H., Kumanyika, S., Kraus, W. E., Fleg, J. L., Redeker, N. S., Meininger, J. C., Banks, J. A., Stuart-Shor, E. M., Fletcher, B. J., Miller, T. D., Hughes, S., Braun, L. T., Kopin, L. A., Berra, K., ... Burke, L. E. (2010). Interventions to promote physical activity and dietary lifestyle changes for cardiovascular risk factor reduction in adults: A scientific statement from the American Heart Association. *Circulation*, *122*(4), 406–441. doi:10.1161/CIR.0b013e3181e8edf1 PMID:20625115

Atchley, M. D., Kroll, N. P., & Etcher, L. A. (2021). Reducing the wait: When time is priceless. *The Nurse Practitioner*, *46*(2), 50–55. doi:10.1097/01.NPR.0000731576.93905.48 PMID:33475331

Aungst, T. D., & Patel, R. (2020). Integrating Digital Health into the Curriculum-Considerations on the Current Landscape and Future Developments. *Journal of Medical Education and Curricular Development*, *7*. doi:10.1177/2382120519901275 PMID:32010795

Babylon. (2021). *About us*. https://www.babylonhealth.com/en-us/about

Bakdash, J. Z., & Drews, F. A. (2012). Using knowledge in the world to improve patient safety: Designing affordances in health care equipment to specify a sequential "Checklist". *Human Factors and Ergonomics in Manufacturing & Service Industries*, *22*(1), 7–20. doi:10.1002/hfm.20289

Ballard, B. D., & Jan, A. (2018). *Cardiovascular Disease.* StatPearls Publishing. https://www.ncbi.nlm.nih.gov/books/NBK535419/

Ball, K., Jeffery, R. W., Abbott, G., McNaughton, S. A., & Crawford, D. (2010). Is healthy behavior contagious: Associations of social norms with physical activity and healthy eating. *The International Journal of Behavioral Nutrition and Physical Activity*, *7*, 86. doi:10.118 6/1479-5868-7-86

Bandura, A. (1978). The self system in reciprocal determinism. *American Psychologist, 33*(4), 344-358.

Bandura, A. (1977). Self-efficacy: Toward a unifying theory of behavioral change. *Psychological Review*, *84*(2), 191–215. doi:10.1037/0033-295X.84.2.191 PMID:847061

Bandura, A. (1998). Health promotion from the perspective of social cognitive theory. *Psychology & Health*, *13*(4), 623–649. doi:10.1080/08870449808407422

Bandura, A. (2004). Health promotion by social cognitive means. *Health Education & Behavior*, *31*(2), 143–164. doi:10.1177/1090198104263660 PMID:15090118

Bandura, A. (2005). The primacy of self-regulation in health promotion. *Applied Psychology*, *54*(2), 245–254. doi:10.1111/j.1464-0597.2005.00208.x

Barak, M. (2017). Cloud pedagogy: Utilizing web-based technologies for the promotion of social constructivist learning in science teaching preparation courses. *Journal of Science Education and Technology*, *26*(5), 459–469. doi:10.100710956-017-9691-3

Bartholomew, L. K., Parcel, G. S., & Kok, G. (1998). Intervention Mapping: A process for developing theory and evidence-based health education programs. *Health Education & Behavior*, *25*(5), 545–563. doi:10.1177/109019819802500502 PMID:9768376

Bartholomew, L. K., Parcel, G. S., Kok, G., Gottlieb, N. H., & Fernandez, M. E. (2011). *Planning health promotion programs: an intervention mapping approach* (3rd ed.). Jossey-Bass.

Bartlett, J. D., Griffin, J., & Thomson, D. (n.d.). *Resources for supporting children's emotional well-being during the COVID-19 pandemic*. https://aisa.or.ke/wp-content/uploads/resources/health-and-wellbeing/wellbeing-resources/resources-for-supporting-childrens-emotional-well-being-during-the-covid-19-pandemic-290320.pdf

Bashshur, R., Shannon, G., Krupinski, E., & Grigsby, J. (2011). The taxonomy of telemedicine. *Telemedicine Journal and e-Health, 17*(6), 484–494. doi:10.1089/tmj.2011.0103 PMID:21718114

Basu Roy, R., & McMahon, G. T. (2012). Video-based cases disrupt deep critical thinking in problem-based learning. *Medical Education, 46*(4), 426–435. doi:10.1111/j.1365-2923.2011.04197.x PMID:22429179

Basu, A., Kuziemsky, C., de Araújo Novaes, M., Kleber, A., Sales, F., Al-Shorbaji, N., Flórez-Arango, J. F., Gogia, S. B., Ho, K., Hunter, I., Iyengar, S., John, O., John, S., Kulatunga, G., Rajput, V. K., Ranatunga, P., & Udayasankaran, J. G. (2021). Telehealth and the COVID-19 pandemic: International perspectives and a health systems framework for telehealth implementation to support critical response. *Yearbook of Medical Informatics, 30*(01), 126–133. doi:10.1055-0041-1726484 PMID:33882598

Batterham, R. W., Hawkins, M., Collins, P. A., Buchbinder, R., & Osborne, R. H. (2016). 2016/03/01/). Health literacy: Applying current concepts to improve health services and reduce health inequalities. *Public Health, 132*, 3–12. doi:10.1016/j.puhe.2016.01.001 PMID:26872738

Bauer, J. M., Bergstrøm, R., & Foss-Madsen, R. (2021). Are you sure, you want a cookie?—The effects of choice architecture on users' decisions about sharing private online data. *Computers in Human Behavior, 120*, 106729. Advance online publication. doi:10.1016/j.chb.2021.106729

Bauzon, J., Alver, A., Ravikumar, V., Devera, A., Mikhael, T., Nauman, R., & Simanton, E. (2021). The Impact of Educational Resources and Perceived Preparedness on Medical Education Performance. *Medical Science Educator, 31*(4), 1–8. doi:10.100740670-021-01306-x PMID:34457974

Beatty, A. L., Doll, J. A., Schopfer, D. W., Maynard, C., Plomondon, M. E., Shen, H., & Whooley, M. A. (2018). Cardiac rehabilitation participation and mortality after percutaneous coronary intervention: Insights from the veterans affairs clinical assessment, reporting, and tracking program. *Journal of the American Heart Association, 7*(19), e010010. doi:10.1161/JAHA.118.010010 PMID:30371315

Becevic, M., Boren, S., Mutrux, R., Shah, Z., & Banerjee, S. (2015). User satisfaction with telehealth: Study of patients, providers, and coordinators. *The HealthcareManager, 34*(4), 337–349. doi:10.1097/HCM.0000000000000081 PMID:26506296

Beleigoli, A. M., Andrade, A. Q., Cancado, A. G., Paulo, M. N. L., Diniz, M. D. H., & Ribeiro, A. L. (2019). Web-based digital health interventions for weight loss and lifestyle habit changes in overweight and obese adults: Systematic review and meta-analysis. *Journal of Medical Internet Research, 21*(1), e298. Advance online publication. doi:10.2196/jmir.9609

Belte, A., Suryawanshi, V., Sharma, R., & Deore, M. (2020). Cancer Disease Prediction Using Machine Learning Over Big Data. International Research Journal of Engineering and Technology, 7(3).

Benight, C. C., & Bandura, A. (2004). Social cognitive theory of posttraumatic recovery: The role of perceived self-efficacy. *Behaviour Research and Therapy, 42*(10), 1129–1148. doi:10.1016/j.brat.2003.08.008 PMID:15350854

Berg, E. A., Picoraro, J. A., Miller, S. D., Srinath, A., Franciosi, J. P., Hayes, C. E., Farrell, P. R., Cole, C. R., & LeLeiko, N. S. (2020). COVID-19—A guide to rapid implementation of telehealth services: A playbook for the pediatric gastroenterologist. *Journal of Pediatric Gastroenterology and Nutrition, 70*(6), 734–740. doi:10.1097/MPG.0000000000002749 PMID:32443021

Berkman, N. D., Davis, T. C., & McCormack, L. (2010). Health literacy: What is it? *Journal of Health Communication, 15*(sup2, S2), 9–19. doi:10.1080/10810730.2010.499985 PMID:20845189

Bernard, R. M., Abrami, P. C., Lou, Y., Borokhovski, E., Wade, A., Wozney, L., Wallet, P. A., Fiset, M., & Huang, B. (2004). How does distance education compare with classroom instruction? A meta-analysis of the empirical literature. *Review of Educational Research, 74*(3), 379–439. doi:10.3102/00346543074003379

Beverly, E. A., & Wray, L. A. (2010). The role of collective efficacy in exercise adherence: A qualitative study of spousal support and type 2 diabetes management. *Health Education Research, 25*(2), 211–223. doi:10.1093/her/cyn032

Bhaskar, S., Bradley, S., Chattu, V. K., Adisesh, A., Nurtazina, A., Kyrykbayeva, S., Sakhamuri, S., Yaya, S., Sunil, T., Thomas, P., Mucci, V., Moguilner, S., Israel-Korn, S., Alacapa, J., Mishra, A., Pandya, S., Schroeder, S., Atreja, A., Banah, M., & Ray, D. (2020). Telemedicine across the globe-position paper from the COVID-19 pandemic health system resilience program (reprogram) international consortium (part 1). *Frontiers in Public Health, 8*(556720), 1–15. doi:10.3389/fpubh.2020.556720 PMID:33178656

Bhavnani, S. P., Parakh, K., Atreja, A., Druz, R., Graham, G. N., Hayek, S. S., Krumholz, H. M., Maddox, T. M., Majmudar, M. D., Rumsfeld, J. S., & Shah, B. R. (2017). 2017 Roadmap for innovation—ACC health policy statement on healthcare transformation in the era of digital health, big data, and precision health: A report of the American College of Cardiology Task Force on Health Policy Statements and Systems of Care. *Journal of the American College of Cardiology, 70*(21), 2696–2718. doi:10.1016/j.jacc.2017.10.018 PMID:29169478

Bichelmeyer, B. A., Marken, J., Harris, T., Misanchuk, M., & Carr-Hixon, E. (2009). Fostering affective development outcomes. In C. M. Reigeluth & A.A. Carr-Chellman (Eds.), Instructional-design theories and models (vol. 3, pp. 249-274). Taylor & Francis.

Bindroo, S., Quintanilla Rodriguez, B. S., & Challa, H. J. (2021, August 13). Renal Failure. StatPearls Publishing.

Bing You, R. G., & Sproul, M. S. (1992). Medical students' perceptions of themselves and residents as teachers. *Medical Teacher, 14*(2-3), 133–138. doi:10.3109/01421599209079479 PMID:1406122

Binyamin, S. S., & Zafar, B. A. (2021). Proposing a mobile apps acceptance model for users in the health area: A systematic literature review and meta-analysis. *Health Informatics Journal, 27*(1). Advance online publication. doi:10.1177/1460458220976737 PMID:33438494

Bissell, T. (2004). The digital divide dilemma: Preserving Native American culture while increasing access to information technology on reservations. *University of Illinois Journal of Law, Technology & Policy, 2004*(1), 129–150.

Bitar, H., & Alismail, S. (2021). The role of ehealth, telehealth, and telemedicine for chronic disease patients during COVID-19 pandemic: A rapid systematic review. *Digital Health, 7*. doi:10.1177/20552076211009396 PMID:33959378

Black Thomas, L. M. (2022). Stress and depression in undergraduate students during the COVID-19 pandemic: Nursing students compared to undergraduate students in non-nursing majors. *Journal of Professional Nursing, 38*, 89–96. doi:10.1016/j.profnurs.2021.11.013 PMID:35042595

Black, A. D., Car, J., Pagliari, C., Anandan, C., Cresswell, K., Bokun, T., McKinstry, B., Procter, R., Majeed, A., & Sheikh, A. (2011). The impact of ehealth on the quality and safety of health care: A systematic overview. *PLoS Medicine, 8*(1), e1000387. doi:10.1371/journal.pmed.1000387 PMID:21267058

Blackmon, S. J. (2018). Beyond cybernation: Technology & teaching in doctoral educational leadership. In L. Hyatt & S. Allen (Eds.), *Advancing doctoral leadership education through technology* (pp. 56–74). Edward Elgar. doi:10.4337/9781786437020.00015

Blackmon, S. J., & Moore, R. L. (2020). A framework to support interdisciplinary engagement with learning analytics. In D. Ifenthaler & D. Gibson (Eds.), *Adoption of data analytics in higher education learning and teaching* (pp. 39–52). Springer. doi:10.1007/978-3-030-47392-1_3

Bloom, B. (1956). Taxonomy of Educational Objectives: The Classification of Educational Goals. Handbook 1 Cognitive Domain.

Bloom, B. S., Engelhart, M. D., Furst, E. J., Hill, W. H., & Krathwohl, D. R. (1956). *Taxonomy of educational objectives: The classification of educational goals*. Longmans.

Bonn, K. L., & Grabowski, B. L. (2001). *Generative learning theory: A practical cousin to constructivism* [Paper presentation]. Joint Mathematics Meetings, New Orleans, LA.

Booksource. (2018). Summer brain drain: Surprising statistics on summer slide. *Booksource Banter Blog*. https://www.booksourcebanter.com/2018/05/04/summer-brain-drain-statistics-summer-slide/

Booksource. (2022). *Reading level chart*. Booksource. https://www.booksource.com/reading-level-chart

Borzecki, A. M., Oliveria, S. A., & Berlowitz, D. R. (2005). Barriers to hypertension control. *American Heart Journal, 149*(5), 785–794. doi:10.1016/j.ahj.2005.01.047 PMID:15894958

Boston University School of Public Health. (2019). *The theory of planned behavior*. https://sphweb.bumc.bu.edu/otlt/mph-modules/sb/behavioralchangetheories/BehavioralChangeTheories3.html

Bosworth, H. B., & Oddone, E. Z. (2002). A model of psychosocial and cultural antecedents of blood pressure control. *Journal of the National Medical Association, 94*(4), 236. PMID:11991336

Brackett, M. A., Elbertson, N. A., & Rivers, S. E. (2015). Applying theory to the development of approaches to SEL. In J. A. Durlak, C. E Domitrovich, R. P., Weissberg, & T. P. Gullotta (Eds.), Handbook of social and emotional learning: Research and practice (pp. 20-32). Guilford Publications.

Bradshaw, J. (1972). Taxonomy of social need. In G. McLachlan (Ed.), *Problems and progress in medical care: Essays on current research, 7th series* (pp. 71–82). Oxford University Press.

Bradshaw, J. (1972). Taxonomy of social need. In G. McLachlan (Ed.), *Problems and progress in medical care: Essays son current research* (pp. 71–82). Oxford University Press.

Branch, R. M., & Kopcha, T. J. (2014). Instructional design models. In J. M. Spector, M. D. Merrill, J. Elen, & M. J. Bishop (Eds.), *Handbook of research on educational communications and technology* (pp. 77–87). Springer New York. doi:10.1007/978-1-4614-3185-5_7

Breton, M., Deville-Stoetzel, N., Gaboury, I., Smithman, M. A., Kaczorowski, J., Lussier, M.-T., Haggerty, J., Motulsky, A., Nugus, P., Layani, G., Paré, G., Evoy, G., Arsenault, M., Paquette, J.-S., Quinty, J., Authier, M., Mokraoui, N., Luc, M., & Lavoie, M.-E. (2021). Telehealth in primary healthcare: A portrait of its rapid implementation during the COVID-19 pandemic. *Healthcare Policy, 17*(1), 73–90. doi:10.12927/hcpol.2021.26576 PMID:34543178

Brinkerhoff, D. A. (2001). Survey of instructional development models. *TechTrends, 45*(1), 48–50. doi:10.1007/BF02763388

Brown, K. W., Ryan, R. M., & Creswell, J. D. (2007). Mindfulness: Theoretical foundations and evidence for its salutary effects. *Psychological Inquiry, 18*(4), 211–237. doi:10.1080/10478400701598298

Bruehlman-Senecal, E., Hook, C. J., Pfeifer, J. H., FitzGerald, C., Davis, B., Delucchi, K. L., Haritatos, J., & Ramo, D. E. (2020). Smartphone app to address loneliness among college students: Pilot randomized controlled trial. *JMIR Mental Health, 7*(10), e21496. doi:10.2196/21496 PMID:33079071

Bryk, A. S., Gomez, L. M., Grunow, A., & LeMahieu, P. G. (2015). *Learning to improve: How schools can get better at getting better*. Harvard Education Press.

Bull, S. (2011). *Technology-based health promotion*. SAGE Publications, Inc.

Burke, L. E., Ma, J., Azar, K. M., Bennett, G. G., Peterson, E. D., Zheng, Y., Riley, W., Stephens, J., Shah, S. H., Suffoletto, B., Turan, T. N., Spring, B., Steinberger, J., & Quinn, C. C. (2015). Current science on consumer use of mobile health for cardiovascular disease prevention: A scientific statement from the American Heart Association. *Circulation*, *132*(12), 1157–1213. doi:10.1161/CIR.0000000000000232 PMID:26271892

Burke, S. M., Carron, A. V., Eys, M. A., Ntoumanis, N., & Estabrooks, P. A. (2006). Group versus individual approach? A meta-analysis of the effectiveness of interventions to promote physical activity. *Sport and Exercise Psychology Review*, *2*(1), 19–35.

Calm for Schools Lesson Plan. (2020). *30 days of mindfulness in the classroom.* https://www.calm.com/schools/resources

Cameron, J. D., Ramaprasad, A., & Syn, T. (2017). An ontology of and roadmap for mHealth research. *International Journal of Medical Informatics*, *100*, 16–25. doi:10.1016/j.ijmedinf.2017.01.007

Campbell, P. C. (2014). Modifying ADDIE: Incorporating new technologies in library instruction. *Public Services Quarterly*, *10*(2), 138–149. doi:10.1080/15228959.2014.904214

Cao, Y., & Koretsky, M. D. (2018). Shared resources: Engineering students' emerging group understanding of thermodynamic work. *Journal of Engineering Education*, *107*(4), 656–689. doi:10.1002/jee.20237

Cardemil, E. V., Millán, F., & Aranda, E. (2019). A new, more inclusive name: The Journal of Latinx Psychology. *Journal of Latina/o Psychology*, *7*(1), 1–5. doi:10.1037/lat0000129

Carlson, S. A., Fulton, J. E., Pratt, M., Yang, Z., & Adams, E. K. (2015). Inadequate physical activity and health care expenditures in the United States. *Progress in Cardiovascular Diseases*, *57*(4), 315–323. doi:10.1016/j.pcad.2014.08.002

Casey, J. A., Schwartz, B. S., Stewart, W. F., & Adler, N. E. (2016). Using electronic health records for population health research: A review of methods and applications. *Annual Review of Public Health*, *37*(1), 61–81. doi:10.1146/annurev-publhealth-032315-021353 PMID:26667605

Castillo-Montoya, M. (2017). Deepening understanding of prior knowledge: What diverse first-generation college students in the U.S. can teach us. *Teaching in Higher Education*, *22*(5), 587–603. doi:10.1080/13562517.2016.1273208

Castillo-Salgado, C. (2010). Trends and directions of global public health surveillance. *Epidemiologic Reviews*, *32*(1), 93–109. doi:10.1093/epirev/mxq008 PMID:20534776

Cavanagh, S., & Chadwick, K. (2005). *Health needs assessment: A practical guide.* Health Development Agency.

Center for Disease Control and Prevention (CDC). (2021). *What Is Health Literacy?* https://www.cdc.gov/healthliteracy/learn/index.html

Centers for Disease Control and Prevention (CDC). (2022). *Disparities in hospitalizations: Racial and ethnic health disparities.* U.S. Department of Health and Human Services. https://www.cdc.gov/coronavirus/2019-ncov/community/health-equity/racial-ethnic-disparities/disparities-hospitalization.html

Centers for Disease Control and Prevention. (2020). *BRFSS prevalence & trends data.* https://www.cdc.gov/brfss/brfssprevalence/index.html

Centers for Disease Control and Prevention. (2021, April 19). *Healthy eating for a healthy weight.* https://www.cdc.gov/healthyweight/healthy_eating/index.html

Chaffee, B. W., & Zimmerman, C. R. (2010). Developing and implementing clinical decision support for use in a computerized prescriber-order-entry system. *American Journal of Health-System Pharmacy*, *67*(5), 391–400. doi:10.2146/ajhp090153 PMID:20172991

Champion, V. L., & Skinner, C. S. (2008). The health belief model. In K. Glanz, B. K., Rimer, & K. Viswanath (Eds.), Health behavior and health education: theory, research, and practice (4th ed., pp. 45-65). Jossey-Bass.

Chan, E. Y., & Kim, J. (2011). Chronic health needs immediately after natural disasters in middle-income countries: The case of the 2008 Sichuan, China earthquake. *European Journal of Emergency Medicine*, *18*(2), 111–114. doi:10.1097/MEJ.0b013e32833dba19 PMID:20679898

Chauhan, R. H., Naik, D. N., Halpati, R. A., Patel, S. J., & Prajapati, M. A. (2008). Disease Prediction using Machine Learning. *Clinical Reports*, 783-7.

Chen, H. J., Liao, L. L., Chang, Y. C., Hung, C. C., & Chang, L. C. (2019). Factors influencing technology integration in the curriculum for Taiwanese health profession educators: A mixed-methods study. *International Journal of Environmental Research and Public Health*, *16*(14), 2602. doi:10.3390/ijerph16142602 PMID:31336610

Chen, J., Zhou, J., Wang, Y., Qi, G., Xia, C., Mo, G., & Zhang, Z. (2020). Blended learning in basic medical laboratory courses improves medical students' abilities in self-learning, understanding, and problem solving. *Advances in Physiology Education*, *44*(1), 9–14. doi:10.1152/advan.00076.2019 PMID:31821032

Cheung, L. (2016). Using an instructional design model to teach medical procedures. *Medical Science Educator*, *26*(1), 175–180. doi:10.100740670-016-0228-9 PMID:27182457

Chew, A. M. K., Ong, R., Lei, H.-H., Rajendram, M., K v, G., Verma, S. K., Fung, D. S. S., Leong, J. J., & Gunasekeran, D. V. (2020). Digital health solutions for mental health disorders during COVID-19. *Frontiers in Psychiatry*, *11*, 898. doi:10.3389/fpsyt.2020.582007 PMID:33033487

Chib, A., van Velthoven, M. H., & Car, J. (2015). mHealth adoption in low-resource environments: A review of the use of mobile healthcare in developing countries. *Journal of Health Communication*, *20*(1), 4–34. doi:10.1080/10810730.2013.864735 PMID:24673171

Chib, A., Wilkin, H., & Hoefman, B. (2013). Vulnerabilities in mHealth implementation: A Ugandan HIV/AIDS SMS campaign. *Global Health Promotion*, *20*(1, suppl), 26–32. doi:10.1177/1757975912462419 PMID:23549699

Choi, Y. S., & Bosch, S. J. (2013). Environmental affordances: Designing for family presence and involvement in patient care. *HERD: Health Environments Research & Design Journal*, *6*(4), 53–75. doi:10.1177/193758671300600404 PMID:24089181

Chunara, R., Zhao, Y., Lawrence, K., Testa, P. A., Nov, O., & Mann, D. M. (2021). Telemedicine and healthcare disparities: A cohort study in a large healthcare system in New York City during COVID-19. *Journal of the American Medical Informatics Association*, *28*(1), 33–41. doi:10.1093/jamia/ocaa217 PMID:32866264

Clark, R. C., & Mayer, R. E. (2016). *e-Learning and the science of instruction: Proven guidelines for consumers and designers of multimedia learning*. John Wiley & Sons, Incorporated.

Cleland, V. J., Ball, K., & Crawford, D. (2010). Social and environmental determinants of health behaviors. In A. Steptoe (Ed.), *Handbook of behavioral medicine: Methods and applications* (pp. 3–18). Springer. doi:10.1007/978-0-387-09488-5_1

Cleo, G., Beller, E., Glasziou, P., Isenring, E., & Thomas, R. (2020). Efficacy of habit-based weight loss interventions: A systematic review and meta-analysis. *Journal of Behavioral Medicine*, *43*(4), 519–532. https://doi.or/10.1007/s10865-019-00100-w

Clinton, H. (2021). *Connecticut Department of Public Health drug overdose monthly report.* https://public.tableau.com/app/profile/heather.clinton/viz/SUDORS_Dashboard_final2/OverdoseDashboard

Coalition of National Health Education Organizations. (2021). 2020 *Health education and promotion terminology report*. http://www.cnheo.org/2020-joint-committee-on-health-education-terminology.html

Coholic, D., Schwabe, N., & Lander, K. (2020). A scoping review of arts-based mindfulness interventions for children and youth. *Child & Adolescent Social Work Journal, 37*(5), 511–526. doi:10.100710560-020-00657-5

Collaboration for Academic, Social and Emotional Learning. (2022). *Our mission and work*. https://casel.org/about-us/our-mission-work/

Collaborative for Academic, Social, and Emotional Learning (CASEL). (2021). *Fundamentals of SEL: What Is the CASEL Framework?* https://casel.org/fundamentals-of-sel/what-is-the-casel-framework/#self-awareness

Conard, S. (2019). Best practices in digital health literacy. *International Journal of Cardiology, 292*, 277–279. doi:10.1016/j.ijcard.2019.05.070 PMID:31230937

Cooper, R. L., Ramesh, A., Juarez, P. D., Edgerton, R., Paul, M., Tabatabai, M., Brown, I. K., & Matthews-Juarez, P. (2020). Systematic review of opioid use disorder treatment training for medical students and residents. *Journal of Health Care for the Poor and Underserved, 31*(5), 26–42. doi:10.1353/hpu.2020.0136 PMID:35061607

Coorey, G. M., Neubeck, L., Mulley, J., & Redfern, J. (2018). Effectiveness, acceptability and usefulness of mobile applications for cardiovascular disease self-management: Systematic review with meta-synthesis of quantitative and qualitative data. *European Journal of Preventive Cardiology, 25*(5), 505–521. doi:10.1177/2047487317750913 PMID:29313363

Cortelyou-Ward, K., Atkins, D. N., Noblin, A., Rotarius, T., White, P., & Carey, C. (2020). Navigating the digital divide: Barriers to telehealth in rural areas. *Journal of Healthcarefor the Poor and Underserved, 31*(4), 1546–1556. doi:10.1353/hpu.2020.0116 PMID:33416736

Crosby, R., & Noar, S. M. (2011). What is a planning model? An introduction to PRECEDE-PROCEED. *Journal of Public Health Dentistry, 71*(s1), S7–S15. doi:10.1111/j.1752-7325.2011.00235.x PMID:21656942

Cross-Denny, B., Betso, A., Cusick, E., Doyle, C., Marbot, M., & Santos-Dempsey, S. (2015). Constructing a deconstruction: Reflections on dismantling racism. *Reflections: Narratives of Professional Helping, 21*(3), 10-17.

Cruz-Martínez, R. R., Noort, P. D., Asbjornsen, R. A., Van Niekerk, J. M., Wentzel, J., Sanderman, R., & Van Gemert-Pijnen, L. (2019). Frameworks, models, and theories used in electronic health research and development to support self-management of cardiovascular diseases through remote monitoring technologies: Protocol for a metaethnography review. *JMIR Research Protocols, 8*(7), e13334. Advance online publication. doi:10.2196/13334 PMID:31313659

Cruz-Martínez, R. R., Wentzel, J., Asbjørnsen, R. A., Noort, P. D., van Niekerk, J. M., Sanderman, R., & van Gemert-Pijnen, J. E. (2020). Supporting self-management of cardiovascular diseases through remote monitoring technologies: Metaethnography review of frameworks, models, and theories used in research and development. *Journal of Medical Internet Research, 22*(5), e16157. doi:10.2196/16157 PMID:32436852

Cusack, L., Del Mar, C. B., Chalmers, I., Gibson, E., & Hoffmann, T. C. (2018). Educational interventions to improve people's understanding of key concepts in assessing the effects of health interventions: A systematic review. *Systematic Reviews, 7*(1), 68. doi:10.118613643-018-0719-4 PMID:29716639

Czerkawski, B. C., & Lyman, E. W. III. (2016). An instructional design framework for fostering student engagement in online learning environments. *TechTrends, 60*(6), 532–539. doi:10.100711528-016-0110-z

Dai, H., Milkman, K. L., & Riis, J. (2014). The fresh start effect: Temporal landmarks motivate aspirational behavior. *Management Science, 60*(10), 2563–2582. doi:10.1287/ mnsc.2014.1901

Dala-Ali, B. M., Lloyd, M. A., & Al-Abed, Y. (2011). The uses of the iPhone for surgeons. *The Surgeon*, *9*(1), 44–48. doi:10.1016/j.surge.2010.07.014 PMID:21195331

Dandavino, M., Snell, L., & Wiseman, J. (2007). Why medical students should learn how to teach. *Medical Teacher*, *29*(6), 558–565. doi:10.1080/01421590701477449 PMID:17922358

Das, A., Agarwal, A., & Das, R. (2021). *Evaluation of Social Human Sentiment Analysis using Machine Learning Algorithms*. Presented in the 2nd International Conference on Computer Engineering & Communication Systems (ICACECS 2021).

Datta, G. (2020). *Mobile Health Apps Conformity Assessment & Certification Guidance Concept Note*. https://www.healthit.gov/isa/sites/isa/files/webform/uscid_webform/2126/Mobile%20Health%20App%20CA%20%26%20Certification%20Guidance%20Concept%20Note%20%20-%20Gora%20Datta.pdf

De Ponti, R., Marazzato, J., Maresca, A. M., Rovera, F., Carcano, G., & Ferrario, M. M. (2020). Pre-graduation medical training including virtual reality during COVID-19 pandemic: A report on students' perception. *BMC Medical Education*, *20*(1), 1–7. doi:10.118612909-020-02245-8 PMID:32977781

D'Eath, M., Barry, M. M., & Sixsmith, J. (2012). *A Rapid Evidence Review of Interventions for Improving Health Literacy*. Academic Press.

Deci, E. L., & Ryan, R. M. (2008). Self-determination theory: A macrotheory of human motivation, development, and health. *Canadian Psychology*, *49*(3), 182–185. doi:10.1037/ a0012801

del Carmen Ortega-Navas, M. (2017). The use of new technologies as a tool for the promotion of health education. *Procedia: Social and Behavioral Sciences*, *237*, 23–29. doi:10.1016/j.sbspro.2017.02.006

Dennick, R. (2016). Constructivism: Reflections on twenty-five years teaching the constructivist approach in medical education. *International Journal of Medical Education*, *7*, 200–205. doi:10.5116/ijme.5763.de11 PMID:27344115

Deterding, S., Dixon, D., Khaled, R., & Nacke, L. (Eds.). (2011). *Proceedings of the 15th international academic MindTrek conference: Envisioning future media environments*. ACM Digital Library. https://dl.acm.org/doi/10.1145/2181037.2181040

Deubel, P. (2003). An investigation of behaviorist and cognitive approaches to instructional multimedia design. *Journal of Educational Multimedia and Hypermedia*, *12*(1), 63–90.

Dewey, J. (1938). *Logic: The theory of inquiry*. Holt.

Dhawan, S. (2020). Online learning: A panacea in the time of COVID-19 crisis. *Journal of Educational Technology Systems*, *49*(1), 5–22. doi:10.1177/0047239520934018

Diabetes Prevention Program Research Group. (2002). Reduction in the incidence of type 2 diabetes with lifestyle intervention or metformin. *The New England Journal of Medicine*, *346*, 393–403. doi:10.1056/NEJMoa012512

Diao, J. A., & Kvedar, J. (2021). *Mobile health technology for diverse populations: challenges and opportunities*. Academic Press.

Diaz, K., Staffileno, B. A., & Hamilton, R. (2021). Nursing student experiences in turmoil: A year of the pandemic and social strife during final clinical rotations. *Journal of Professional Nursing*, *37*(5), 978–984. doi:10.1016/j.profnurs.2021.07.019

Dicianno, B. E., Parmanto, B., Fairman, A. D., Crytzer, T. M., Yu, D. X., Pramana, G., Coughenour, D., & Petrazzi, A. A. (2015). Perspectives on the evolution of mobile (mHealth) technologies and application to rehabilitation. *Physical Therapy*, *95*(3), 397–405. doi:10.2522/ptj.20130534 PMID:24925075

Dick, W., Carey, L., & Carey, J. O. (2015). *The systematic design of instruction*. Pearson.

Ding, D., Lawson, K. D., Kolbe-Alexander, T. L., Finkelstein, E. A., Katzmarzyk, P. T., van Mechelen, W., & Pratt, M. (2016). The economic burden of physical inactivity: A global analysis of major non-communicable diseases. *Lancet, 388*(10051), 1311–1324. doi:10.10 16/S0140-6736(16)30383-X

Dippel, C. (2014). Forced coexistence and economic development: Evidence from NativeAmerican reservations. *Econometrica, 82*(6), 2131–2165. doi:10.3982/ECTA11423

Dowell, A., Crampton, P., & Parkin, C. (2001). The first sunrise: An experience of cultural immersion and community health needs assessment by undergraduate medical students in New Zealand. *Medical Education, 35*(3), 242–249. doi:10.1046/j.1365-2923.2001.00772.x PMID:11260447

Drenkard, K., Sakallaris, B., Deyo, P., Abdillahi, S., & Hahn, H. (2021). University COVID -19 Surveillance Testing Center: Challenges and Opportunities for Schools of Nursing. *Journal of Professional Nursing, 37*(5), 948–953. doi:10.1016/j.profnurs.2021.07.004

Driscoll, M. P. (2005). *Psychology of learning for instruction* (3rd ed.). Pearson Allyn and Bacon.

Duffy, F. M. (2009). Paradigms, mental models, and mindsets: Triple barriers to transformational change in school systems. *Journal of Educational Leadership Preparation, 4*(3), 357–376.

Duffy, J., & Hoskins, L. (2003). The Quality-Caring Model©: Blending dual paradigms. *Advances in Nursing Science, 26*(1), 79–90. doi:10.1097/00012272-200301000-00010 PMID:12611432

Duffy, T. M., & Cunningham, D. J. (2007). Constructivism: Implications for the design and delivery of instruction. In D. H. Jonassen (Ed.), *Handbook of research for educational communications and technology* (pp. 1–31). The Association for Educational Communications and Technology.

Dunn, P., & Cianflone, D. (2020). Special Issue on Digital Health Literacy. *International Journal of Cardiology, 299*, 301–302. doi:10.1016/j.ijcard.2019.08.055 PMID:31493913

Dunn, P., & Conard, S. (2018). Improving health literacy in patients with chronic conditions: A call to action. *International Journal of Cardiology, 273*, 249–251. doi:10.1016/j.ijcard.2018.08.090 PMID:30193793

Dunn, P., Margaritis, V., & Anderson, C. L. (2017). Understanding Health Literacy Skills in Patients with Cardiovascular Disease and Diabetes. *Qualitative Report, 22*(1), 33–46. doi:10.46743/2160-3715/2017.2548

Durlak, J. A., Weissberg, R. P., Dymnicki, A. B., Taylor, R. D., & Schellinger, K. B. (2011). The impact of enhancing students' social and emotional learning: A meta-analysis of school-based universal interventions: Social and emotional learning. *Child Development, 82*(1), 405–432. doi:10.1111/j.1467-8624.2010.01564.x PMID:21291449

Dustin, D. L., Bricker, K. S., & Schwab, K. A. (2009). People and nature: Toward an ecological model of health promotion. *Leisure Sciences, 32*(1), 3–14. doi:10.1080/01490400903430772

Dwivedi, Y. K., Shareef, M. A., Simintiras, A. C., Lal, B., & Weerakkody, V. (2016). A generalised adoption model for services: A cross-country comparison of mobile health (m-health). *Government Information Quarterly, 33*(1), 174–187. doi:10.1016/j.giq.2015.06.003

Eady, M., & Lockyer, L. (2013). Tools for learning: Technology and teaching. *Learning to Teach in the Primary School, 71.*

Eapen, Z. J., Turakhia, M. P., McConnell, M. V., Graham, G., Dunn, P., Tiner, C., Rich, C., Harrington, R. A., Peterson, E. D., & Wayte, P. (2016). Defining a mobile health roadmap for cardiovascular health and disease. *Journal of the American Heart Association, 5*(7), e003119. doi:10.1161/JAHA.115.003119 PMID:27405809

Eckel, R. H., Jakicic, J. M., Ard, J. D., de Jesus, J. M., Houston Miller, N., Hubbard, V. S., Lee, I.-M., Lichtenstein, A. H., Loria, C. M., Millen, B. E., Nonas, C. A., Sacks, F. M., Smith, S. C. Jr, Svetkey, L. P., Wadden, T. A., & Yanovski, S. Z. (2014). 2013 AHA/ACC guideline on lifestyle management to reduce cardiovascular risk: A report of the American College of Cardiology/American Heart Association Task Force on Practice Guidelines. *Journal of the American College of Cardiology*, *63*(25, 25 Part B), 2960–2984. doi:10.1016/j.jacc.2013.11.003 PMID:24239922

Edelman, A. (2021, May 23). *Congress could spend big on broadband. Tribal nations say it can't come soon enough.* NBC Universal News Group. https://www.nbcnews.com/politics/joe-biden/congress-could-spend-big-broadband-tribal-nations-say-it-can-n1267923

Edgenuity. (2018). *Edgenuity Courseware: Reviewer's guide.* Edgenuity, Inc.

Eide, E. R., Showalter, M. H., & Goldhaber, D. D. (2010). The relation between children's health and academic achievement. *Children and Youth Services Review*, *32*(2), 231–238. doi:10.1016/j.childyouth.2009.08.019

English, R. E., & Reigeluth, C. M. (1996). Formative research on sequencing instruction with the elaboration theory. *Educational Technology Research and Development*, *44*(1), 23–42. doi:10.1007/BF02300324

Ernest, P. (1999). *Social constructivism as a philosophy of mathematics: Radical constructivism rehabilitated. A 'historical paper'*. Available at www. people. ex.ac.uk/PErnest

Ertmer, P. A., York, C. S., & Gedik, N. (2009). Learning from the pros: How experienced designers translate instructional design models into practice. *Educational Technology*, *49*(1), 19–27.

Etando, A., Amu, A. A., Haque, M., Schellack, N., Kurdi, A., Alrasheedy, A. A., Timoney, A., Mwita, J. C., Rwegerera, G. M., Patrick, O., Niba, L. L., Boahen-Boaten, B. B., Tabi, F. B., Amu, O. Y., Acolatse, J., Incoom, R., Sefah, I. A., Guantai, A. N., Opanga, S., ... Godman, B. (1722). Challenges and Innovations Brought about by the COVID-19 Pandemic Regarding Medical and Pharmacy Education Especially in Africa and Implications for the Future. *Healthcare (Basel, Switzerland)*, *9*(12), 1722. Advance online publication. doi:10.3390/healthcare9121722

Eysenbach, G. (2001). What is e-health? *Journal of Medical Internet Research*, *3*(2), e20. doi:10.2196/jmir.3.2.e20 PMID:11720962

Fahad, P. K., & Pallavi, M. S. (2018, April). Prediction of human health using machine learning and big data. In *2018 International Conference on Communication and Signal Processing (ICCSP)* (pp. 195-199). IEEE. 10.1109/ICCSP.2018.8524352

Fardanesh, H. (2006). *A classification of constructivist instructional design models based on learning and teaching approaches.* https://files.eric.ed.gov/fulltext/ED491713.pdf

Farrish, K. (2020). *Healthcareand education suffer when there's no internet access.* Connecticut Investigative Team. http://c-hit.org/2020/08/14/health-care-and-education-suffer-when-theres-no-internet-access/

Fatehi, F., Gray, L. C., & Russell, A. W. (2017). Mobile health (mHealth) for diabetes care: Opportunities and challenges. *Diabetes Technology & Therapeutics*, *19*(1), 1–3. doi:10.1089/dia.2016.0430 PMID:28099051

FDA. (2020). *What is Digital Health?* https://www.fda.gov/medical-devices/digital-health-center-excellence/what-digital-health

Federal Communications Commission (FCC). (2021, Feb 1). *Fourteenth broadband deployment report.* https://www.fcc.gov/reports-research/reports/broadband-progress-reports/fourteenth-broadband-deployment-report

Feeney, B. C., & Collins, N. L. (2015). A new look at social support: A theoretical perspective on thriving through relationships. *Personality and Social Psychology Review*, *19*(2), 113–147. doi:10.1177/1088868314544222

Fiddian-Green, A., Kim, S., Gubrium, A. C., Larkey, L. K., & Peterson, J. C. (2019). Restor(y)ing health: A conceptual model of the effects of digital storytelling. *Health Promotion Practice*, *20*(4), 502–512. doi:10.1177/1524839918825130 PMID:30736703

Fiordelli, M., Diviani, N., & Schulz, P. J. (2013). Mapping mHealth research: A decade of evolution. *Journal of Medical Internet Research*, *15*(5), e95–e95. doi:10.2196/jmir.2430 PMID:23697600

Fiorella, L., & Mayer, R. E. (2015). *Learning as a generative activity*. Cambridge University Press. doi:10.1017/CBO9781107707085

Fishbein, M., & Ajzen, I. (2010). *Predicting and changing behavior: The reasoned action approach*. ProQuest Ebook Central. https://ebookcentral.proquest.com

Fishbein, M. (2008). A reasoned action approach to health promotion. *Medical Decision Making*, *28*(6), 834–844. doi:10.1177/0272989X08326092 PMID:19015289

Fish, M. T., & Saul, A. D. (2019). The gamification of meditation: A randomized-controlled study of a prescribed mobile mindfulness meditation application in reducing college students' depression. *Simulation & Gaming*, *50*(4), 419–435. doi:10.1177/1046878119851821

Fogel, A. L., & Kvedar, J. C. (2018). Artificial intelligence powers digital medicine. *NPJ Digital Medicine*, *1*(1), 1–4. doi:10.103841746-017-0012-2 PMID:31304291

Fogg, B. (2009). A behavior model for persuasive design. *Proceedings of the 4th International Conference on Persuasive Technology (Persuasive '09)*. 10.1145/1541948.1541999

Fong, S. F., Sakai, D. H., Kasuya, R. T., Kramer, K., Wong, V. S., Haning, W., Asano, I., Uyehara-Lock, J. H., Thompson, K., Omori, J. S., Hirose-Wong, S. M., & Horio, D. T. (2016). Medical School Hotline: Liaison Committee on Medical Education Accreditation, Part IV: Pre-clerkship Education. *Hawai'i Journal of Medicine & Public Health: a Journal of Asia Pacific Medicine & Public Health*, *75*(2), 48–51. PMID:26918209

Food and Drug Administration. (2020). *What is Digital Health?* https://www.fda.gov/medical-devices/digital-health-center-excellence/what-digital-health

Ford, C. L., & Airhihenbuwa, C. O. (2010). Critical race theory, race equity, and public health: Toward antiracism praxis. *American Journal of Public Health*, *100*(S1), S30–S35. doi:10.2105/AJPH.2009.171058 PMID:20147679

Ford, C. L., & Airhihenbuwa, C. O. (2018). Commentary: Just what is critical race theory and what's it doing in a progressive field like public health? *Ethnicity & Disease*, *28*(Suppl 1), 223. doi:10.18865/ed.28.S1.223 PMID:30116090

Forthofer, M., Wilcox, S., Kinnard, D., Hutto, B., & Sharpe, P. A. (2019). Sumter county on the move! Evaluation of a walking group intervention to promote physical activity within existing social networks. *Journal of Physical Activity & Health*, *16*(1), 22–28. doi:10.1123/jpah.2017-0603

Fowler, L. R., Gillard, C., & Morain, S. R. (2020). Readability and accessibility of terms of service and privacy policies for menstruation-tracking smartphone applications. *Health Promotion Practice*, *21*(5), 679–683. doi:10.1177/1524839919899924 PMID:32037887

France, D., Powell, V., Mauchline, A. L., Welsh, K., Park, J., Whalley, W. B., & Rewhorn, S. (2016). Ability of students to recognize the relationship between using mobile apps for learning during fieldwork and the development of graduate attributes. *Journal of Geography in Higher Education*, *40*(2), 182–192. doi:10.1080/03098265.2016.1154931

Franko, O. I. (2011). Smartphone apps for orthopaedic surgeons. *Clinical Orthopaedics and Related Research*, *469*(7), 2042–2048. doi:10.100711999-011-1904-0 PMID:21547414

Free, C., Phillips, G., Felix, L., Galli, L., Patel, V., & Edwards, P. (2010). The effectiveness of M-health technologies for improving health and health services: A systematic review protocol. *BMC Research Notes*, *3*(1), 1–7. doi:10.1186/1756-0500-3-250 PMID:20925916

Frehywot, S., Vovides, Y., Talib, Z., Mikhail, N., Ross, H., Wohltjen, H., Bedada, S., Korhumel, K., Koumare, A. K., & Scott, J. (2013). E-learning in medical education in resource constrained low-and middle-income countries. *Human Resources for Health*, *11*(1), 1–15. doi:10.1186/1478-4491-11-4 PMID:23379467

Frenk, J., Chen, L., Bhutta, Z. A., Cohen, J., Crisp, N., Evans, T., Fineberg, H., Garcia, P., Ke, Y., Kelley, P., Kistnasamy, B., Meleis, A., Naylor, D., Pablos-Mendez, A., Reddy, S., Scrimshaw, S., Sepulveda, J., Serwadda, D., & Zurayk, H. (2010). Health professionals for a new century: Transforming education to strengthen health systems in an interdependent world. *Lancet*, *376*(9756), 1923–1958. doi:10.1016/S0140-6736(10)61854-5 PMID:21112623

Friedman, J., & Akre, S. (2021). COVID-19 and the drug overdose crisis: Uncovering the deadliest months in the United States, January–July 2020. *American Journal of Public Health*, *111*(7), 1284–1291. doi:10.2105/AJPH.2021.306256 PMID:33856885

Fung, B. (2013). *How Chattanooga beat Google Fiber by half a decade.* https://www.washingtonpost.com/news/the-switch/wp/2013/09/17/how-chattanooga-beat-google-fiber-by-half-a-decade/

Gagné, R. M. (1984). Learning outcomes and their effects: Useful categories of human performance. *The American Psychologist*, *39*(4), 377–385. doi:10.1037/0003-066X.39.4.377

Gagné, R. M., Biggs, L. J., & Wager, W. W. (1992). *Principles of instructional design* (4th ed.). Harcourt Brace Jovanovich, Publishers.

Ganasegeran, K., Renganathan, P., Rashid, A., & Al-Dubai, S. A. R. (2017). The m-Health revolution: Exploring perceived benefits of WhatsApp use in clinical practice. *International Journal of Medical Informatics*, *97*, 145–151. doi:10.1016/j.ijmedinf.2016.10.013 PMID:27919374

Gardner, H. (2002). *Frames of Mind: The Theory of Multiple Intelligences*. Basic Books.

Garfan, S., Alamoodi, A. H., Zaidan, B. B., Al-Zobbi, M., Hamid, R. A., Alwan, J. K., Ahmaro, I. Y. Y., Khalid, E. T., Jumaah, F. M., Albahri, O. S., Zaidan, A. A., Albahri, A. S., Al-qaysi, Z T., Ahmed, M. A., Shuwandy, M. L., Salih, M. M., Zughoul, O., Mohammed, K. I., & Momani, F. (2021). Telehealth utilization during the COVID-19 pandemic: A systematic review. *Computers in Biology and Medicine, 138*. doi:10.1016/j.compbiomed.2021.104878

Garrison, D. R. (2000). Theoretical challenges for distance education in the 21st century: A shift from structural to transactional issues. *International Review of Research in Open and Distance Learning*, *1*(1), 6–21. doi:10.19173/irrodl.v1i1.2

Garrison, D. R., Anderson, T., & Archer, W. (2000). Critical inquiry in a text-based environment: Computer conferencing in higher education. *The Internet and Higher Education*, *2*(2-3), 87–105. doi:10.1016/S1096-7516(00)00016-6

Gentry, S., & Gentry, B. (2017). Chronic obstructive pulmonary disease: Diagnosis and management. *American Family Physician*, *95*(7), 433–441. PMID:28409593

Gergen, K. J. (1999). *An invitation to social construction*. Sage Publications.

Ghersin, Z. J., Yager, P., Cummings, B. M., Hersh, C., Cayer, M., Callans, K. M., Zablah, J. E., Gallagher, T., Abrego, S., Bonilla, J., Sanchez Vela, O., Guzman, L., Aguilar, A., & Hartnick, C. J. (2020). A multidisciplinary, video-based, curriculum for management of the intubated and surgical airway patient for a pediatric hospital in El Salvador. *International Journal of Pediatric Otorhinolaryngology*, *128*, 109732. doi:10.1016/j.ijporl.2019.109732 PMID:31644996

GhoseA.GuoX.LiB.DangY. (2021). *Empowering patients using smart mobile health platforms: Evidence from a randomized field experiment. Forthcoming at MIS Quarterly, NYU Stern School of Business Forthcoming*. https://ssrn.com/abstract=377318

Ghose, A., Guo, X., Li, B., & Dang, Y. (2021). *Empowering patients using smart mobile health platforms: Evidence from a randomized field experiment*. Forthcoming at MIS Quarterly.

Ginsberg, J., Mohebbi, M. H., Patel, R. S., Brammer, L., Smolinski, M. S., & Brilliant, L. (2009). Detecting influenza epidemics using search engine query data. *Nature, 457*(7232), 1012–1014. doi:10.1038/nature07634 PMID:19020500

Ginzburg, S. (2018). Curriculum Inventory in Context: Use of Self-Directed Learning in U.S. and Canadian Medical Schools. *AAMC, 5*(5).

Glanz, K., Rimer, B. K., & Viswanath, K. (2008). *Health behavior and health education: theory, research, and practice* (4th ed.). Jossey-Bass.

Glanz, K., Rimer, B. K., & Viswanath, K. (Eds.). (2015). *Health behavior: Theory, research, and practice*. John Wiley & Sons, Incorporated.

Gleason, A. W. (2015). mHealth—Opportunities for transforming global health care and barriers to adoption. *Journal of Electronic Resources in Medical Libraries, 12*(2), 114–125. doi:10.1080/15424065.2015.1035565

Goddard, A., Sullivan, E., Fields, P., & Mackey, S. (2021). The future of telehealth in school- based health centers: Lessons from COVID-19. *Journal of Pediatric Health Care, 35*(3), 304–309. https://doi.org/10.1016/j.pedhc.2020.11.008

Gómez-Olmedo, A. M., Valor, C., & Carrero, I. (2020). Mindfulness in education for sustainable development to nurture socioemotional competencies: A systematic review and meta-analysis. *Environmental Education Research, 26*(11), 1527–1555. doi:10.1080/13504622.2020.1777264

Goodman, B. E., Barker, M. K., & Cooke, J. E. (2018). Best practices in active and student-centered learning in physiology classes. *Advances in Physiology Education, 42*(3), 417–423. doi:10.1152/advan.00064.2018 PMID:29972063

Goodson, P. (2010). *Theory in health promotion research and practice: Thinking outside the box*. Jones and Bartlett.

Gorin, A. A., Powers, T. A., Gettens, K., Cornelius, T., Koestner, R., Mobley, A. R., Pescatello, L. S., & Huedo-Medina, T. B. (2020). A randomized controlled trial of a theory-based weight loss program for couples. *Health Psychology, 39*(2), 137–146. doi:10.1037/hea000080 8

Gorin, A. A., Raynor, H. A., Fava, J., Maguire, K., Robichaud, E., Trautvetter, J., Crane, M., & Wing, R. R. (2013). Randomized controlled trial of a comprehensive home environment-focused weight-loss program for adults. *Health Psychology, 32*, 128–137. doi:10.1037/a0026959

Graff, C. J., Kaljo, K., Treat, R. W., & Dielentheis, K. (2021). The Adaptive Learner: How Faculty and Medical Students' Perceptions of Learning Needs and Desires Differ. *WMJ: Official Publication of the State Medical Society of Wisconsin, 120*(1), 8–16. PMID:33974759

Grampurohit, S., & Sagarnal, C. (2020, June). Disease prediction using machine learning algorithms. In *2020 International Conference for Emerging Technology (INCET)* (pp. 1-7). IEEE.

Grant, M. M. (2019). Difficulties in defining mobile learning: Analysis, design characteristics, and implications. *Educational Technology Research and Development, 67*(2), 361–388. doi:10.100711423-018-09641-4

Greaves, C. J., Sheppard, K. E., Abraham, C., Hardeman, W., Roden, M., Evans, P. H., & Schwarz, P.The IMAGE Study Group. (2011). Systematic review of reviews of intervention components associated with increased effectiveness in dietary and physical activity interventions. *BMC Public Health, 11*, 119. Advance online publication. doi:10.1186/1471-2458-11-119

Gredler, M. E. (1997). Learning and instruction. *Theory into Practice.*

Green, B. B., Cook, A. J., Ralston, J. D., Fishman, P. A., Catz, S. L., Carlson, J., Carrell, D., Tyll, L., Larson, E. B., & Thompson, R. S. (2008). Effectiveness of home blood pressure monitoring, Web communication, and pharmacist care on hypertension control: A randomized controlled trial. *Journal of the American Medical Association, 299*(24), 2857–2867. doi:10.1001/jama.299.24.2857 PMID:18577730

Greenberg, J. S. (2010). Health education as freeing. In J. M. Black, S. Furney, H. M. Graf, & A. E. Nolte (Eds.), *Philosophical foundations of health education* (pp. 210–205). Jossey-Bass.

Greenberg, M. T., Domitrovich, C. E., Weissberg, R. P., & Durlak, J. A. (2017). Social and emotional learning as a public health approach to education. *The Future of Children, 27*(1), 13–32. doi:10.1353/foc.2017.0001

Green, L. W., Glanz, K., Hochbaum, G. M., Kok, G., Kreuter, M. W., Lewis, F. M., Lorig, K., Morisky, D., Rimer, B. K., & Rosenstock, I. M. (1994). Can we build on, or must we replace, the theories and models in health education? *Health Education Research, 9*(3), 397–404. doi:10.1093/her/9.3.397 PMID:10150456

Green, L. W., & Kreuter, M. W. (2005). *Health program planning: An educational and ecological approach*. McGraw-Hill.

Green, L. W., Richard, L., & Potvin, L. (1996). Ecological foundations of health promotion. *American Journal of Health Promotion, 10*(4), 270–281. doi:10.4278/0890-1171-10.4.270 PMID:10159708

Grimley, D., Prochaska, J. O., Velicer, W. F., Blais, L. M., & DiClemente, C. C. (1994). The transtheoretical model of change. In T. M. Brinthaupt & R. P. Lipka (Eds.), *Changing the self: philosophies, techniques, and experiences* (pp. 201–228). SUNY Press. https://books.google.com/books?hl=en&lr=&id=nhrTvXVhBLMC&pgis=1

Gueldner, B. A., Feuerborn, L. L., & Merrell, K. W. (2020). Social and emotional learning in the classroom, second edition: Promoting mental health and academic success. Guilford Publications.

Guo, C., Ashrafian, H., Ghafur, S., Fontana, G., Gardner, C., & Prime, M. (2020). Challenges for the evaluation of digital health solutions—A call for innovative evidence generation approaches. *NPJ Digital Medicine, 3*(1), 1–14. doi:10.103841746-020-00314-2 PMID:32904379

Guo, X., Sun, Y., Wang, N., Peng, Z., & Yan, Z. (2013). The dark side of elderly acceptance of preventive mobile health services in China. *Electronic Markets, 23*(1), 49–61. doi:10.100712525-012-0112-4

Gustafson, K. L., & Branch, R. M. (2002). *Survey of instructional development models* (4th ed.). ERIC Clearinghouse on Information & Technology.

Gustafson, K., & Branch, R. (1997). Revisioning models of instructional development. *Educational Technology Research and Development, 45*(3), 73–89. doi:10.1007/BF02299731

Guze, P. A. (2015). Using Technology to Meet the Challenges of Medical Education. *Transactions of the American Clinical and Climatological Association, 126*, 260–270. PMID:26330687

Haber, R. J., Bardach, N. S., Vedanthan, R., Gillum, L. A., Haber, L. A., & Dhaliwal, G. (2006). Preparing fourth-year medical students to teach during internship. *Journal of General Internal Medicine, 21*(5), 518–520. doi:10.1111/j.1525-1497.2006.00441.x PMID:16704402

Haex, R., Thoma-Lürken, T., Zwakhalen, S., & Beurskens, A. (2020). The needs of key-stakeholders for evaluating client's experienced quality of home care: A qualitative approach. *Journal of Patient-Reported Outcomes*, *4*(1), 96. doi:10.118641687-020-00260-3 PMID:33169288

Haffajee, R. L., Bohnert, A. S., & Lagisetty, P. A. (2018). Policy pathways to address provider workforce barriers to buprenorphine treatment. *American Journal of Preventive Medicine*, *54*(6), S230–S242. doi:10.1016/j.amepre.2017.12.022 PMID:29779547

Hagen, J. W., Skenandore, A. H., Scow, B. M., Schanen, J. G., & Clary, F. H. (2012). Adolescent pregnancy prevention in a rural Native American community. *Journal of Family Social Work*, *15*(1), 19–33.

Hallberg, D., & Salimi, N. (2020). Qualitative and Quantitative Analysis of Definitions of e-Health and m-Health. *Healthcare Informatics Research*, *26*(2), 119–128. doi:10.4258/hir.2020.26.2.119 PMID:32547809

Hamilton, C.-C. L., Gross, C.-C. B., Adams, D., Bradshaw, C. P., Cantor, P., Gurwitch, R., Jagers, R., Murry, V. M., & Wong, M. (n.d.). *How has the pandemic affected students' social- emotional well-being? A review of the evidence to Date*. https://files.eric.ed.gov/fulltext/ED614131.pdf

Hamilton, A. M. (2020). A genealogy of critical race and digital studies: Past, present, and future. *Sociology of Race and Ethnicity (Thousand Oaks, Calif.)*, *6*(3), 292–301.

Han, K. J., Subramanian, R., & Cameron, G. T. (2019). Listen before you leap: Sri Lankan health professionals' perspectives on m-health. *Health Informatics Journal*, *25*(3), 858–866. doi:10.1177/1460458217725903 PMID:28825329

Hanover, J., & Perry, R. (2011). The business value of automating evidence-based medicine: Southeast Alabama Medical Center. *IDC Health Insights,* 1–9.

Hao, X., Peng, X., Ding, X., Qin, Y., Lv, M., Li, J., & Li, K. (2022). Application of digital education in undergraduate nursing and medical interns during the COVID-19 pandemic: A systematic review. *Nurse Education Today*, *108*, 105183. doi:10.1016/j.nedt.2021.105183 PMID:34741918

Harrington, R. A., Califf, R. M., Balamurugan, A., Brown, N., Benjamin, R. M., Braund, W. E., Hipp, J., Konig, M., Sanchez, E., & Joynt Maddox, K. E. (2020). Call to action: rural health: a presidential advisory from the American Heart Association and American Stroke Association. *Circulation*, *141*(10), e615–e644. doi:10.1161/CIR.0000000000000753 PMID:32078375

Hartlep, N. D. (2009). *Critical Race Theory an examination of its past, present, and future implications*. https://files.eric.ed.gov/fulltext/ED506735.pdf

Hashemi, A., Nourbakhsh, S., Tehrani, P., & Karimi, A. (2018). Remote telemonitoring of cardiovascular patients: Benefits, barriers, new suggestions. *Artery Research*, *22*(C), 57–63. doi:10.1016/j.artres.2018.04.001

Hays, H., Carroll, M., Ferguson, S., Fore, C., & Horton, M. (2014). The success of telehealthcarein the Indian Health Service. *AMA Journal of Ethics*, *16*(12), 986–996. https://doi.org/10.1001/virtualmentor.2014.16.12.stas1-1412

Health Resources & Services Administration (HRSA). (2021a, Sept). *What is telehealth?* https://www.hrsa.gov/rural-health/telehealth/what-is-telehealth

Health Resources & Services Administration (HRSA). (2021b, Oct). *Telehealth programs*. https://www.hrsa.gov/rural-health/telehealth

Heath, C., Luff, P., & Sanchez Svensson, M. (2007). Video and qualitative research: Analysing medical practice and interaction. *Medical Education*, *41*(1), 109–116. doi:10.1111/j.1365-2929.2006.02641.x PMID:17209899

Heijmans, M., Waverijn, G., Rademakers, J., van der Vaart, R., & Rijken, M. (2015). Functional, communicative and critical health literacy of chronic disease patients and their importance for self-management. *Patient Education and Counseling*, *98*(1), 41–48. doi:10.1016/j.pec.2014.10.006 PMID:25455794

Heinsch, M., Wyllie, J., Carlson, J., Wells, H., Tickner, C., & Kay-Lambkin, F. (2021). Theories informing ehealth implementation: Systematic review and typology classification. *Journal of Medical Internet Research*, *23*(5), e18500. Advance online publication. doi:10.2196/18500 PMID:34057427

Hempel, G., Weissenbacher, A., & Stehr, S. N. (2021). COVID-19: eine Chance zur Digitalisierung der Lehre?: Erfahrungsbericht und Ergebnisse einer Umfrage zur digitalen Lehre im Bereich Anästhesiologie, Intensiv-, Notfall-, Schmerz- und Palliativmedizin an der Universität Leipzig [COVID-19: a chance for digitalization of teaching?: Report of experiences and results of a survey on digitalized teaching in the fields of anesthesiology, intensive care, emergency, pain, and palliative medicine at the University of Leipzig]. *Der Anaesthesist*, 1–9. Advance online publication. doi:10.100700101-021-01016-4 PMID:34338817

Hendricks, M., Nair, G., Staunton, C., Pather, M., Garrett, N., Baadjies, D., Kidd, M., & Moodley, K. (2018). *Impact of an educational video as a consent tool on knowledge about cure research among patients and caregivers at HIV clinics in South Africa*. Academic Press.

Hersh, W., Margolis, A., Quirós, F., & Otero, P. (2010). Building a health informatics workforce in developing countries. *Health Affairs*, *29*(2), 274–277. doi:10.1377/hlthaff.2009.0883 PMID:20348073

Hess, K., McAuliffe, E. L., Gleckman-Krut, M., & Shapiro, S. (2022). Learning from 2020: How the Challenges of Remote Teaching Reinforce the Need for Care-Informed Pedagogy. *Teaching Sociology*, *50*(1), 3–16. https://doi org.sacredheart.idm.oclc.org/10.1177/0092055X211060344

Hess, A. N. (2016). A case study of job-embedded learning. *portal. Portal (Baltimore, Md.)*, *16*(2), 327–347. doi:10.18438/eblip29526

Hill, J. R., Wiley, D., Nelson, L. M., & Han, S. (2004). Exploring research on Internet-based learning: From infrastructure to interactions. In D. H. Jonassen (Ed.), *Handbook of research on educational communications and technology* (2nd ed., pp. 433–460). Lawrence Erlbaum Associates.

Hirko, K. A., Kerver, J. M., Ford, S., Szafranski, C., Beckett, J., Kitchen, C., & Wendling, A. L. (2020). Telehealth in response to the COVID-19 pandemic: Implications for rural health disparities. *Journal of the American Medical Informatics Association*, *27*(11), 1816–1818. https://doi.org/10.1093/jamia/ocaa156

Hirumi, A. (2021). IAMSE 2021—Plenary Session: Top 10 Ways an Instructional Designer Can Help You Define the New Normal. *Medical Science Educator*, *31*(S1), 1–8. doi:10.100740670-021-01400-0 PMID:34567833

Holland, K. M., Jones, C., Vivolo-Kantor, A. M., Idaikkadar, N., Zwald, M., Hoots, B., Yard, E., D' Inverno, A., Swedo, E., Chen, M. S., Petrosky, E., Board, A., Martinez, P., Stone, D. M., Law, R., Coletta, M. A., Adjemian, J., Thomas, C., Puddy, R. W., ... Houry, D. (2021). Trends in U.S. emergency department visits for mental health, overdose, and violence outcomes before and during the COVID-19 pandemic. *JAMA Psychiatry*, *78*(4), 372–379. doi:10.1001/jamapsychiatry.2020.4402 PMID:33533876

Honeycutt, A. A., Wile, K., Dove, C., Hawkins, J., & Orenstein, D. (2015). Strategic planning for chronic disease prevention in rural America: Looking through a PRISM lens. *Journal of Public Health Management and Practice*, *21*(4), 392–399.

Hoofman, J., & Secord, E. (2021). The Effect of COVID-19 on Education. *Pediatric Clinics of North America*, *68*(5), 1071–1079. doi:10.1016/j.pcl.2021.05.009 PMID:34538299

Hoque, R., & Sorwar, G. (2017). Understanding factors influencing the adoption of mHealth by the elderly: An extension of the UTAUT model. *International Journal of Medical Informatics*, *101*, 75–84. doi:10.1016/j.ijmedinf.2017.02.002 PMID:28347450

Houben, S., Frost, M., & Bardram, J. E. (2015, February). Collaborative affordances of hybrid patient record technologies in medical work. In *Proceedings of the 18th ACM Conference on Computer Supported Cooperative Work & Social Computing* (pp. 785-797). 10.1145/2675133.2675164

Howlett, N., Trivedi, D., Troop, N. A., & Chater, A. M. (2019). Are physical activity interventions for healthy inactive adults effective in promoting behavior change and maintenance, and which behavior change techniques are effective? A systematic review and meta-analysis. *Translational Behavioral Medicine*, *9*(1), 147–157. doi:10.1093/tbm/ iby010

Hsieh, C.-H., Tsai, H.-H., Yin, J.-W., Chen, C.-Y., Yang, J. C.-S., & Jeng, S.-F. (2004). Teleconsultation with the mobile camera-phone in digital soft-tissue injury: A feasibility study. *Plastic and Reconstructive Surgery*, *114*(7), 1776–1782. doi:10.1097/01.PRS.0000142402.07896.21 PMID:15577348

Huang, C. L. (2021). Article. *Hu Li Za Zhi*, *68*(5), 4–6. doi:10.6224/JN.202110_68(5).01 PMID:34549401

Huberty, J., Green, J., Glissmann, C., Larkey, L., Puzia, M., & Lee, C. (2019). Efficacy of the mindfulness meditation mobile app "Calm" to reduce stress among college students: Randomized controlled trial. *JMIR mHealth and uHealth*, *7*(6), e14273. doi:10.2196/14273 PMID:31237569

Hughes, J. (n.d.). *Communicating with Generation Z: Everything You Need to Know*. Keystone Academic. https://www.keystoneacademic.com/news/communicating-with-generation-z-everything-you-need-to-know

Huhn, A. S., Hobelmann, J. G., Strickland, J. C., Oyler, G. A., Bergeria, C. L., Umbricht, A., & Dunn, K. E. (2020). Differences in availability and use of medications for opioid use disorder in residential treatment settings in the United States. *JAMA Network Open*, *3*(2), e1920843–e1920843. doi:10.1001/jamanetworkopen.2019.20843 PMID:32031650

Humble, J. R., Tolley, E. A., Krukowski, R. A., Womack, C. R., Motley, T. S., & Bailey, J. E. (2016). Use of and interest in mobile health for diabetes self-care in vulnerable populations. *Journal of Telemedicine and Telecare*, *22*(1), 32–38. doi:10.1177/1357633X15586641 PMID:26026179

Hwabamungu, B., & Williams, Q. (2010, October). m-Health adoption and sustainability prognosis from a care givers' and patients' perspective. In *Proceedings of the 2010 Annual Research Conference of the South African Institute of Computer Scientists and Information Technologists* (pp. 123-131). 10.1145/1899503.1899517

Hyman, J. A., Moser, M. T., & Segala, L. N. (2014). Electronic reading and digital library technologies: Understanding learner expectation and usage intent for mobile learning. *Educational Technology Research and Development*, *62*(1), 35–52. doi:10.100711423-013-9330-5

Ibacache, K. (2019). Use of language-learning apps as a tool for foreign language acquisition by academic libraries employees. *Information Technology and Libraries*, *38*(3), 22–33. doi:10.6017/ital.v38i3.11077

Ickovics, J. R., Carroll-Scott, A., Peters, S. M., Schwartz, M., Gilstad-Hayden, K., & McCaslin, C. (2014). Health and academic achievement: Cumulative effects of health assets on standardized test scores among urban youth in the United States. *The Journal of School Health*, *84*(1), 40–48. doi:10.1111/josh.12117 PMID:24320151

Interactions, A. (2021). *E-Learning development with SAM*. Allen Interactions. Retrieved from: https://www.alleninteractions.com/services/custom-learning/sam/elearning-development

International Work Group for Indigenous Affairs (IWGIA). (2021, Mar 18). *The indigenous world 2021: The United States of America*. https://www.iwgia.org/en/usa/4253-iw-2021-usa.html

IQVIA. (2017). *Grows as Innovation, Evidence and Adoption of Mobile Health Apps Accelerate*. https://www.iqvia.com/newsroom/2017/11/impact-of-digital-health-grows-as-innovation-evidence-and-adoption-of-mobile-health-apps-accelerate

IQVIA. (2017). *Grows as Innovation, Evidence and Adoption of Mobile Health Apps Accelerate*. https://www.iqvia.com/newsroom/2017/11/impact-of-digital-health-grows-asinnovation-evidence-and-adoption-of-mobile-health-apps-accelerate/

Irby, D. M., Cooke, M., & O'Brien, B. C. (2010). Calls for reform of medical education by the Carnegie Foundation for the Advancement of Teaching: 1910 and 2010. *Academic Medicine*, *85*(2), 220–227. doi:10.1097/ACM.0b013e3181c88449 PMID:20107346

Iribarren, S. J., Cato, K., Falzon, L., & Stone, P. W. (2017). What is the economic evidence for mHealth? A systematic review of economic evaluations of mHealth solutions. *PLoS One*, *12*(2), e0170581. Advance online publication. doi:10.1371/journal.pone.0170581

Isaza-Restrepo, A., Gómez, M. T., Cifuentes, G., & Argüello, A. (2018). The virtual patient as a learning tool: A mixed quantitative qualitative study. *BMC Medical Education*, *18*(1), 297. doi:10.118612909-018-1395-8 PMID:30522478

Jahangiry, L., Farhangi, M. A., Shab-Bidar, S., Rezaei, F., & Pashaei, T. (2017). Web-based physical activity interventions: A systematic review and meta-analysis of randomized controlled trials. *Public Health*, *152*, 36–46. doi:10.1016/j.puhe.2017.06.005

Jakicic, J. M., Winters, C., Lang, W., & Wing, R. R. (1999). *Effects of intermittent exercise and use of home exercise equipment on adherence, weight loss, and fitness in overweight women: A randomized trial*. https://doi.org/ doi:10.1001/jama.282.16.1554

Jetty, A., Moore, M. A., Coffman, M., Petterson, S., & Bazemore, A. (2018). Rural family physicians are twice as likely to use telehealth as urban family physicians. *Telemedicine and eHealth, 24*(4), 268-276.

Johannesson, M., Ostling, R., & Ranehill, E. (2010). The effect of competition on physical activity: A randomized trial. *B.E. The B.E. Journal of Economic Analysis & Policy Pol*, *10*(1). Advance online publication. doi:10.2202/1935-1682.2555

Joint Committee on Health Education and Promotion Terminology. (2021). *Joint committee on health education and promotion terminology report*. http://www.cnheo.org/2020-joint-committee-on-health-education-terminology.html

Jokinen, A., Stolt, M., & Suhonen, R. (2021). Ethical issues related to eHealth: An integrative review. *Nursing Ethics*, *28*(2), 253–271. doi:10.1177/0969733020945765 PMID:32930041

Jonassen, D. (1999). Designing constructivist learning environments. In C. M. Reigeluth (Ed.), Instructional design theories and models (vol. 2, pp. 215-239). Lawrence Erlbaum Associates.

Jonassen, D. H., Tessmer, M., & Hannum, W. H. (1999). *Task analysis methods for instructional design*. Lawrence Erlbaum Associates.

Jonassen, D., Cernusca, D., & Ionas, G. (2007). Constructivism and instructional design: The emergence of the learning sciences and design research. In R. A. Reiser & J. V. Dempsey (Eds.), *Trends and issues in instructional design and technology* (2nd ed., pp. 45–52). Pearson.

Kahangamage, U., & Leung, R. C. K. (2020). Remodelling and engineering design subject to enhance students' learning outcomes. *International Journal of Technology and Design Education*, *30*(4), 799–814. doi:10.100710798-019-09519-3

Kahn, E. B., Ramsey, L. T., Brownson, R. C., Heath, G. W., Howze, E. H., Powell, K. E., Stone, E. J., Rajab, M. W., & Corso, P. (2002). The effectiveness of interventions to increase physical activity: Review and update. *American Journal of Preventive Medicine*, *34*(12), 1996–2001. doi:10.10160749-3797(02)00434-8

Kaini, S., & Motie, L. Z. (2021). Virtual vs Online: Insight from Medical Students. Comment on "Effectiveness of virtual medical teaching during the COVID-19 crisis: Systematic review.". *JMIR Medical Education*, *7*(2), e27020. doi:10.2196/27020 PMID:33988518

Kaium, M. A., Bao, Y., Alam, M. Z., Hasan, N., & Hoque, M. R. (2019). Understanding the insight of factors affecting mHealth adoption: A systematic review. *International Journal of Research in Business and Social Science, 8*(6), 181-200.

Kanselaar, G. (2002). Constructivism and socio-constructivism. *Constructivism and Socio-Constructivism*, 1–7.

Kaplan, B. (2020). Revisiting health information technology ethical, legal, and social issues and evaluation: Telehealth/telemedicine and COVID-19. *International Journal of Medical Informatics, 143*. doi:10.1016/j.ijmedinf.2020.104239

Kaplan, R. M., & Simon, H. J. (1990). Compliance in medical care: Reconsideration of self-predictions. *Annals of Behavioral Medicine*, *12*(2), 66–71. doi:10.120715324796abm1202_2

Karunamuni, N., & Weerasekera, R. (2019). Theoretical foundations to guide mindfulness meditation: A path to wisdom. *Current Psychology (New Brunswick, N.J.)*, *38*(3), 627–646. doi:10.100712144-017-9631-7

Kassavou, A., Turner, A., & French, D. P. (2013). Do interventions to promote walking in groups increase physical activity? A meta-analysis. *The International Journal of Behavioral Nutrition and Physical Activity*, *10*, 18. doi:10.1186/1479-5868-10-18

Kaufman, R., & Guerra-Lopez, I. (2013). *Needs assessment for organizational success*. ASTD Press.

Kaur, J., & Mann, K. S. (2017, December). AI based healthcare platform for real time, predictive and prescriptive analytics using reactive programming. *Journal of Physics: Conference Series*, *933*(1), 012010.

Kazanidis, I., Pellas, N., Fotaris, P., & Tsinakos, A. (2018). Facebook and Moodle integration into instructional media design courses: A comparative analysis of students' learning experiences using the Community of Inquiry (CoI) model. *International Journal of Human-Computer Interaction*, *34*(10), 932–942. doi:10.1080/10447318.2018.1471574

Kazemi, D. M., Borsari, B., Levine, M. J., Shehab, M., Nelson, M., Dooley, B., Stinson, B., Fang, F., & Li, S. (2019). Real-time demonstration of a mHealth app designed to reduce college students hazardous drinking. *Psychological Services*, *16*(2), 255–259. doi:10.1037er0000310 PMID:30407059

Kazevman, G., Mercado, M., Hulme, J., & Somers, A. (2021). Prescribing phones to address health equity needs in the COVID-19 era: The phone-connect program. *Journal of Medical Internet Research*, *23*(4), e23914. https://doi.org/10.2196/23914

Keating, A. (2020). The history of the birth control pill. *Journal of Undergraduate Social Work Research*, *4*(2), 13–23.

Keifenheim, K. E., Teufel, M., Ip, J., Speiser, N., Leehr, E. J., Zipfel, S., & Herrmann-Werner, A. (2015). Teaching history taking to medical students: A systematic review. *BMC Medical Education*, *15*(1), 159. doi:10.118612909-015-0443-x PMID:26415941

Keller, J. M. (2009). *Motivational design for learning and performance: The arcs model approach*. ProQuest Ebook Central. https://ebookcentral.proquest.com

Kernot, J., Lewis, L. K., Olds, T., & Maher, C. (2019). Effectiveness of a Facebook-delivered physical activity intervention for postpartum women: A randomized controlled trial. *Journal of Physical Activity & Health, 16*(2), 125–133. doi:10.1123/jpah.2017-0573

Keyser, B. B., & Broadbear, J. T. (2010). The paradigm shift toward thinking for thinking: Perspectives, barriers, solutions, and accountability. In J. M. Black, S. Furney, H. M. Graf, & A. E. Nolte (Eds.), *Philosophical foundations of health education* (pp. 109–118). Jossey-Bass.

Khlaif, Z. N., Salha, S., Fareed, S., & Rashed, H. (2021). The hidden shadow of coronavirus on education in developing countries. *Online Learning, 25*(1), 269–285. doi:10.24059/olj.v25i1.2287

Kim, H. Y. (2011). International graduate students' difficulties: Graduate classes as a community of practices. *Teaching in Higher Education, 16*(3), 281–292. doi:10.1080/13562517.2010.524922

Kip, H., & van Gemert-Pijnen, L. J. (2018). Holistic development of eheatlh technology. In eHealth research, theory and development (pp. 131-166). Routledge.

Kirkpatrick, J. D., & Kayser, W. (2016). *Kirkpatrick's four levels of training evaluation.* Association For Talent Development. https://login.pallas2.tcl.sc.edu/login?url=https://search.ebscohost.com/login.aspx?direct=true&db=e025xna&AN=1364594&site=ehost-live

Kirkpatrick, J. D., & Kirkpatrick, W. K. (2016). *Kirkpatrick's four levels of training evaluation.* Association for Talent Development.

Klainin-Yobas, P., Kowitlawakul, Y., Lopez, V., Tang, C. T., Hoek, K. E., Gan, G. L., Lei, F., Rawtaer, I., & Mahendran, R. (2019). The effects of mindfulness and health education programs on the emotional state and cognitive function of elderly individuals with mild cognitive impairment: A randomized controlled trial. *Journal of Clinical Neuroscience, 68*, 211–217. doi:10.1016/j.jocn.2019.05.031 PMID:31303397

Kluge, E.-H. W. (2011). e-Health promises and challenges: Some ethical considerations. *Studies in Health Technology and Informatics, 164*, 148–153. PMID:21335703

Knowles, M. S., Holton, E. F., & Swanson, R. A. (1998). *The Adult Learner: the Definitive Classic in Adult Education and Human Resource Development.* Gulf Publishing Company.

Koehler, M. J., & Mishra, P. (2009). What is technological pedagogical content knowledge? *Contemporary Issues in Technology & Teacher Education, 9*, 60–70.

Koivisto, J., & Hamari, J. (Eds.). (2019). *GamiFIN conference.* https://trepo.tuni.fi/bitstream/han dle/10024/117608/Gamification_of_physical_activity_2019.pdf?sequence=2

Koivunen, M., & Saranto, K. (2018). Nursing professionals' experiences of the facilitators and barriers to the use of telehealth applications: A systematic review of qualitative studies. *Scandinavian Journal of Caring Sciences, 32*(1), 24–44. https://doi.org/10.1111/scs.12445

Kok, G., Gottlieb, N. H., Peters, G. Y., Mullen, P. D., Parcel, G. S., Ruiter, R. A. C., Fernandez, M. E., Markham, C., & Bartholomew, L. K. (2016). A taxonomy of beahaviour change methods: An intervention mapping approach. *Health Psychology Review, 10*(3), 297–312. doi:10.1080/17437199.2015.1077155

Kononowicz, A. A., Woodham, L. A., Edelbring, S., Stathakarou, N., Davies, D., Saxena, N., Tudor Car, L., Carlstedt-Duke, J., Car, J., & Zary, N. (2019). Virtual patient simulations in health professions education: Systematic review and meta-analysis by the digital health education collaboration. *Journal of Medical Internet Research, 21*(7), e14676. doi:10.2196/14676 PMID:31267981

Krathwohl, D. R. (2002). A revision of Bloom's taxonomy: An overview. *Theory into Practice*, *41*(4), 212–218. doi:10.120715430421tip4104_2

Krebs, P., & Duncan, D. T. (2015). Health app use among US mobile phone owners: A national survey. *JMIR mHealth and uHealth*, *3*(4), e4924. doi:10.2196/mhealth.4924 PMID:26537656

Kreps, G. L., & Neuhauser, L. (2010). New directions in eHealth communication: Opportunities and challenges. *Patient Education and Counseling*, *78*(3), 329–336. doi:10.1016/j.pec.2010.01.013 PMID:20202779

Kroll, N. L., Sanchez-Jones, T., Atchley, M. D., & Etcher, L. A. (2021). COVID-19 and the golden years. *The Nurse Practitioner*, *46*(6), 37–42. doi:10.1097/01.NPR.0000743320.82081.6a PMID:34004640

Kruse, C. S., Bouffard, S., Dougherty, M., & Parro, J. S. (2016). Telemedicine use in rural Native American communities in the era of the ACA: A systematic literature review. *Journal of Medical Systems*, *40*(6). https://doi.org/10.1007/s10916-016-0503-8

Kruse, C. S., Karem, P., Shifflett, K., Vegi, L., Ravi, K., & Brooks, M. (2018). Evaluating barriers to adopting telemedicine worldwide: A systematic review. *Journal of Telemedicine and Telecare*, *24*(1), 4–12.

Kumar Basak, S., Wotto, M., & Bélanger, P. (2018). e-Learning, m-learning and d-learning: Conceptual definition and comparative analysis. *E-Learning and Digital Media*, *15*(4), 191–216. doi:10.1177/2042753018785180

Labonté, R. (2016). Health promotion in an age of normative equity and rampant inequality. *International Journal of Health Policy and Management*, *5*(12), 675–682. doi:10.15171/ijhpm.2016.95 PMID:28005546

Ladson-Billings, G., & Tate, W. F. (2016). Toward a Critical Race Theory of education. In *Critical Race Theory in Education* (pp. 10–31). Routledge.

Lakshin, G., Banek, S., Keese, D., Rolle, U., & Schmedding, A. (2021). Telemedicine in pediatric surgery in Germany during the COVID-19 pandemic. *Pediatric Surgery International*, *37*(3), 389–395. https://doi.org/10.1007/s00383-020-04822-w

Laskaris, D., Kalogiannakis, M., & Heretakis, E. (2017). "Interactive evaluation" of an e-learning course within the context of blended education. *International Journal of Technology Enhanced Learning*, *9*(4), 339–353. doi:10.1504/IJTEL.2017.087793

Lattie, E. G., Adkins, E. C., Winquist, N., Stiles-Shields, C., Wafford, Q. E., & Graham, A. K. (2019). Digital mental health interventions for depression, anxiety, and enhancement of psychological well-being among college students: Systematic review. *Journal of Medical Internet Research*, *21*(7), e12869. doi:10.2196/12869 PMID:31333198

Lave, J., & Wenger, E. (1991). Legitimate peripheral participation. *Situated Learning: Legitimate Peripheral Participation, 1*, 29-43.

Law, L. M., & Wason, J. M. (2014). Design of telehealth trials–introducing adaptive approaches. *International Journal of Medical Informatics*, *83*(12), 870–880.

Leahey, T. M., Kumar, R., Weinberg, B. M., & Wing, R. R. (2012). Teammates and social influence affect weight loss outcomes in a team-based weight loss competition. *Obesity (Silver Spring, Md.)*, *20*, 1413–1418. doi:10.1038/oby.2012.18

Lee, J., & Jang, S. (2014). A methodological framework for instructional design model development: Critical dimensions and synthesized procedures. *Educational Technology Research and Development*, *62*(6), 743–765. doi:10.100711423-014-9352-7

Lee, M. H., Wu, H. C., Tseng, C. M., Ko, T. L., Weng, T. J., & Chen, Y. F. (2018). Health education and symptom flare management using a video-based m-health system for caring women with IC/BPS. *Urology, 119*, 62–69. doi:10.1016/j.urology.2018.05.027 PMID:29894774

Lee, R., & Chitnis, C. (2018, December). Improving Health-Care Systems by Disease Prediction. In *2018 International Conference on Computational Science and Computational Intelligence (CSCI)* (pp. 726-731). IEEE. 10.1109/CSCI46756.2018.00145

Lee, S. H., Nurmatov, U. B., Nwaru, B. I., Mukherjee, M., Grant, L., & Pagliari, C. (2016). Effectiveness of mHealth interventions for maternal, newborn and child health in low–and middle–income countries: Systematic review and meta–analysis. *Journal of Global Health, 6*(1), 010401. doi:10.7189/jogh.06.010401 PMID:26649177

Lee, S., Black, D., & Held, M. L. (2019). Factors associated with telehealth service utilization among rural populations. *Journal of Healthcarefor the Poor and Underserved, 30*(4), 1259–1272. https://doi.org/10.1353/hpu.2019.0104

Lee, Y., Kozar, K. A., & Larsen, K. R. T. (2003). The technology acceptance model: Past, present, and future. *Communications of the Association for Information Systems, 12*, 50. Advance online publication. doi:10.17705/1CAIS.01250

Leh, A. S. (2005). Lessons learned from service learning and reverse mentoring in faculty development: A case study in technology training. *Journal of Technology and Teacher Education, 13*(1), 25–41.

Lemberger-Truelove, M. E., Carbonneau, K. J., Atencio, D. J., Zieher, A. K., & Palacios, A. F. (2018). Self-regulatory growth effects for young children participating in a combined social and emotional learning and mindfulness-based intervention. *Journal of Counseling and Development, 96*(3), 289–302. doi:10.1002/jcad.12203

Leung, L., & Chen, C. (2019). E-health/m-health adoption and lifestyle improvements: Exploring the roles of technology readiness, the expectation-confirmation model, and health-related information activities. *Telecommunications Policy, 43*(6), 563–575. doi:10.1016/j.telpol.2019.01.005

Lewis, P. J. (2016). Brain Friendly teaching – Reducing Learners' Cognitive Load. *Academic Radiology, 23*(7), 877-880.

Lieneck, C., Weaver, E., & Maryon, T. (2021). Outpatient telehealth implementation in the United States during the COVID-19 global pandemic: A systematic review. *Medicina, 57*(5), 462. doi:10.3390/medicina57050462

Liew, M. S., Zhang, J., See, J., & Ong, Y. L. (2019). Usability challenges for health and wellness mobile apps: Mixed-methods study among mHealth experts and consumers. *JMIR mHealth and uHealth, 7*(1), e12160. doi:10.2196/12160 PMID:30698528

Lillibridge, S. R., Noji, E. K., & Burkle, F. M. Jr. (1993). Disaster assessment: The emergency health evaluation of a population affected by a disaster. *Annals of Emergency Medicine, 22*(11), 1715–1720. doi:10.1016/S0196-0644(05)81311-3 PMID:8214862

Linn, M. C. (1995). Designing computer learning environments for engineering and computer science: The scaffolded knowledge integration framework. *Journal of Science Education and Technology, 4*(2), 103–126. doi:10.1007/BF02214052

Liu, Z., & Wassyng, A. (Eds.). (2012). *Foundations of Health Informatics Engineering and Systems: First International Symposium, FHIES 2011, Johannesburg, South Africa, August 29-30, 2011. Revised Selected Papers (Vol. 7151)*. Springer. 10.1007/978-3-642-32355-3

Lloyd-Jones, D. M., Hong, Y., Labarthe, D., Mozaffarian, D., Appel, L. J., Van Horn, L., Greenlund, K., Daniels, S., Nichol, G., Tomaselli, G. F., Arnett, D. K., Fonarow, G. C., Ho, P. M., Lauer, M. S., Masoudi, F. A., Robertson, R. M., Roger, V., Schwamm, L. H., Sorlie, P., ... Rosamond, W. D. (2010). Defining and setting national goals for cardiovascular health promotion and disease reduction: The American Heart Association's strategic Impact Goal through 2020 and beyond. *Circulation, 121*(4), 586–613. doi:10.1161/CIRCULATIONAHA.109.192703 PMID:20089546

Locke, E. A., & Latham, G. P. (2006). New directions in goal-setting theory. *Current Directions in Psychological Science, 15*(5), 265–268. doi:10.1111/j.1467-8721.2006.00449.x

Lucchini, R. G., Hashim, D., Acquilla, S., Basanets, A., Bertazzi, P. A., Bushmanov, A., Crane, M., Harrison, D. J., Holden, W., Landrigan, P. J., Luft, B. J., Mocarelli, P., Mazitova, N., Melius, J., Moline, J. M., Mori, K., Prezant, D., Reibman, J., Reissman, D. B., ... Todd, A. C. (2017). A comparative assessment of major international disasters: The need for exposure assessment, systematic emergency preparedness, and lifetime health care. *BMC Public Health, 17*(1), 1–12. doi:10.118612889-016-3939-3 PMID:28061835

Ludden, G. D. S., van Rompay, T. J. L., Kelders, S. M., & van Gemert-Pijnen, J. E. W. C. (2015). How to increase reach and adherence of web-based interventions: A design research viewpoint. *Journal of Medical Internet Research, 17*(7), e172. Advance online publication. doi:10.2196 /jmir.4201

Lupton, D. (2014). Apps as artefacts: Towards a critical perspective on mobile health and medical apps. *Societies (Basel, Switzerland), 4*(4), 606–622. doi:10.3390oc4040606

Luszczynska, A., & Schwarzer, R. (2005). Social cognitive theory. In M. Conner & P. Norman (Eds.), Predicting health behaviour: Research and practice with social cognition models (pp. 127-169). Open University Press.

Lyles, C. R., Wachter, R. M., & Sarkar, U. (2021). Focusing on digital health equity. *Journal of the American Medical Association, 326*(18), 1795–1796.

Lyon, A. R., & Koerner, K. (2016). User-centered design for psychosocial intervention development and implementation. *Clinical Psychology: Science and Practice, 23*(2), 180–200. doi:10.1111/cpsp.12154 PMID:29456295

Machine Learning in Python. (n.d.). https://scikit-learn.org/

Madden, E. F. (2019). Intervention stigma: How medication-assisted treatment marginalizes patients and providers. *Social Science & Medicine, 232*, 324–331. doi:10.1016/j.socscimed.2019.05.027 PMID:31125801

Madigan, S., Racine, N., Cooke, J. E., & Korczak, D. J. (2021). COVID-19 and telemental health: Benefits, challenges, and future directions. *Canadian Psychology, 62*(1), 5–11. doi:10.1037/cap0000259

Magid, D. J., Olson, K. L., Billups, S. J., Wagner, N. M., Lyons, E. E., & Kroner, B. A. (2013). A pharmacist-led, American Heart Association Heart360 Web-enabled home blood pressure monitoring program. *Circulation: Cardiovascular Quality and Outcomes, 6*(2), 157–163. doi:10.1161/CIRCOUTCOMES.112.968172 PMID:23463811

Magnan, R. E., Shorey Fennell, B. R., & Brady, J. M. (2017). Health decision making and behavior: The role of affect-laden constructs. *Social & Personality Psychology Compass, 11*(8). doi:10.1111/spc3.12333

Magnani, J. W., Mujahid, M. S., Aronow, H. D., Cené, C. W., Dickson, V. V., Havranek, E., Morgenstern, L. B., Paasche-Orlow, M. K., Pollak, A., & Willey, J. Z. (2018). Health literacy and cardiovascular disease: fundamental relevance to primary and secondary prevention: a scientific statement from the American Heart Association. *Circulation, 138*(2), e48–e74. doi:10.1161/CIR.0000000000000579 PMID:29866648

Maher, C. F., Ferguson, M., Vandelanotte, C., Plotnikoff, R., De Bourdeaudhuij, I., Thomas, S., Nelson-Field, K., & Olds, T. (2015). A web-based, social networking physical activity intervention for insufficiently active adults delivered via Facebook app: Randomized controlled trial. *Journal of Medical Internet Research, 17*(7), e174. Advance online publication. doi:10.2196/jmir.4086

Maiman, L. A., & Becker, M. H. (1974). The health belief model: Origins and correlates in psychological theory. In M. H. Becker (Ed.), *The health belief model and personal health behavior* (pp. 9–26). Charles B. Slack. doi:10.1177/109019817400200404

Mao, C. M., & Hovick, S. R. (2020). Adding Affordances and Communication Efficacy to the Technology Acceptance Model to Study the Messaging Features of Online Patient Portals among Young Adults. *Health Communication*, 1–9. PMID:33243017

Mao, J. Y., Vredenburg, K., Smith, P. W., & Carey, T. (2005). The state of user-centered design practice. *Communications of the ACM, 48*(3), 105–109. doi:10.1145/1047671.1047677

Margolis, K. L., Asche, S. E., Bergdall, A. R., Dehmer, S. P., Groen, S. E., Kadrmas, H. M., Kerby, T. J., Klotzle, K. J., Maciosek, M. V., Michels, R. D., O'Connor, P. J., Pritchard, R. A., Sekenski, J. L., Sperl-Hillen, J. A. M., & Trower, N. K. (2013). Effect of home blood pressure telemonitoring and pharmacist management on blood pressure control: A cluster randomized clinical trial. *Journal of the American Medical Association, 310*(1), 46–56. doi:10.1001/jama.2013.6549 PMID:23821088

Martin, B. L., & Reigeluth, C. M. (1999). Affective education and the affective domain: Implications for instructional-design theories and models. In C. M. Reigeluth (Ed.), Instructional design theories and models (vol. 2, pp. 485-509). Lawrence Erlbaum Associates.

Martinelli, S. M., Chen, F., Isaak, R. S., Huffmyer, J. L., Neves, S. E., & Mitchell, J. D. (2021). Educating Anesthesiologists During the Coronavirus Disease 2019 Pandemic and Beyond. *Anesthesia and Analgesia, 132*(3), 585–593. doi:10.1213/ANE.0000000000005333 PMID:33201006

Martínez-Pérez, B., De La Torre-Díez, I., & López-Coronado, M. (2013). Mobile health applications for the most prevalent conditions by the World Health Organization: Review and analysis. *Journal of Medical Internet Research, 15*(6), e2600. doi:10.2196/jmir.2600 PMID:23770578

Mateo, G. F., Granado-Font, E., Ferre-Grau, C., & Montana-Carreras, X. (2015). Mobile phone apps to promote weight loss and increase physical activity: A systematic review and meta-analysis. *Journal of Medical Internet Research, 17*(11), e253. Advance online publication. doi:10.2196/jmir.4836

Matplotlib Library in Python. (n.d.). https://matplotlib.org/

Matsumoto, M., Koike, S., Kashima, S., & Awai, K. (2015). Geographic distribution of radiologists and utilization of teleradiology in Japan: A longitudinal analysis based on National Census Data. *PLoS One, 10*(9), e0139723. doi:10.1371/journal.pone.0139723 PMID:26421721

Mayer, R. E. (2008). Applying the science of learning: Evidence-based principles for the design of multimedia instruction. *The American Psychologist, 63*(8), 760–769. doi:10.1037/0003-066X.63.8.760 PMID:19014238

Mayer, R. E., & Chandler, P. (2001). When learning is just a click away: Does simple user interaction foster deeper understanding of multimedia messages? *Journal of Educational Psychology, 93*(2), 390–397. doi:10.1037/0022-0663.93.2.390

McAuley, E., & Blissmer, B. (2000). Self-efficacy determinants and consequences of physical activity. *Exercise and Sport Sciences Reviews, 28*(2), 85–88.

McEwan, D., Rhodes, R. E., & Beauchamp, M. R. (2020). What happens when the party is over? Sustaining physical activity behaviors after intervention cessation. *Behavioral Medicine (Washington, D.C.)*, *48*(1), 1–9. doi:10.1080/08964289.2020.1750335

McGuire, W. J. (1981). Behavioral medicine, public health and communication theories. *Health Education*, *12*(3), 8–13. doi:10.1080/00970050.1981.10618148 PMID:6792134

McLaughlin, J. E., Wolcott, M., Hubbard, D., Umstead, K., & Rider, T. R. (2019). A qualitative review of the design thinking framework in health professions education. *BMC Medical Education*, *19*(1), 98. doi:10.118612909-019-1528-8 PMID:30947748

McLeroy, K. R., Bibeau, D., Steckler, A., & Glanz, K. (1988). An ecological perspective on health promotion programs. *Health Education Quarterly*, *15*(4), 351–377. doi:10.1177/109019818801500401 PMID:3068205

McMillan, C., Loads, D., & McQueen, H. A. (2018). From students to scientists: The impact of interactive engagement in lectures. *New Directions in the Teaching of Physical Sciences*, (13).

McQueen, S., McKinnon, V., VanderBeek, L., McCarthy, C., & Sonnadara, R. (2019). Video-based assessment in surgical education: A scoping review. *Journal of Surgical Education*, *76*(6), 1645–1654. doi:10.1016/j.jsurg.2019.05.013 PMID:31175065

Mehall, S. (2021). Purposeful interpersonal interaction and the point of diminishing returns for graduate learners. *The Internet and Higher Education*, *48*, 100774. Advance online publication. doi:10.1016/j.iheduc.2020.100774

Meier, C. A., Fitzgerald, M. C., & Smith, J. M. (2013). eHealth: Extending, enhancing, and evolving health care. *Annual Review of Biomedical Engineering*, *15*(1), 359–382. doi:10.1146/annurev-bioeng-071812-152350 PMID:23683088

Mental Health First Aid. (2022). *About MHFA*. https://www.mentalhealthfirstaid.org/about/

Merriam, S. B., & Bierema, L. L. (2014). *Adult learning: Linking theory and practice*. Jossey-Bass.

Meyers, W. A. (2019). C if for cookie: Is the EU's new 'cookie law' good enough to protect my data? *International Lawyer*, *52*(3), 491–514.

Mezuk, B., & Allen, J. (2021). Rethinking the goals of diabetes prevention programs. *Diabetes Care*, *44*(11), 2457–2459. doi:10.2337/dci21-0038

Michie, S., & Prestwich, A. (2010). Are interventions theory-based? Development of a theory coding scheme. *Health Psychology: Official Journal of the Division of Health Psychology, American Psychological Association*, *29*(1), 1–8. doi:10.1037/a0016939 PMID:20063930

Michie, S., Richardson, M., Johnston, M., Abraham, C., Francis, J., Hardeman, W., Eccles, M. P., Cane, J., & Wood, C. E. (2013). The behavior change technique taxonomy (v1) of 93 hierarchically clustered techniques: Building an international consensus for the reporting of behavior change interventions. *Annals of Behavioral Medicine*, *46*(1), 81–95. doi:10.1 00712160-013-9486-6

Michie, S., Yardley, L., West, R., Patrick, K., & Greaves, F. (2017). Developing and evaluating digital interventions to promote behavior change in health and health care: Recommendations resulting from an international workshop. *Journal of Medical Internet Research*, *19*(6), e232. doi:10.2196/jmir.7126 PMID:28663162

Miller, W. R., & Rollnick, S. (2002). *Motivational interviewing: Preparing people for change*. Book Review.

Mills, K. A., & Godley, A. (2017). Race and racism in digital media: What can Critical Race Theory contribute to research on techno-cultures? In *Handbook of writing, literacies, and education in digital cultures*. Routledge. https://acuresearchbank.acu.edu.au/download/301a941263cff02cedb052d909d0ef4cdb109b0549084c9102e2f5c49cd7d221/152464/AM_Mills_2017_Race_and_racism_in_digital_media.pdf

Milsom, K. M., Jones, C., Kearney-Mitchell, P., & Tickle, M. (2009). A comparative needs assessment of the dental health of adults attending dental access centres and general dental practices in Halton & St Helens and Warrington PCTs 2007. *British Dental Journal*, *206*(5), 257–261. doi:10.1038j.bdj.2009.165 PMID:19287420

Molenda, M. (2003). In search of the elusive ADDIE model. *Performance Improvement*, *42*(5), 34–36. doi:10.1002/pfi.4930420508

Molenda, M. H. (2020). *The elements of instruction: A framework for the age of emerging technologies*. Routledge. doi:10.4324/9781315194721

Monaco, A., Palmer, K., Faber, N. H. R., Kohler, I., Silva, M., Vatland, A., van Griensven, J., Votta, M., Walsh, D., & Clay, V. (2021). Digital health tools for managing noncommunicable diseases during and after the COVID-19 pandemic: Perspectives of patients and caregivers. *Journal of Medical Internet Research*, *23*(1), e25652. doi:10.2196/25652 PMID:33464206

Monroe, C. M., Geraci, M., Turner-McGrievy, G., Wallace, K., Jake-Schoffman, D. E., Bucko, A., & Brazendale, K. (2019, June). *Leveraging a social network approach via gamification and mobile technology to increase physical activity among adults: a cluster randomized controlled trial* [Conference presentation]. International Society of Behavioral Nutrition and Physical Activity Annual Meeting, Prague, Czech Republic.

Monroe, C. M., Bassett, D. R. Jr, Fitzhugh, E. C., Raynor, H. A., & Thompson, D. L. (2017). Effect of adding online social support tools to an adult walking program: A pilot randomized controlled trial. *Health Promotion Practice*, *18*(1), 84–92. doi:10.1177/1524839915626 674

Monroe, C. M., Geraci, M., Larsen, C. A., & West, D. S. (2019). Feasibility and efficacy of a novel technology-based approach to harness social networks for weight loss: The NETworks pilot randomized controlled trial. *Obesity Science & Practice*, *5*(4), 354–365. doi:10. 1002/osp4.352

Monroe, C. M., Thompson, D. L., Bassett, D. R. Jr, Fitzhugh, E. C., & Raynor, H. A. (2015). Usability of mobile phones in physical activity-related research: A systematic review. *American Journal of Health Education*, *46*, 196–206. doi:10.1080/19325037.2015.1044141

Morgan, H. (2020). Best practices for implementing remote learning during a pandemic. *The Clearing House: A Journal of Educational Strategies, Issues and Ideas*, *93*(3), 135–141. doi:10.1080/00098655.2020.1751480

Morrison, M. (2006). *SWOT Analysis*. https://www.rapidbi.com/history-of-the-swot-analysis/

Morrison, G. R., Ross, S. M., Kalman, H. K., & Kemp, J. E. (2013). *Designing effective instruction*. Wiley & Sons, Inc.

Morrison, L. G. (2015). Theory-based strategies for enhancing the impact and usage of digital health behaviour change interventions: A review. *Digital Health*, *1*. doi:10.1177/2055207615595335 PMID:29942544

Morris, T. H. (2020). Transformative learning through mindfulness: Exploring the mechanism of change. *Australian Journal of Adult Learning*, *60*(1), 44–65.

Moss, R. J., Süle, A., & Kohl, S. (2019). eHealth and mHealth. *European Journal of Hospital Pharmacy. Science and Practice*, *26*(1), 57–58. doi:10.1136/ejhpharm-2018-001819 PMID:31157099

Mustafa, A., & Rahimi Azghadi, M. (2021). Automated Machine Learning for Healthcare and Clinical Notes Analysis. *Computers*, *10*(2), 24. doi:10.3390/computers10020024

Nacinovich, M. (2011). Defining mhealth. *Journal of Communication in Healthcare*, *4*(1), 1–3. doi:10.1179/175380611X12950033990296

Nadal, C., Sas, C., & Doherty, G. (2020). Technology acceptance in mobile health: Scoping review of definitions, models, and measurement. *Journal of Medical Internet Research*, *22*(7), e17256. doi:10.2196/17256 PMID:32628122

National Alliance on Mental Illness. (2021). *COVID-19 resource and information guide.* https://nami.org/Support-Education/NAMI-HelpLine/COVID-19-Information-and-Resources/COVID-19-Resource-and-Information-Guide#q18

National Council on Disability. (2017). *Mental health on college campuses: investments, accommodations needed to address student needs.* ncd.gov/sites/default/files/NCD_Mental_Health_Report_508.pdf

National Human Genome Research Institute (NHGRI). (2020, Dec 22). *The human genome project.* https://www.genome.gov/human-genome-project

National Institute for Standards and Measures. (2021). *Malcolm Baldridge National Quality Award.* https://www.nist.gov/baldrige/baldrige-award

National Research Council. (1997). Privacy and Security Concerns Regarding Electronic Health Information. In *For the Record Protecting Electronic Health Information*. National Academies Press.

Ng, L., Seow, K. C., MacDonald, L., Correia, C., Reubenson, A., Gardner, P., Spence, A. L., Bunzli, S., & De Oliveira, B. (2021). eLearning in Physical Therapy: Lessons Learned From Transitioning a Professional Education Program to Full eLearning During the COVID-19 Pandemic. *Physical Therapy*, *101*(4), pzab082. doi:10.1093/ptj/pzab082

Nisha, N., Iqbal, M., & Rifat, A. (2019). The changing paradigm of health and mobile phones: An innovation in the health care system. *Journal of Global Information Management*, *27*(1), 19–46. doi:10.4018/JGIM.2019010102

Nixon, E. K., & Lee, D. (2001). Rapid prototyping in the instructional design process. *Performance Improvement Quarterly*, *14*(3), 95–116. doi:10.1111/j.1937-8327.2001.tb00220.x

Noesgaard, S.S., & Ørngreen, R. (2015). The effectiveness of e-learning: An explorative and integrative review of the definitions, methodologies and factors that promote e-Learning effectiveness. *Electronic Journal of e-Learning*, *13*(4), 278-290.

Noetel, M., Griffith, S., Delaney, O., Sanders, T., Parker, P., del Pozo Cruz, B., & Lonsdale, C. (2021). Video improves learning in higher education: A systematic review. *Review of Educational Research*, *91*(2), 204–236. doi:10.3102/0034654321990713

Norman, D. (2013). *The design of everyday things*. Basic books.

Nutbeam, D. (2008). The evolving concept of health literacy. *Social Science & Medicine*, *67*(12), 2072–2078. doi:10.1016/j.socscimed.2008.09.050 PMID:18952344

Nutbeam, D. O. N. (1998). Health promotion glossary. *Health Promotion International*, *13*(4), 349–364. doi:10.1093/heapro/13.4.349

O'Brien Pott, M., Blanshan, A. S., Huneke, K. M., Baasch Thomas, B. L., & Cook, D. A. (2020). What influences choice of continuing medical education modalities and providers? A National Survey of U.S. physicians, nurse practitioners, and physician assistants. *Academic Medicine*, *96*(1), 93–100. doi:10.1097/ACM.0000000000003758 PMID:32969838

O'Connor, S. M. (2020). *Exploring eHealth implementation: understanding factors affecting engagement and enrolment in consumer digital health* (Doctoral dissertation). University of Glasgow.

OECD. (2010). *Improving health sector efficiency, the role of information and communication technologies*. OECD.

Oehler, R. L., Smith, K., & Toney, J. F. (2010). Infectious diseases resources for the iPhone. *Clinical Infectious Diseases*, *50*(9), 1268–1274. doi:10.1086/651602 PMID:20233061

Office of the Vice President for Research. (n.d.). *ASPIRE*. https://sc.edu/about/offices_and_divi sions/research/internal_funding_awards/faculty/aspire/

Ogedegbe, G., Ravenell, J., Adhikari, S., Butler, M., Cook, T., Francois, F., ... Horwitz, L. I. (2020). Assessment of racial/ethnic disparities in hospitalization and mortality in patients with COVID-19 in New York City. *JAMA Network Open*, *3*(12), e2026881–e2026881.

Oh, H., Rizo, C., Enkin, M., Jadad, A., Powell, J., & Pagliari, C. (2005). What is ehealth (3): A Systematic review of published definitions. *Journal of Medical Internet Research*, *7*(1), e1. doi:10.2196/jmir.7.1.e1 PMID:15829471

Oinas-Kukkonen, H., & Harjumaa, M. (2009). Persuasive systems design: Key issues, process model, and system features. *Communications of the Association for Information Systems*, *24*. Advance online publication. doi:10.17705/1CAIS.02428

Okunogbe, A., Nugent, R., Spencer, G., Ralston, J., & Wilding, J. (2021). Economic impacts of overweight and obesity: Current and future estimates for eight countries. *BMJ Global Health*, *6*(10), e006351. Advance online publication. doi:10.1136/bmjgh-2021-006351

Otto, L., Harst, L., Timpel, P., Wollschlaeger, B., Richter, P., & Schlieter, H. (2020). Defining and delimitating telemedicine and related terms - An ontology-based classification. *Studies in Health Technology and Informatics*, *268*, 113–122. https://doi-org.pallas2.tcl.sc.edu/10.3233/SHTI200010 PMID:32141883

Oyedotun, T. D. (2020). Sudden change of pedagogy in education driven by COVID-19: Perspectives and evaluation from a developing country. *Research in Globalization*, *2*(100029), 100029. Advance online publication. doi:10.1016/j.resglo.2020.100029

Padilla Rodríguez, B. C., Armellini, A., & Traxler, J. (2021). The forgotten ones: How rural teachers in Mexico are facing the COVID-19 pandemic. *Online Learning*, *25*(1), 253–268. doi:10.24059/olj.v25i1.2453

Pagliari, C., Sloan, D., Gregor, P., Sullivan, F., Detmer, D., Kahan, J. P., Oortwijn, W., & MacGillivray, S. (2005). What Is eHealth (4): A scoping exercise to map the field. *Journal of Medical Internet Research*, *7*(1), e9. doi:10.2196/jmir.7.1.e9 PMID:15829481

Palfrey, C. (2018). The future of health promotion. In *The Future for Health Promotion* (1st ed., pp. 25–54). Bristol University Press., doi:10.2307/j.ctt22rbkdc.6

Pan, Scott, & Phillips. (2021). Using Learning Experience Design to Optimize Digital Instruction During COVID-19 and Beyond. *Academic Medicine, 96*(5). doi:10.1097/ACM.0000000000003889

Panch, T., Szolovits, P., & Atun, R. (2018). Artificial intelligence, machine learning and health systems. *Journal of Global Health*, *8*(2), 020303. doi:10.7189/jogh.08.020303 PMID:30405904

Papadopoulos, D. (2020). Effect of a social-emotional learning-based program on self-esteem and self-perception of gifted kindergarten students: A pilot study. *Journal for the Education of Gifted Young Scientists*. doi:10.17478/jegys.779438

Papandrea, P. (2019). Addressing the HIPAA-potamus sized gap in wearable technology regulation. *Minnesota Law Review*. https://minnesotalawreview.org/wp-content/uploads/2019/12/Papandrea_FINAL_MLR104-Updated.pdf

Parimbelli, E., Bottalico, B., Losiouk, E., Tomasi, M., Santosuosso, A., Lanzola, G., Quaglini, S., & Bellazzi, R. (2018). Trusting telemedicine: A discussion on risks, safety, legal implications and liability of involved stakeholders. *International Journal of Medical Informatics*, *112*, 90–98. https://doi.org/10.1016/j.ijmedinf.2018.01.012

Patel, M. S., Small, D. S., Harrison, J. D., Fortunato, M. P., Oon, A. L., Rareshide, C. A. L., Reh, G., Szwartz, G., Guszcza, J., Steier, D., Kalra, P., & Hilbert, V. (2019). Effectiveness of behaviorally designed gamification interventions with social incentives for increasing physical activity among overweight and obese adults across the United States: The STEP UP randomized clinical trial. JAMA Internal Medicine, 179(12), 1624-1632. https://doi.org/ed.2019.3505 doi:10.1001/jamainternm

Patel, M. S., Benjamin, E. J., Volpp, K. G., Fox, C. S., Small, D. S., Massaro, J. M., Lee, J. J., Hilbert, V., Valentino, M., Taylor, D. H., Manders, E. S., Mutalik, K., Zhu, J., Wang, W., & Murabito, J. M. (2017). Effect of a game-based intervention designed to enhance social incentives to increase physical activity among families: The BE FIT randomized clinical trial. *JAMA Internal Medicine*, *177*(11), 1586–1593. doi:10.1001/jamainternmed.2017.3458

PatientBond. (2021). *Psychographics: The Key to Motivating Healthcare Consumer Behaviors*. https://www.patientbond.com/psychographics

Patrick, K., Hekler, E., & Estrin, D. (2016). Rapid rate of technological development and its implications for research on digital behavior change interventions. *American Journal of Preventive Medicine*.

Paul, M., & Das, A. (2017). Health informatics as a service (HIAAS) for developing countries. In Internet of Things and big data technologies for next generation healthcare (pp. 251–279). Springer. doi:10.1007/978-3-319-49736-5_11

Paul, M., & Das, A. (2017). Service Level Agreements for Smart Healthcare in Cloud. *International Journal of Grid and High Performance Computing*, *9*(4), 57–70.

Pedersen, C., Halvari, H., & Williams, G. C. (2018). Worksite intervention effects on motivation, physical activity, and health: A cluster randomized controlled trial. *Psychology of Sport and Exercise*, *35*, 171–180. doi:10.1016/j.psychsport.2017.11.004

Peisachovich, E., Da Silva, C., Penhearow, N. J., Sombilon, E. V., & Koh, M. (2020). Implementing virtual simulated person methodology to support the shift to online learning: Technical report. *Cureus*, *12*(6). Advance online publication. doi:10.7759/cureus.8864 PMID:32754403

Pennel, C. L., McLeroy, K. R., Burdine, J. N., & Matarrita-Cascante, D. (2015). Nonprofit hospitals' approach to community health needs assessment. *American Journal of Public Health*, *105*(3), e103–e113. doi:10.2105/AJPH.2014.302286 PMID:25602862

Perera, C. (2012). The evolution of e-health–mobile technology and m-health. *Journal of Mobile Technology in Medicine*, *1*(1), 1–2. doi:10.7309/jmtm.1

Persky, A. M., & Robinson, J. D. (2017). Moving from novice to expertise and its implications for instruction. *American Journal of Pharmaceutical Education*, *81*(9), 6065. doi:10.5688/ajpe6065 PMID:29302087

Pew Research Center. (2021a, April 7). *Internet/broadband fact sheet*. https://www.pewresearch. org/internet/fact-sheet/internet-broadband/

Pew Research Center. (2021b, April 7). *Internet/broadband fact sheet*. https://www.pewresearch. org/internet/fact-sheet/mobile/

Pfefferbaum, B., & North, C. S. (2020). Mental health and the Covid-19 pandemic. *The New England Journal of Medicine*, *383*(6), 510–512. Advance online publication. doi:10.1056/NEJMp2008017 PMID:32283003

Phelps, P., Rodríguez, M. M. D., de la Caridad Alvarez, M., & Johnson, J. L. (2021). Shifts in attitudes and intentions to practice following medication-assisted treatment training. *The Journal of Physician Assistant Education: the Official Journal of the Physician Assistant Education Association*, *32*(3), 182–184. doi:10.1097/JPA.0000000000000368 PMID:34224540

Pierce, R. P., & Stevermer, J. J. (2020). Disparities in use of telehealth at the onset of the COVID-19 public health emergency. *Journal of Telemedicine and Telecare*.

Pieterse, M., Kip, H., & Cruz-Martínez, R. R. (2018). The complexity of ehealth implemetation: A theoretical and pracitcal perspective. In eHealth research, theory and development (pp. 247-270). Routledge.

Popham, W. J. (2017). Objectives. In D. J. Flinders & S. T. Thornton (Eds.), *The curriculum reader* (5th ed., pp. 115–128). Routledge.

Popkin, B. M., Du, S., Green, W. D., Beck, M. A., Algaith, T., Herbst, C. H., Alsukait, R. F., Alluhidan, M., Alazemi, N., & Shekar, M. (2020). Individuals with obesity and COVID-19: A global perspective on the epidemiology and biological relationships. *Obesity Reviews*, *21*, e13128. Advance online publication. doi:10.1111/obr.13128

Porter, C. M. (2016). Revisiting Precede–Proceed: A leading model for ecological and ethical health promotion. *Health Education Journal*, *75*(6), 753–764. doi:10.1177/0017896915619645

Posner, G. J., & Strike, K. A. (1976). A categorization scheme for principles of sequencing content. *Review of Educational Research*, *46*(4), 665–690. doi:10.3102/00346543046004665

Pratt, A., Nunes, J., & Nunes, J. (2012). *Interactive design: An introduction to the theory and application of user-centered design*. Quarto Publishing Group USA.

Prawat, R. S., & Floden, R. E. (1994). Philosophical perspectives on constructivist views of learning. *Educational Psychologist*, *29*(1), 37–48. doi:10.120715326985ep2901_4

Prober, C. G., & Norden, J. G. (2021). Learning Alone or Learning Together: Is It Time to Reevaluate Teacher and Learner Responsibilities? *Academic Medicine*, *96*(2), 170–172. doi:10.1097/ACM.0000000000003741 PMID:32910002

Prochaska, J. O., Redding, C. A., & Evers, K. E. (2008). The transtheoretical model of stages of change. In K. Glanz, B.K. Rimer, & K. Viswanath (Eds.), Health behavior and health education: theory, research, and practice (4th ed., pp. 45-65). Jossey-Bass. Publications, Inc.

Prochaska, J. O., & DiClemente, C. C. (1983). Stages and processes of self-change of smoking: Toward an integrative model of change. *Journal of Consulting and Clinical Psychology*, *51*(3), 390–395. doi:10.1037/0022-006X.51.3.390 PMID:6863699

Prochaska, J. O., & DiClemente, C. C. (1986). Toward a comprehensive model of change. In N. Miller & R. W. Heather (Eds.), *Treating addictive behaviors* (pp. 3–27). Plenum Publishing Corporation. doi:10.1007/978-1-4613-2191-0_1

Prochaska, J. O., & Norcross, J. C. (2001). Stages of change. *Psychotherapy (Chicago, Ill.)*, *38*(4), 443–448. doi:10.1037/0033-3204.38.4.443

Prochaska, J. O., Redding, C. A., & Evers, K. E. (2008). The transtheoretical model and stages of change. In K. Glanz, B. K. Rimer, & K. Viswanath (Eds.), *Health behavior and health education: Theory, research, and practice*. Jossey Bass.

PromotePrevent. (2013). *Who we are*. http://www.promoteprevent.org/about

Puskar, K. R., & Bernardo, L. M. (2007). Mental health and academic achievement: Role of school nurses. *Journal for Specialists in Pediatric Nursing*, *12*(4), 215–223. doi:10.1111/j.1744-6155.2007.00117.x PMID:17956370

Qasim, A., & Patel, J. (2021). *ANCA Positive Vasculitis.* StatPearls Publishing. https://www.ncbi.nlm.nih.gov/books/NBK554372/

Quaosar, G. A. A., Hoque, M. R., & Bao, Y. (2018). Investigating factors affecting elderly's intention to use m-health services: An empirical study. *Telemedicine Journal and e-Health, 24*(4), 309–314. doi:10.1089/tmj.2017.0111 PMID:28976824

Qudah, B., & Luetsch, K. (2019). The influence of mobile health applications on patient-healthcare provider relationships: A systematic, narrative review. *Patient Education and Counseling, 102*(6), 1080–1089. doi:10.1016/j.pec.2019.01.021 PMID:30745178

Qureshi, M., Farooq, A., & Qureshi, M. (2021). *Current ehealth challenges and recent trends in ehealth applications.* https://arxiv.org/ftp/arxiv/papers/2103/2103.01756.pdf

Qureshi, Q. A., Shah, B., Kundi, G. M., Nawaz, A., Miankhel, A. K., Chishti, K. A., & Qureshi, N. A. (2013). Infrastructural barriers to e-health implementation in developing countries. *European Journal of Sustainable Development, 2*(1), 163–163.

Rahman, S., Ramakrishnan, T., & Ngamassi, L. (2019). Impact of social media use on student satisfaction in higher education. *Higher Education Quarterly, 74*(3), 304–319. doi:10.1111/hequ.12228

Raj Westwood, A. (2021). Is hybrid telehealth model the next step for private healthcare in India? *Health Services Insights*, 1–4. doi:10.1177/11786329211043301

Ranga, J. (2018). Multipurpose use of explain everything iPad app for teaching chemistry courses. *Journal of Chemical Education, 95*(5), 895–898. doi:10.1021/acs.jchemed.7b00676

Rannikmäe, M., Holbrook, J., & Soobard, R. (2020). Social Constructivism—Jerome Bruner. In B. Akpan & T. J. Kennedy (Eds.), *Science Education in Theory and Practice. Springer Texts in Education.* Springer. doi:10.1007/978-3-030-43620-9_18

Ratycz, M. C., Papadimos, T. J., & Vanderbilt, A. A. (2018). Addressing the growing opioid and heroin abuse epidemic: A call for medical school curricula. *Medical Education Online, 23*(1), 1466574. doi:10.1080/10872981.2018.1466574 PMID:29708863

Ratz, T., & Lippke, S. (2021). Health Behavior Change. In *Reference Module in Neuroscience and Biobehavioral Psychology*. Elsevier. doi:10.1016/B978-0-12-818697-8.00068-6

Ray, R., & Gibbons, A. (2021, November). *Why are states banning Critical Race Theory?* Brookings. https://www.brookings.edu/blog/fixgov/2021/07/02/why-are-states-banning-critical-race-theory/

Rebar, A. L., Dimmock, J. A., Jackson, B., Rhodes, R. E., Kates, A., Starling, J., & Vandelanotte, C. (2016). A systematic review of the effects of non-conscious regulatory processes in physical activity. *Health Psychology, 10*(4), 395–407. doi:10.1080/ 17437199.2016.1183505

Reigeluth, C. M., & Moor, J. (1999). Cognitive education and the cognitive domain. In C. M. Reigeluth (Ed.), Instructional design theories and models (vol. 2, pp. 5-29). Lawrence Erlbaum Associates.

Reigeluth, C. M., & An, Y. (2021). *Merging the instructional design process with learner-centered theory: The holistic 4D model*. Routledge.

Reynolds, R., & Harel Caperton, I. (2009, April). *Development of high school and community college students' contemporary learning abilities in Globaloria-West Virginia in the first pilot year*. Paper presented at the annual convention of the American Education Research Association, San Diego, CA.

Reynolds, R. (2016). Defining, designing for, and measuring "social constructivist digital literacy" development in learners: A proposed framework. *Educational Technology Research and Development, 64*(4), 735–762. doi:10.100711423-015-9423-4

Rhim, H. C., & Han, H. (2020). Teaching online: Foundational concepts of online learning and practical guidelines. *Korean Journal of Medical Education, 32*(3), 175–183. doi:10.3946/kjme.2020.171 PMID:32894921

Richard-Amato, P. A. (2003). *Making it happen: From interactive to participatory language teaching: Theory and practice*. Pearson.

Richard, L., Gauvin, L., & Raine, K. (2011). Ecological models revisited: Their uses and evolution in health promotion over two decades. *Annual Review of Public Health, 32*, 307–326. doi:10.1146/annurev-publhealth-031210-101141

Richey, R. C., Klein, J. D., & Tracey, M. W. (2011). *The instructional design knowledge base: Theory, research, and practice*. Routledge.

Riegel, B., Moser, D. K., Buck, H. G., Dickson, V. V., Dunbar, S. B., Lee, C. S., Lennie, T. A., Lindenfeld, J., Mitchell, J. E., Treat-Jacobson, D. J., & Webber, D. E. (2017). Self-care for the prevention and management of cardiovascular disease and stroke: A scientific statement for healthcare professionals from the American Heart Association. *Journal of the American Heart Association, 6*(9), e006997. doi:10.1161/JAHA.117.006997 PMID:28860232

Riley, A. R., Chen, Y. H., Matthay, E. C., Glymour, M. M., Torres, J. M., Fernandez, A., & Bibbins-Domingo, K. (2020). Excess death among Latino people in California during the COVID-19 pandemic. *SSM Population Health, 15*. doi:10.1016/j.ssmph.2021.100860

Riley, W. T., Rivera, D. E., Atienza, A. A., Nilsen, W., Allison, S. M., & Mermelstein, R. (2011). Health behavior models in the age of mobile interventions: Are our theories up to the task? *Translational Behavioral Medicine, 1*(1), 53–71. doi:10.100713142-011-0021-7 PMID:21796270

Ritchey, M. D., Maresh, S., McNeely, J., Shaffer, T., Jackson, S. L., Keteyian, S. J., Brawner, C. A., Whooley, M. A., Chang, T., Stolp, H., Schieb, L., & Wright, J. (2020). Tracking cardiac rehabilitation participation and completion among Medicare beneficiaries to inform the efforts of a national initiative. *Circulation: Cardiovascular Quality and Outcomes, 13*(1), e005902. doi:10.1161/CIRCOUTCOMES.119.005902 PMID:31931615

Ritz, L. T., & Buss, A. R. (2016). A framework for aligning instructional design strategies with affordances of CAVE immersive virtual reality systems. *TechTrends, 60*(6), 549–566. doi:10.100711528-016-0085-9

Rivera, V., Aldridge, M. D., Ornstein, K., Moody, K. A., & Chun, A. (2021). Racial and socioeconomic disparities in access to telehealth. *Journal of the American Geriatrics Society, 69*(1), 44–45. https://doi.org/10.1111/jgs.16904

Roane, H. S., & Betz, A. M. (2012). Behavior Analysis. In V. S. Ramachandran (Ed.), *Encyclopedia of Human Behavior* (2nd ed., pp. 267–273). Academic Press. doi:10.1016/B978-0-12-375000-6.00059-8

Robinson, E., Fleming, A., & Higgs, S. (2014). Social norms and weight loss prompting healthier eating: Testing the use of health and social norm based messages. *Health Psychology, 33*(9), 1057–1064. doi:10.1037/a0034213

Robinson, E., Thomas, J., Aveyard, P., & Higgs, S. (2014). What everyone else is eating: A systematic review and meta-analysis of the effect of informational eating norms on eating behavior. *Journal of the Academy of Nutrition and Dietetics, 114*(3), 414–429. doi:10.1016/j.jand.2013.11.009

Rodrigues, R. J. (2008). *Compelling issues for adoption of e-health. In The Commonwealth Health Ministers Reference Book*. Henley Media Group Ltd.

Rogers, T., Milkman, K. L., & Volpp, K. G. Commitment devices: Using initiatives to change behavior. (2014). *JAMA*, *311*(20), 2065-2066. https://doi.org/ doi:10.1001/jama.2014.3485

Roger, V. L., Sidney, S., Fairchild, A. L., Howard, V. J., Labarthe, D. R., Shay, C. M., Tiner, A. C., Whitsel, L. P., Rosamond, W. D., & Committee, A. H. A. A. C. (2020). Recommendations for cardiovascular health and disease surveillance for 2030 and beyond: A policy statement from the American Heart Association. *Circulation*, *141*(9), e104–e119. doi:10.1161/CIR.0000000000000756 PMID:31992050

Rogoff, B. (1990). *Apprenticeship in thinking*. Oxford University Press.

Rose, E. (2004). Instructional Design and Curriculum Development: Deconstructing the Difference. *Educational Technology*, *44*(2), 3–12. https://www.jstor.org/stable/44428883

Rosenstock, I. M. (1974). The historic origins of the health belief model. In M. H. Becker (Ed.), *The health belief model and personal health behavior* (pp. 1–8). Charles B. Slack.

Rosenstock, I. M., Strecher, V. J., & Becker, M. H. (1988). Social learning theory and the health belief model. *Health Education Quarterly*, *15*(2), 175–183. doi:10.1177/109019818801500203 PMID:3378902

Rose, P. R. (2020). *Health equity, diversity, and inclusion: Context, controversies, and solutions*. Jones & Bartlett Learning.

Roth, G. A., Mensah, G. A., Johnson, C. O., Addolorato, G., Ammirati, E., Baddour, L. M., Barengo, N. C., Beaton, A. Z., Benjamin, E. J., Benziger, C. P., Bonny, A., Brauer, M., Brodmann, M., Cahill, T. J., Carapetis, J., Catapano, A. L., Chugh, S. S., Cooper, L. T., Coresh, J., ... Fuster, V. (2020). Global burden of cardiovascular diseases and risk factors, 1990–2019: Update from the GBD 2019 study. *Journal of the American College of Cardiology*, *76*(25), 2982–3021. doi:10.1016/j.jacc.2020.11.010 PMID:33309175

Rouleau, G., Gagnon, M. P., Côté, J., Payne-Gagnon, J., Hudson, E., Dubois, C. A., & Bouix-Picasso, J. (2019). Effects of e-Learning in a continuing education context on nursing care: Systematic review of systematic qualitative, quantitative, and mixed-studies reviews. *Journal of Medical Internet Research*, *21*(10), e15118. doi:10.2196/15118 PMID:31579016

Rowlands, G., Protheroe, J., Winkley, J., Richardson, M., Seed, P. T., & Rudd, R. (2015). A mismatch between population health literacy and the complexity of health information: An observational study. *The British Journal of General Practice*, *65*(635), e379–e386. doi:10.3399/bjgp15X685285 PMID:26009533

Rubenstein, E. (2016). Knowing how to help: Providing health information in public libraries. *Journal of Consumer Health on the Internet*, *20*(3), 114–129. doi:10.1080/15398285.2016.1198111

Rudolph, M., Barr, M. S., Kuhn, T., Hersh, W. R., & McDonald, C. J. (2008). *e-Health and its impact on medical practice*. https://www.acponline.org/advocacy/where_we_stand/policy/ehealth.pdf

Rudolph, M., Barr, M. S., Kuhn, T., Hersh, W. R., & McDonald, C. J. (2008). *E-health and its impact on medical practice*. https://www.acponline.org/advocacy/where_we_stand/policy/ehealth.pdf

Ruggeri, K., Farrington, C., & Brayne, C. (2013). A global model for effective use and evaluation of e-learning in health. *Telemedicine Journal and e-Health*, *19*(4), 312–321. doi:10.1089/tmj.2012.0175 PMID:23472702

Rushing, S. C., & Stephens, D. (2011). Use of media technologies by Native American teens and young adults in the Pacific Northwest: Exploring their utility for designing culturally appropriate technology-based health interventions. *The Journal of Primary Prevention*, *32*(3), 135–145.

Safdari, R., Shams Abadi, A. R., & Pahlevany Nejad, S. (2018). Improve health of the elderly people with M-health and technology. *Iranian Journal of Aging*, *13*(3), 288–299. doi:10.32598ija.13.3.288

Safie, N., & Aljunid, S. (2013). E-learning initiative capacity building for healthcare workforce of developing countries. *Journal of Computational Science*, *9*(5), 583–591. doi:10.3844/jcssp.2013.583.591

Salinas, C. Jr. (2020). The complexity of the "x" in Latinx: How Latinx/a/o students relate to, identify with, and understand the term Latinx. *Journal of Hispanic Higher Education*, *19*(2), 149–168.

Salinas, C. Jr, & Lozano, A. (2019). Mapping and recontextualizing the evolution of the term Latinx: An environmental scanning in higher education. *Journal of Latinos and Education*, *18*(4), 302–315.

Salinas, M., Salinas, N., Duffy, J. R., & Davidson, J. (2020). Do caring behaviors in the quality caring model promote the human emotion of feeling cared for in hospitalized stroke patients and their families? *Applied Nursing Research*, *55*, 151299. doi:10.1016/j.apnr.2020.151299 PMID:32518006

Sallis, J. F., & Owen, N. (2015). Ecological models of health behavior. In Health behavior: Theory, research, and practice (5th ed., pp- 43-64). John Wiley & Sons Incorporated.

Sallis, J. F. (2018). Needs and challenges related to multilevel interventions: Physical activity examples. *Health Education & Behavior*, *45*(5), 661–667. doi:10.1177/109019811879 6458

Sallis, J. F., Grossman, R. M., Pinski, R. B., Patterson, T. L., & Nader, P. R. (1987). The development of scales to measure social support for diet and exercise behaviors. *Preventive Medicine*, *16*, 825–836. doi:10.1016/0091-7435(87)90022-3

Salmoirago-Blotcher, E., Druker, S., Frisard, C., Dunsiger, S. I., Crawford, S., Meleo-Meyer, F., Bock, B., & Pbert, L. (2018). Integrating mindfulness training in school health education to promote healthy behaviors in adolescents: Feasibility and preliminary effects on exercise and dietary habits. *Preventive Medicine Reports*, *9*, 92–95. doi:10.1016/j.pmedr.2018.01.009 PMID:29527459

Salvador, J. G., Bhatt, S. R., Jacobsohn, V. C., Maley, L. A., Alkhafaji, R. S., Rishel Brakey, H., Myers, O. B., & Sussman, A. L. (2020). Feasibility and acceptability of an online ECHO intervention to expand access to medications for treatment of opioid use disorder, psychosocial treatments and supports. *Substance Abuse*, *42*(4), 1–8. PMID:32814005

Salvi, D., Ottaviano, M., Muuraiskangas, S., Martínez-Romero, A., Vera-Muñoz, C., Triantafyllidis, A., Cabrera Umpiérrez, M. F., Arredondo Waldmeyer, M. T., Skobel, E., Knackstedt, C., Liedes, H., Honka, A., Luprano, J., Cleland, J. G. F., Stut, W., & Deighan, C. (2018). An m-Health system for education and motivation in cardiac rehabilitation: The experience of HeartCycle guided exercise. *Journal of Telemedicine and Telecare*, *24*(4), 303–316. doi:10.1177/1357633X17697501 PMID:28350282

Samuel-Hodge, C. D., Holder-Cooper, J. C., Gizlice, Z., Davis, G., Steele, S. P., Keyserling, T. C., Kumanyika, S. K., Brantely, P. J., & Svetkey, L. P. (2017). Family partners in lifestyle support (PALS): Family-based weight loss for African American adults with type 2 diabetes. *Obesity (Silver Spring, Md.)*, *25*, 45–55. doi:10.1002/oby.21700

Sandars, J., Correia, R., Dankbaar, M., de Jong, P., Goh, P. S., Hege, I., Masters, K., Oh, S., Patel, R., Premkumar, K., Webb, A., & Pusic, M. (2020). Twelve tips for rapidly migrating to online learning during the COVID-19 pandemic. *MedEdPublish*, *9*(1), 3068.

Sanders, C. K., & Scanlon, E. (2021). The digital divide is a human rights issue: Advancing social inclusion through social work advocacy. *Journal of Human Rights and Social Work*, 1–14. Advance Online Publication. doi:10.1007/s41134-020-00147-9

Sangrà, A., Vlachopoulos, D., & Cabrera, N. (2012). Building an inclusive definition of e-learning: An approach to the conceptual framework. *The International Review of Research in Open and Distributed Learning*, *13*(2), 145. doi:10.19173/irrodl.v13i2.1161

Santo, K., Richtering, S. S., Chalmers, J., Thiagalingam, A., Chow, C. K., & Redfern, J. (2016). Mobile phone apps to improve medication adherence: A systematic stepwise process to identify high-quality apps. *JMIR mHealth and uHealth*, *4*(4), e6742. doi:10.2196/mhealth.6742 PMID:27913373

Sapra, A., Bhandari, P., & Wilhite Hughes, A. (2021). Diabetes Mellitus (Nursing). StatPearls Publishing.

Sapthiang, S., Van Gordon, W., & Shonin, E. (2019). Health school-based mindfulness interventions for improving mental health: A systematic review and thematic synthesis of qualitative studies. *Journal of Child and Family Studies*, *28*(10), 2650–2658. doi:10.100710826-019-01482-w

Sava, S. (2012). Methods of Needs Analysis in Educational Context. In *Needs Analysis and Programme Planning in Adult Education* (1st ed., pp. 59–119). Verlag Barbara Budrich. doi:10.2307/j.ctvbkjvs2.8

Scarapicchia, T. M. F., Amireault, S., Faulkner, G., & Sabiston, C. M. (2017). Social support and physical activity participation among healthy adults: A systematic review of prospective studies. *International Review of Sport and Exercise Psychology*, *10*(1), 50–83. doi:10.1080/17 50984X.2016.1183222

Scharff, D. P., Mathews, K. J., Jackson, P., Hoffsuemmer, J., Martin, E., & Edwards, D. (2010). More than Tuskegee: Understanding mistrust about research participation. *Journal of Healthcarefor the Poor and Underserved*, *21*(3), 879–897. https://doi.org/10.1353/hpu.0.0323

Schartzstein, R., & Roberts, D. (2017). Saying Goodbye to Lectures in Medical School – Paradigm Shift or Passing Fad? *The New England Journal of Medicine*, *377*(7), 605–607. doi:10.1056/NEJMp1706474 PMID:28813217

Schelbert, L. (2003). Pathways of human understanding: An inquiry into Western and North American Indian worldview structures. *American Indian Culture and Research Journal*, *27*(1), 61–75.

Schiro, M. (2013). Curriculum theory: Conflicting visions and enduring concerns. *Sage (Atlanta, Ga.)*.

Schmidt, U., & Zank, H. (2005). What is loss aversion? *Journal of Risk and Uncertainty*, *30*(20), 157–167. doi:10.100711166-005-6564-6

Schonfeld, D. J., & Gurwitch, R. H. (2009). Addressing disaster mental health needs of children: Practical guidance for pediatric emergency health care providers. *Clinical Pediatric Emergency Medicine*, *10*(3), 208–215. doi:10.1016/j.cpem.2009.06.002

Schunk, D. H. (1991). Self-efficacy and academic motivation. *Educational Psychologist*, *26*(3), 207–231. doi:10.120715326985ep2603&4_2

Scikit-Library. (2021). https://scikit-learn.org/

Scott, R., & Mars, M. (2019). Here we go again—'Digital health'. *Journal of the International Society for Telemedicine and EHealth*, *7*, e1. doi:10.29086/JISfTeH.7.e1

Sekhar, M. S., & Vyas, N. (2013). Defensive medicine: A Bane to Healthcare. *Annals of Medical and Health Sciences Research*, *3*(2), 295–296. 9248.113688 doi:10.4103/2141-

Servey, J. T., Hartzell, J. D., & McFate, T. (2020). A faculty development model for academic leadership education across a health care organization. *Journal of Medical Education and Curricular Development*, *7*. Advance online publication. doi:10.1177/2382120520948878 PMID:32851193

Seval, N., Eaton, E., & Springer, S. A. (2020, January). Beyond antibiotics: A practical guide for the infectious disease physician to treat opioid use disorder in the setting of associated infectious diseases. *Open Forum Infectious Diseases*, *7*(1), ofz539. doi:10.1093/ofid/ofz539 PMID:31993454

Seymour-Walsh, A. E., Bell, A., Weber, A., & Smith, T. (2020). Adapting to a new reality: COVID-19 coronavirus and online education in the health professions. *Rural and Remote Health*, *20*(2), 6000. doi:10.22605/RRH6000 PMID:32456441

Sezgin, E. (2021). Can we use commercial mobile apps instead of research mobile apps in healthcare research? *Frontiers in Public Health*, *9*, 685439. doi:10.3389/fpubh.202 1.685439

Shabani, K., Khatib, M., & Ebadi, S. (2010). Vygotsky's zone of proximal development: Instructional implications and teachers' professional development. *English Language Teaching*, *3*(4), 237–248. doi:10.5539/elt.v3n4p237

Shah, D., Patel, S., & Bharti, S. K. (2020). Heart disease prediction using machine learning techniques. *SN Computer Science*, 684-687.

Shah, S. M. A., Mohammad, D., Qureshi, M. F. H., Abbas, M. Z., & Aleem, S. (2021). Prevalence, Psychological Responses and Associated Correlates of Depression, Anxiety and Stress in a Global Population, During the Coronavirus Disease (COVID-19) Pandemic. *Community Mental Health Journal*, *57*(1), 101–110. doi:10.100710597-020-00728-y PMID:33108569

Shank, P. (2018). *Manage memory for deeper learning: 21 evidence-based and easy-to-apply tactics that support memory while learning and beyond.* Learning Peaks LLC.

Sharma, B., & John, S. (2020). Hepatic Cirrhosis. StatPearls Publishing.

Sharma, M., & Romas, J. A. (2012). *Theoretical foundations of health education and health promotion* (2nd ed.). Jones & Bartlett Learning.

Shaw, T., McGregor, D., Brunner, M., Keep, M., Janssen, A., & Barnet, S. (2017). What is ehealth (6)? Development of a conceptual model for ehealth: Qualitative study with key informants. *Journal of Medical Internet Research*, *19*(10), e324. doi:10.2196/jmir.8106 PMID:29066429

Sheehy, R. (2019). This is Not Your Grandfather's Medical School: Novel Tools to Enhance Medical Education. *Missouri Medicine*, *116*(5), 371–375. PMID:31645786

Shetty, V. (2016, November 22). *Machine Learning in layman's terms*. Academic Press.

Shiels, M. S., Haque, A. T., Haozous, E. A., Albert, P. S., Almeida, J. S., García-Closas, M., . . . de González, A. B. (2021). Racial and ethnic disparities in excess deaths during the COVID-19 pandemic, March to December 2020. *Annals of Internal Medicine*. doi:10.7326/M21-2134

Short, C. E., Rebar, A. L., Plotnikoff, R. C., & Vandelanotte, C. (2015). Designing engaging online behaviour change interventions: A proposed model of user engagement. *The European Health Psychologist*, *17*(1), 32–38.

Showell, C., & Nøhr, C. (2012). How should we define ehealth, and does the definition matter? *Studies in Health Technology and Informatics*, *180*, 881–884. PMID:22874319

Shum, S. B. (2012). *Learning analytics.* https://iite.unesco.org/pics/publications/en/files/3214711.pdf

Shunk, D. H. (2000). Learning: introduction, issues, and historical perspectives. In *Learning theories: An educational perspective* (pp. 1–29). Upper Saddle River, NJ: Pearson Education.

Silva, B. M., Rodrigues, J. J., de la Torre Díez, I., López-Coronado, M., & Saleem, K. (2015). Mobile-health: A review of current state in 2015. *Journal of Biomedical Informatics*, *56*, 265–272. doi:10.1016/j.jbi.2015.06.003 PMID:26071682

Silva, M. A., Perez, O. F. R., Añez, L. M., & Paris, M. (2021). Telehealth treatment engagement with Latinx populations during the COVID-19 pandemic. *The Lancet. Psychiatry*, *8*(3), 176–178.

Simoni, J. M., Ronen, K., & Aunon, F. M. (2018). Health behavior theory to enhance ehealth intervention research in HIV: Rationale and review. *Current HIV/AIDS Reports*, *15*(6), 423–430. doi:10.100711904-018-0418-8 PMID:30511186

Simons-Morton, B. G., Greene, W. H., & Gottlieb, N. H. (1995). *Introduction to health education and health promotion* (2nd ed.). Waveland Press.

Simpson, D., Marcdante, K., Souza, K. H., Anderson, A., & Holmboe, E. (2018). Job Roles of the 2025 Medical Educator. *Journal of Graduate Medical Education*, *10*(3), 243–246. doi:10.4300/JGME-D-18-00253.1 PMID:29946376

Simpson, R., & Katsanis, E. (2020). The immunological case for staying active during the COVID-19 pandemic. *Brain, Behavior, and Immunity*, *87*, 6–7. doi:10.1016/j.bbi.2020. 04.041

Singh, A., Avula, A., & Zahn, E. (2021). *Acute bronchitis*. StatPearls Publishing. https://www.ncbi.nlm.nih.gov/books/NBK448067/

Singh, V., & Thurman, A. (2019). How many ways can we define online learning? A systematic literature review of definitions of online learning (1988-2018). *American Journal of Distance Education*, *33*(4), 289–306. doi:10.1080/08923647.2019.1663082

Skinner, B. F. (1966). The phylogeny and ontogeny of behavior. *Science*, *153*(3741), 1205–1213. doi:10.1126cience.153.3741.1205 PMID:5918710

Skyttner, L. (2001). *General systems theory: Ideas and applications*. World Scientific Publishing. doi:10.1142/4307

Smith, P. L., & Ragan, T. J. (1996). Impact of R.M. Gagné's work on instructional theory. *Proceedings of Selected Research and Development Presentation, National Convention of the Association of Educational Communications and Technology*.

Smith, B. J., Tang, K. C., & Nutbeam, D. (2006). WHO health promotion glossary: New terms. *Health Promotion International*, *21*(4), 340–345. doi:10.1093/heapro/dal033 PMID:16963461

Smith, B., & Magnani, J. W. (2019). New technologies, new disparities: The intersection of electronic health and digital health literacy. *International Journal of Cardiology*, *292*, 280–282. doi:10.1016/j.ijcard.2019.05.066 PMID:31171391

Smith, E., & Boscak, A. (2021). A virtual emergency: Learning lessons from remote medical student education during the COVID-19 pandemic. *Emergency Radiology*, *28*(3), 445–452. doi:10.100710140-020-01874-2 PMID:33420528

Smith, P. L., & Ragan, T. J. (2005). *Instructional design* (3rd ed.). Wiley & Sons.

Snowball, J. D., & McKenna, S. (2017). Student-generated content: An approach to harnessing the power of diversity in higher education. *Teaching in Higher Education*, *22*(5), 604–618. doi:10.1080/13562517.2016.1273205

Solberg Nes, L. (2020). Digital Health in Cardiology: Time for Action. *Cardiology*, *145*(2), 106–109. doi:10.1159/000504797 PMID:31825946

Solomon, K. T., Bandara, S., Reynolds, I. S., Krawczyk, N., Saloner, B., Stuart, E., & Connolly, E. (2022). Association between availability of medications for opioid use disorder in specialty treatment and use of medications among patients: A state-level trends analysis. *Journal of Substance Abuse Treatment*, *132*, 108424. doi:10.1016/j.jsat.2021.108424 PMID:34144299

Song, Y., Ding, Y., Ren, X., Liu, B., & Ma, H. (2021). Experience in online teaching and examining of histological experiments based on digital slices, Rain Class and QQ group class. *Chin J Histochem Cytochem.*, *1*, 102–106. doi:10.16705/j.cnki.1004-1850.2021.01.017

South Carolina Department of Education. (2015). *College- and career-ready standards for English language arts*. https://ed.sc.gov/scdoe/assets/file/programs-services/59/documents/ELA2015SCCCRStandards.pdf

South Carolina Department of Education. (2021a). *Free and lower-cost Internet response to Covid-19.* https://ed.sc.gov/districts-schools/shared-services/free-and-lower-cost-internet-in-response-to-covid-9/

South Carolina Department of Education. (2021b). *Social emotional learning.* https://ed.sc.gov/districts-schools/special-education-services/social-emotional-learning/

South Carolina Department of Education. (2021c). *PersonalizeSC: Social and emotional learning.* https://personalizesc.ed.sc.gov/pscg-competencies/social-and-emotional-learning/

South Carolina Department of Education. (2021d). *PSCG & CASEL competency crosswalk PDF.* https://personalizesc.ed.sc.gov/competencies-based-ed/sc-competencies-prototype/casel-competencies-pscg-competencies-crosswalk/

Sovacool, B. K., & Hess, D. J. (2017). Ordering theories: Typologies and conceptual frameworks for sociotechnical change. *Social Studies of Science, 47*(5), 703–750. doi:10.1177/0306312717709363 PMID:28641502

Spencer, L. M., Schooley, M. W., Anderson, L. A., Kochtitzky, C. S., DeGroff, A. S., Devlin, H. M., & Mercer, S. L. (2013). Seeking best practices: A conceptual framework for planning and improving evidence-based practices. *Preventing Chronic Disease, 10*, 130186. doi:10.5888/pcd10.130186 PMID:24331280

Spring, B., Ockene, J. K., Gidding, S. S., Mozaffarian, D., Moore, S., Rosal, M. C., Brown, M. D., Vafiadis, D. K., Cohen, D. L., Burke, L. E., & Lloyd-Jones, D. (2013). Better population health through behavior change in adults: A call to action. *Circulation, 128*(19), 2169–2176. doi:10.1161/01.cir.0000435173.25936.e1 PMID:24100544

Spring, B., Pfammatter, A. F., Hoffman, S. A., Pellegrini, C., McFadden, H. G., Siddique, J., Hedeker, D., & Collins, L. (2019). Determining the optimal 6-month weight loss treatment package: Results of the opt-in study. *Annals of Behavioral Medicine, 53*, S443–S443.

Stefaniak, J. (2020). The utility of design thinking to promote systemic instructional design practices in the workplace. *TechTrends, 64*(2), 202–210. doi:10.100711528-019-00453-8

Stefaniak, J. E. (2021). *Needs assessment for learning and performance: Theory, process, and practice*. Routledge.

Stefaniak, J. E., Mi, M., & Afonso, N. (2015). Triangulating perspectives: A needs assessment to develop an outreach program for vulnerable and underserved populations. *Performance Improvement Quarterly, 28*(1), 49–68. doi:10.1002/piq.21186

Stefaniak, J., & Xu, M. (2020). An examination of the systemic reach of instructional design models: A systematic review. *TechTrends, 64*(5), 710–719. doi:10.100711528-020-00539-8

Steinhubl, S. R., Muse, E. D., & Topol, E. J. (2013). Can mobile health technologies transform health care? *Journal of the American Medical Association, 310*(22), 2395–2396. doi:10.1001/jama.2013.281078 PMID:24158428

Steinhubl, S. R., Muse, E. D., & Topol, E. J. (2015). The emerging field of mobile health. *Science Translational Medicine, 7*(283), 283rv3. Advance online publication. doi:10.1126citranslmed.aaa3487 PMID:25877894

Stiff, J. B., & Mongeau, P. A. (2016). *Persuasive communication* (3rd ed.). Guilford Publications

Stone, P., Brooks, R., Brynjolfsson, E., Calo, R., Etzioni, O., Hager, G., ... Teller, A. (2016). *Artificial intelligence and life in 2030: the one hundred year study on artificial intelligence*. Academic Press.

Strauss, V. (2013). *Howard Gardner: 'Multiple intelligences' are not 'learning styles'*. https://www.washingtonpost.com/news/answer-sheet/wp/2013/10/16/howard-gardner-multiple-intelligences-are-not-learning-styles/

Stroebe, W. (2000). *Social psychology and health* (2nd ed.). Open University Press.

Su, B., Zhang, T., Yan, L., Huang, C., Cheng, X., Cai, C., & Cui, D. (2021). Online Medical Teaching in China During the COVID-19 Pandemic: Tools, Modalities, and Challenges. *Frontiers in Public Health, 9*, 797694. doi:10.3389/fpubh.2021.797694 PMID:34988057

Substance Abuse and Mental Health Services Administration. (2021). *Coping tips for traumatic events and disasters.* https://www.samhsa.gov/find-help/disaster-distress-helpline/coping-tips

Sulzer, S. H., Prevedel, S., Barrett, T., Voss, M. W., Manning, C., & Madden, E. F. (2021). Professional education to reduce provider stigma toward harm reduction and pharmacotherapy. *Drugs Education Prevention & Policy, 28*(2), 1–11. doi:10.1080/09687637.2021.1936457

Sutton, S. (2005). Stage theories of health behavior. In M. Conner & P. Norman (Eds.), Predicting health behaviour: Research and practice with social cognition models (pp. 29-80). Open University Press.

Sutton, S. (2001). Back to the drawing board? A review of applications of the transtheoretical model to substance use. *Addiction (Abingdon, England), 96*(1), 175–186. doi:10.1046/j.1360-0443.2001.96117513.x PMID:11177528

Sweller, J., Ayres, P., Kalyuga, S., Sweller, J., Ayres, P., & Kalyuga, S. (2011). *Cognitive load theory.* Springer. doi:10.1007/978-1-4419-8126-4

Tabakin, A. L., Patel, H. V., & Singer, E. A. (2021). Lessons learned from the COVID-19 pandemic: A call for a national video-based curriculum for urology residents. *Journal of Surgical Education, 78*(1), 324–326. doi:10.1016/j.jsurg.2020.07.013 PMID:32741691

Tabak, R. G., Khoong, E. C., Chambers, D. A., & Brownson, R. C. (2012). Bridging Research and Practice. *American Journal of Preventive Medicine, 43*(3), 337–350. doi:10.1016/j.amepre.2012.05.024 PMID:22898128

Taber, J. M., Leyva, B., & Persoskie, A. (2015). Why do people avoid medical care? A qualitative study using national data. *Journal of General Internal Medicine, 30*(3), 290–297. doi:10.100711606-014-3089-1 PMID:25387439

Talbot, J. A., Burgess, A. R., Thayer, D., Parenteau, L., Paluso, N., & Coburn, A. F. (2018). Patterns of telehealth use among rural Medicaid beneficiaries. *The Journal of Rural Health.* doi:10.1111/jrh.12324

Tamim, S. R. (2012). *An exploration of how health professionals create ehealth and mhealth education interventions* (Publication No. 3529980) [Doctoral Dissertation, University of Memphis]. ProQuest Dissertations & Thesis Global.

Tebeje, T. H., & Klein, J. (2020). 2021/02/01). Applications of e-health to support person-centered health care at the time of COVID-19 pandemic. *Telemedicine Journal and e-Health, 27*(2), 150–158. doi:10.1089/tmj.2020.0201 PMID:32746750

Teixeria, P. J., Carraca, E. V., Markland, D., Silva, M. N., & Ryan, R. M. (2012). Exercise, physical activity, and self-determination theory: A systematic review. *The International Journal of Behavioral Nutrition and Physical Activity, 9*, 78. doi:0.1186/1479-5868-9-78

Tessmer, M., & Richey, R. C. (1997). The role of context in learning and instructional design. *Educational Technology Research and Development, 45*(2), 85–115. doi:10.1007/BF02299526

Tetrault, J. M., Krause, R., Roessler, E., Heimer, R., Powell, M. L., Drew, S., & Edens, E. (n.d.). *Addiction treatment: Clinical skills for healthcare providers.* https://www.coursera.org/lecture/addiction-treatment/how-do-you-talk-about-addiction-YVN5U

The Carnegie Classification of Institutions of Higher Education. (n.d.). *About Carnegie classification.* https://carnegieclassifications.iu.edu/

Thomas, K. L., Shah, B. R., Elliot-Bynum, S., Thomas, K. D., Damon, K., Allen LaPointe, N. M., Calhoun, S., Thomas, L., Breathett, K., Mathews, R., Anderson, M., Califf, R. M., & Peterson, E. D. (2014). Check it, change it: A community-based, multifaceted intervention to improve blood pressure control. *Circulation: Cardiovascular Quality and Outcomes*, *7*(6), 828–834. doi:10.1161/CIRCOUTCOMES.114.001039 PMID:25351480

Timmreck, T. C., Cole, G. E., Gordon, J., & Butterwoth, D. D. (2010). Health education and health promotion: A look at the jungle of supportive fields, philosophies, and theoretical foundations. In J. M. Black, S. Furney, H. M. Graf, & A. E. Nolte (Eds.), *Philosophical foundations of health education* (pp. 67–78). Jossey-Bass.

Topol, E. J. (2015). *The patient will see you now: The future of medicine is in your hands*. Basic Books.

Topol, E. J. (2019). High-performance medicine: The convergence of human and artificial intelligence. *Nature Medicine*, *25*(1), 44–56. doi:10.103841591-018-0300-7 PMID:30617339

Transforming and Scaling Up Health Professionals' Education and Training: World Health Organization Guidelines. (n.d.). *World Health Organization*. https://www.ncbi.nlm.nih.gov/books/NBK298950/

Triantafyllidis, A., Kondylakis, H., Votis, K., Tzovaras, D., Maglaveras, N., & Rahimi, K. (2019). Features, outcomes, and challenges in mobile health interventions for patients living with chronic diseases: A review of systematic reviews. *International Journal of Medical Informatics*, *132*, 103984. doi:10.1016/j.ijmedinf.2019.103984 PMID:31605884

Triemstra, J. D., Haas, M., Bhavsar-Burke, I., Gottlieb-Smith, R., Wolff, M., Shelgikar, A. V., Samala, R. V., Ruff, A. L., Kuo, K., Tam, M., Gupta, A., Stojan, J., Gruppen, L., & Ellinas, H. (2021). Impact of the COVID-19 Pandemic on the Clinical Learning Environment: Addressing Identified Gaps and Seizing Opportunities. *Academic Medicine*, *96*(9), 1276–1281. doi:10.1097/ACM.0000000000004013 PMID:34432665

Trochim, W. M., Cabrera, D. A., Milstein, B., Gallagher, R. S., & Leischow, S. J. (2006). Practical challenges of systems thinking and modeling in public health. *American Journal of Public Health*, *96*(3), 538–546. doi:10.2105/AJPH.2005.066001 PMID:16449581

Trost, S. G., Owen, N., Bauman, A. E., Sallis, J. F., & Brown, W. (2002). Correlates of adults' participation in physical activity: Review and update. *Medicine and Science in Sports and Exercise*, *4*(1), 1996–2001. doi:10.1249/01.MSS.0000038974.76900.92

Tsai, J.-M., Cheng, M.-J., Tsai, H.-H., Hung, S.-W., & Chen, Y.-L. (2019). Acceptance and resistance of telehealth: The perspective of dual-factor concepts in technology adoption. *International Journal of Information Management*, *49*, 34–44. doi:10.1016/j.ijinfomgt.2019.03.003

Tucker, A., Maass, A., Bain, D., Chen, L., Azzam, M., Dawson, H., & Johnston, A. (2010). Augmentation of venous, arterial and microvascular blood supply in the leg by isometric neuromuscular stimulation via the peroneal nerve. *The International Journal of Angiology*, *19*(01), e31–e37. doi:10.1055-0031-1278361 PMID:22477572

Tuong, W., Larsen, E. R., & Armstrong, A. W. (2014). Videos to influence: A systematic review of effectiveness of video-based education in modifying health behaviors. *Journal of Behavioral Medicine*, *37*(2), 218–233. doi:10.100710865-012-9480-7 PMID:23188480

Tyler, R. W. (2017). Basic principles of curriculum and instruction. In D. J. Flinders & S. T. Thornton (Eds.), *The curriculum reader* (5th ed., pp. 73–82). Routledge.

U.S. Census Bureau. (2021a). *2020 Population and Housing State Data*. https://www.ce nsus.gov/library/visualizations/interactive/2020-population-and-housing-state-data.html

U.S. Census Bureau. (2021b). *QuickFacts*. https://www.census.gov/quickfacts/fact/table /columbiacitysouthcarolina,US/RHI125219

U.S. Department of Health & Human Services. (2018). *2018 Physical activity guidelines advisory committee scientific report*. https://health.gov/sites/default/files/2019-09/PAG_Advisory_Committee_Report.pdf

Van Dyke, M. E., Mendoza, M. C., Li, W., Parker, E. M., Belay, B., Davis, E. M., ... Clarke, K. E. (2021). Racial and ethnic disparities in COVID-19 incidence by age, sex, and period among persons aged< 25 years—16 US jurisdictions, January 1–December 31, 2020. *Morbidity and Mortality Weekly Report*, *70*(11), 382.

van Gemert-Pijnen, L. J., Kip, H., Kelders, S. M., & Sanderman, R. (2018). Introducing ehealth. In eHealth research, theory and development (pp. 3-26). Routledge. doi:10.4324/9781315385907-1

van Gemert-Pijnen, J. E., Nijland, N., van Limburg, M., Ossebaard, H. C., Kelders, S. M., Eysenbach, G., & Seydel, E. R. (2011). A holistic framework to improve the uptake and impact of ehealth technologies. *Journal of Medical Internet Research*, *13*(4), e111. doi:10.2196/jmir.1672 PMID:22155738

van Merriënboer, J. J., Clark, R. E., & De Croock, M. B. (2002). Blueprints for complex learning: The 4C/ID-model. *Educational Technology Research and Development*, *50*(2), 39–61.

van Rooij, T., & Marsh, S. (2016). eHealth: Past and future perspectives. *Personalized Medicine*, *13*(1), 57–70. doi:10.2217/pme.15.40 PMID:29749870

Van Wyk, T., Mahomed-Asmail, F., & Swanepoel, D. W. (2019). Supporting hearing health in vulnerable populations through community care workers using mHealth technologies. *International Journal of Audiology*, *58*(11), 790–797. doi:10.1080/14992027.2019.1649478 PMID:31419388

Vance, K., Howe, W., & Dellavalle, R. P. (2009). Social internet sites as a source of public health information. *Dermatologic Clinics*, *27*(2), 133–136. doi:10.1016/j.det.2008.11.010 PMID:19254656

Vargas, T. (2017, May 15). Guinea pigs or pioneers? How Puerto Rican women were used to test the birth control pill. *Washington Post*. https://link.gale.com/apps/doc/A491755323/ITOF?u=24034&sid=bookmark-ITOF&xid=4ad4241c

Varkevisser, R. D. M., van Stralen, M. M., Kroeze, W., Ket, J. C. F., & Steenhuis, I. H. M. (2019). Determinants of weight loss maintenance: A systematic review. *Obesity (Silver Spring, Md.)*, *20*, 171–211. doi:10.1111/obr.12772

Venkatesh, M., Morris, Davis, & Davis. (2003). User acceptance of information technology: Toward a unified view. *Management Information Systems Quarterly*, *27*(3), 425. doi:10.2307/30036540

Verstuyf, J., Patrick, H., Vansteenkiste, M., & Teixeira, P. (2012). Motivational dynamics of eating regulation: A self-determination theory perspective. *The International Journal of Behavioral Nutrition and Physical Activity*, *9*(1), 21. doi:10.1186/1479-5868-9-21

Vest, J. R., & Gamm, L. D. (2009). A critical review of the research literature on Six Sigma, Lean and StuderGroup's Hardwiring Excellence in the United States: The need to demonstrate and communicate the effectiveness of transformation strategies in healthcare. *Implementation Science; IS*, *4*(1), 1–9. doi:10.1186/1748-5908-4-35 PMID:19570218

Villachica, S. W., Marker, A., & Taylor, K. (2010). But what do they really expect? Employer perceptions of the skills of entry-level instructional designers. *Performance Improvement Quarterly*, *22*(4), 33–51. doi:10.1002/piq.20067

Virtanen, L., Kaihlanen, A. M., Laukka, E., Gluschkoff, K., & Heponiemi, T. (2021). Behavior change techniques to promote healthcare professionals' eHealth competency: A systematic review of interventions. *International Journal of Medical Informatics*, *149*, 104432. doi:10.1016/j.ijmedinf.2021.104432 PMID:33684712

Vo, L., Albrecth, S. S., & Kershaw, K. N. (2019). Multilevel interventions to prevent and reduce obesity. *Current Opinion in Endocrine and Metabolic Research, 4*, 62–69. doi:10.101 6/j.coemr.2018.11.002

Vos, T., Abajobir, A. A., Abate, K. H., Abbafati, C., Abbas, K. M., Abd-Allah, F., Abdulkader, R. S., Abdulle, A. M., Abebo, T. A., Abera, S. F., Aboyans, V., Abu-Raddad, L. J., Ackerman, I. N., Adamu, A. A., Adetokunboh, O., Afarideh, M., Afshin, A., Agarwal, S. K., Aggarwal, R., ... Murray, C. J. L. (2017). Global, regional, and national incidence, prevalence, and years lived with disability for 328 diseases and injuries for 195 countries, 1990–2016: A systematic analysis for the Global Burden of Disease Study 2016. *Lancet, 390*(10100), 1211–1259. doi:10.1016/S0140-6736(17)32154-2 PMID:28919117

Vygotsky (1978). *Mind in society: The development of higher psychological processes.* Harvard University Press.

Vygotsky, L. S. (1962). *Thought and language.* MIT Press. doi:10.1037/11193-000

Vygotsky, L. S. (1978). *Mind in society: The development of higher psychological processes.* Harvard University Press.

Walker, J. L., & Mascardi, J. (2015). Personal epistemologies and teaching. In H. Fives & M. G. Gill (Eds.), *International handbook of research on teachers' beliefs* (pp. 319–335). Routledge.

Wang, C. J., Liu, T. T., Car, J., & Zuckerman, B. (2020). Design, adoption, implementation, scalability, and sustainability of telehealth programs. *Pediatric Clinics of North America, 67*(4), 675–682.

Waters, E., & Sroufe, L. A. (1983). Social competence as a developmental construct. *Developmental Review, 3*, 79–97.

Watkins, J. B., & Eisenberg, D. (2012). Increased demand for mental health services on college campuses: Perspectives from administrators. *Qualitative Social Work, 11*(3), 319–337. doi:10.1177/1473325011401468

Watson, M. C. (2002). Normative needs assessment: Is this an appropriate way in which to meet the new public health agenda? *International Journal of Health Promotion and Education, 40*(1), 4–8. doi:10.1080/14635240.2002.10806189

Wegermann, K., Wilder, J. M., Parish, A., Niedzwiecki, D., Gellad, Z. F., Muir, A. J., & Patel, Y. A. (2021). Racial and socioeconomic disparities in utilization of telehealth in patients with liver disease during COVID-19. *Digestive Diseases and Sciences*, 1–7.

Weinstein, N. D. (2007). Misleading tests of health behavior theories. *Annals of Behavioral Medicine, 33*(1), 1–10. doi:10.120715324796abm3301_1 PMID:17291165

Weissberg, R. P., Durlak, J. A., Domitrovich, C. E., & Gullotta, T. P. (2015). Social emotional learning: Past, present, and future. In J. A. Durlak, C. E Domitrovich, R. P., Weissberg, & T. P. Gullotta (Eds.), Handbook of social and emotional learning: Research and practice (pp. 3-19). Guilford Publications.

Welle, H. M., Russel, R. D., & Kittleson, M. J. (2010). Philosophical trends in health education: Implications for the 21st century. In J. M. Black, S. Furney, H. M. Graf, & A. E. Nolte (Eds.), *Philosophical foundations of health education* (pp. 79–93). Jossey-Bass.

Westby, A., Nissly, T., Gieseker, R., Timmins, K., & Justesen, K. (2021). Achieving equity in telehealth: "centering at the margins" in access, provision, and reimbursement. *Journal of the American Board of Family Medicine, 34*(Supplement), S29–S32.

West, D. S., Coulon, S. M., Monroe, C. M., & Wilson, D. K. (2016). Evidence-based lifestyle interventions for obesity and type 2 diabetes: The Look AHEAD intensive lifestyle intervention as exemplar. *The American Psychologist, 71*(7), 614–627. doi:10.1037/a0040394

West, R. E. (2018). *Foundations of learning and instructional design technology* (1st ed.). EdTech Books.

Westwood, A. R. (2021). Telehealth and maternity: Has the onset of the pandemic changed the way we utilise telemedicine forever? *British Journal of Midwifery*, *29*(6), 352–355. https://doi.org/10.12968/bjom.2021.29.6.352

WHO. (2019). *WHO guideline: recommendations on digital interventions for health system strengthening*. World Health Organization.

WHO. (2021). *Global strategy on digital health 2020–2025*. World Health Organization. https://www.who.int/docs/default-source/documents/gs4dhdaa2a9f352b0445bafbc79ca799dce4d.pdf?sfvrsn=f112ede5_38

Willgoose, C. E. (2010). Health education as a basic. In J. M. Black, S. Furney, H. M. Graf, & A. E. Nolte (Eds.), *Philosophical foundations of health education* (pp. 17–27). Jossey-Bass.

Williams, T. (2020). The benefits of using video in healthcare. *Health Tech Digital*. https://www.healthtechdigital.com/the-benefits-of-using-video-in-healthcare/

Williams, E. P., Mesidor, M., Winters, K., Dubbert, P. M., & Wyatt, S. B. (2015). Overweight and obesity: Prevalence, consequences, and causes of a growing public health problem. *Current Obesity Reports*, *4*, 363–370. doi:10.100713679-015-0169-4

Wilson, P. M., Rodgers, W. M., Loitz, C. C., & Scime, G. (2006). "It's who I am…Really!" The importance of integrated regulation in exercise contexts. *Journal of Applied Biobehavioral Research*, *11*(2), 79–104. doi:10.1111/j.1751-9861.2006.tb00021.x

Wing, R. R., & Jeffery, R. W. (1999). Benefits of recruiting participants with friends and increasing social support for weight loss and maintenance. *Journal of Consulting and Clinical Psychology*, *67*(1), 132–138. doi:10.1037/0022-006X.67.1.132

Wisniewski, H., Liu, G., Henson, P., Vaidyam, A., Hajratalli, N. K., Onnela, J.-P., & Torous, J. (2019). Understanding the quality, effectiveness and attributes of top-rated smartphone health apps. *Evidence-Based Mental Health*, *22*(1), 4–9. doi:10.1136/ebmental-2018-300069 PMID:30635262

Wittrock, M. C. (1992). Generative learning processes of the brain. *Educational Psychologist*, *27*(4), 531–541. doi:10.120715326985ep2704_8

Woltmann, E., Grogan-Kaylor, A., Perron, B., Georges, H., Kilbourne, A. M., & Bauer, M. S. (2012). Comparative effectiveness of collaborative chronic care models for mental health conditions across primary, specialty, and behavioral health care settings: Systematic review and meta-analysis. *The American Journal of Psychiatry*, *169*(8), 790–804. doi:10.1176/appi.ajp.2012.11111616 PMID:22772364

Wong, B. M., & Headrick, L. A. (2020). Application of continuous quality improvement to medical education. *Medical Education*, *55*(1), 72–81. doi:10.1111/medu.14351 PMID:32790930

Wong, R. Y. (2020). Medical education during COVID-19: Lessons from a pandemic. *BCMJ*, *62*(5), 170–171.

World Health Organization. (1998). *Health promotion glossary*. https://www.who.int/publications/i/item/WHO-HPR-HEP-98.1

World Health Organization. (2011). *mHealth: New Horizons for Health through Mobile Technologies: Based on the Findings of the Second Global Survey on eHealth (Global Observatory for eHealth Series, Volume 3)*. https://www.who.int/goe/publications/goe_mhealth_web.pdf

World Health Organization. (2013). *Annex 1, Definition and list of health professionals*. From.

World Health Organization. (2016a). *Global difusion of ehealth: Making universal health coverage achievable. Report of the third global survey on eHealth*. World Health Organization.

World Health Organization. (2016b). *From innovation to implementation: eHealth in the WHO European region*. World Health Organization.

World Health Organization. (2020). *Health Clusters*. https://healthcluster.who.int/publications/i/item/9789240004726

World Health Organization. (2021a). *Obesity and overweight*. https://www.who.int/news-room/f act-sheets/detail/obesity-and-overweight

World Health Organization. (2021b). *Physical activity*. https://www.who.int/news-room/fact-she ets/detail/physical-activity

World Health Organization. (2022). *Constitution of the World Health Organization*. https://www.who.int/about/governance/constitution

World Health Organization. (2022). *Improving the mental and brain health of children and adolescents*. https://www.who.int/activities/improving-the-mental-and-brain-health-of-children-and-adolescents

Wu, R. C., Morra, D., Quan, S., Lai, S., Zanjani, S., Abrams, H., & Rossos, P. G. (2010). The use of smartphones for clinical communication on internal medicine wards. *Journal of Hospital Medicine*, *5*(9), 553–559. doi:10.1002/jhm.775 PMID:20690190

Wu, Y. L., & Wu, H. C. (2015). Higher education learning experiences among Vietnamese immigrant women in Taiwan. *Adult Education Quarterly*, *65*(2), 133–151. doi:10.1177/0741713614566673

Yang, C., Bear, G. G., & May, H. (2018). Multilevel associations between school-wide social–emotional learning approach and student engagement across elementary, middle, and high schools. *School Psychology Review*, *47*(1), 45–61. doi:10.17105/SPR-2017-0003.V47-1

Yang, X., & Kovarik, C. L. (2021). A systematic review of mobile health interventions in China: Identifying gaps in care. *Journal of Telemedicine and Telecare*, *27*(1), 3–22. doi:10.1177/1357633X19856746 PMID:31319759

Yarabarla, M. S., Ravi, L. K., & Sivasangari, A. (2019, April). Breast cancer prediction via machine learning. In *2019 3rd International Conference on Trends in Electronics and Informatics (ICOEI)* (pp. 121-124). IEEE. 10.1109/ICOEI.2019.8862533

Yeates, P., Moult, A., Lefroy, J., Walsh-House, J., Clews, L., McKinley, R., & Fuller, R. (2020). Understanding and developing procedures for video-based assessment in medical education. *Medical Teacher*, *42*(11), 1250–1260. doi:10.1080/0142159X.2020.1801997 PMID:32749915

York, C. S., & Ertmer, P. A. (2016). Examining instructional design principles applied by experienced designers in practice. *Performance Improvement Quarterly*, *29*(2), 169–192. doi:10.1002/piq.21220

Youm, J., & Corral, J. (2019). Technological Pedagogical Content Knowledge Among Medical Educators: What Is Our Readiness to Teach With Technology? *Academic Medicine*, *94*(11S), S69–S72. doi:10.1097/ACM.0000000000002912 PMID:31365390

Zakrajsek, T. (2018). Reframing the lecture versus active learning debate: Suggestions for a new way forward. *Educ Health Prof*, *1*(1), 1–3. doi:10.4103/EHP.EHP_14_18

Zhang, J., Brackbill, D., Yang, S., Becker, J., Herbert, N., & Centola, D. (2016). Support or competition? How online social networks increase physical activity: A randomized controlled trial. *Preventive Medicine Reports*, *4*, 453–458. doi:10.1016/j.pmedr.2016.08.008

Zhou, D., Gomez, R., Wright, N., Rittenbruch, M., & Davis, J. (2020). A design-led conceptual framework for developing school integrated STEM programs: The Australian context. *International Journal of Technology and Design Education*. doi:10.100710798-020-09619-5

Zobair, K. M., Sanzogni, L., Houghton, L., & Islam, M. Z. (2021). Forecasting care seekers satisfaction with telemedicine using machine learning and structural equation modeling. *PLoS One*, *16*(9), 1–31. https://doi.org/https://doi.org/10.1371/journal.pone.0257300

About the Contributors

Suha R. Tamim is a Clinical Assistant Professor in the Department of Instruction and Teacher Education at the University of South Carolina, USA. She earned her Doctorate in Instructional Design and Technology from the University of Memphis, Tennessee, USA, where she taught courses in instructional design. She earned her Master of Public Health from the American University of Beirut, Lebanon where she taught courses in health education and worked on several health education projects. Her research interests revolve around systems thinking and the design of learning environments, with a focus on constructivist, online, and health-related environments. She is an active member of the Association for Educational Communications and Technology, previously serving as president of the Systems Thinking and Change division. She is also active in the Carnegie Project on the Education Doctorate, previously chairing the Dissertation in Practice Awards committee. She currently serves as a co-editor in chief for Impacting Education: Journal of Transforming Professional Practice. She is also co-editor of the book Systems Thinking for Instructional Designers: Catalyzing Organizational Change.

* * *

Anjali Agarwal is currently working as a developer in Tata Consultancy Services. Anjali is awarded Master of Computer Applications from Amity University Kolkata in 2021 and has graduated with a Bachelor of Computer Applications in 2018 from Techno India University. She received a scholarship during her Master's program. Her primary research interests include Data Science, Machine Learning, Computer Vision, Cloud Computing, and Natural Language Processing. Ms. Agarwal worked on an international project in close collaboration with Mobility Labs Sweden and was engaged in developing AI technologies such as a power wheelchair using facial features for people with neuromotor disorder Duchenne's Myodystrophy.

Ravish Bansal is awarded Doctor of Medicine from St. Martinus University and has done his Clinical Clerkship at Pontiac General Hospital, Michigan, US. Dr. Bansal has also served the local community of curacao by organising free medical health relief camps in association with his fellow medical students and university. His primary research interests include New-Age Medicine, Medical-Technology Symbiosis, Ancient Medicine, Natural Treatment, and Ayurveda. Dr. Bansal has also been engaged with few doctors about new age medicine and treatment.

Stephanie J. Blackmon has a Ph.D. in Higher Education and is an Associate Professor of Higher Education in the William & Mary School of Education. Her research focuses on college and university teaching and learning, with a current emphasis on experiential learning; technology integration in college and university classrooms; and technology, trust, and privacy, which includes the areas of cybersecurity and learning analytics respectively.

Ralph Brooks holds a BS and MS in Chemical Engineering from Yale and Lehigh University, respectively. He joined the Yale AIDS Program in 2008, after a decade in commercial vaccine and pharmaceutical research and development. He has served as data manager for the AIDS program's HIV/HCV coinfection treatment initiatives, as well as for several of Yale's HIV and TB prevention and treatment projects in South Africa, including an IPT trial, and is also developing and managing the Data System for a RCT focused on HIV and HCV prevention services in persons recently released from the justice systems in CT and TX. In these projects, he has developed innovative data management approaches and tools combining surveillance data from jurisdiction health departments with clinical data from local primary care clinics, especially around care and treatment cascades for HIV and HCV infected individuals, that result in greatly expanded capability.

Gáramis Campusano currently works for the Center for the Advancement of Teaching (CAT) at Florida International University as their educational technology specialist. In this role, he is responsible for supporting the CAT team as well as faculty and staff on a wide range of tech-related projects and endeavors. He relies heavily on his 8 years of teaching experience in higher ed to support initiatives around the institution and spends a great deal of time developing student-centered curriculum and educational technology programming. He has a BA in English and an MA in Linguistics both from FIU.

Bronwyn Cross-Denny is associate professor of health science, college co-director of research education and consultation, and global health faculty fellow in the College of Health Professions at Sacred Heart University. She founded the Master of Social Work program and was responsible for the development and initial accreditation with integrated social work practice as the curriculum model. Dr. Cross-Denny earned a Ph.D. in social work and M.S.W. with concentrations in clinical practice and research from Fordham University. She is a Licensed Clinical Social Worker.

Hadi Danawi, trained in Public Health with a Ph.D. in Epidemiology from the University of Texas at Houston and a master degree in Environmental Health from the American University of Beirut, has an international exposure to various Public Health issues in the U.S. Middle East and Africa. Dr. Danawi is passionate about creating positive social change and truly believes his research interests should be multidisciplinary as is Public Health. With 25 years of experience including teaching, research and service, Dr. Danawi currently serves as a full-time faculty at Walden University, College of Health Sciences teaching and mentoring doctoral dissertations.

Ajanta Das is Professor in the Institute of Information Technology, Amity University Kolkata. Dr. Das has graduated in B.Sc. (Mathematics) in 1993 from Bethune College, University of Calcutta, and received MCA degree from Jadavpur University in 1996. She is having altogether twenty-five years of experience including seven years of Industry experience. She started her career with Industry and is proud to work for reputed, famous, pioneer companies like, Tata Steel, Jamshedpur, India and Lexis Nexis Inc., Boston, USA. She is experienced with development and release of new real-life projects in Industry. Later, she joined academics and started teaching and research simultaneously. In 2009, Dr. Das has been awarded PhD (Engg.) from Jadavpur University. Notably, she had also been associated with Birla Institute of Technology, Mesra, for more than eleven years and Heritage Institute of Technology at the beginning of her academic career. She had guided three PhD scholars in Birla Institute of Technology, Mesra. Her major interest of teaching includes database, software engineering and distributed computing. Her field of Specialization is Distributed Computing. Her focused research area includes Grid Computing, Cloud Computing, Internet of Things, Big Data Management, Wireless Sensor Network, Block Chain and Machine Learning. Currently one scholar is continuing PhD and many other graduates, post graduate students are carrying out research projects under her supervision.

Patrick Dunn, PhD, MS, MBA, FAHA, is the Program Director for Connected Heart Health and the architect of the Intelligent Health Solutions for the American Heart Association's Center of Excellence for Health Technology and Innovation. He also is Contributing Faculty in the College of Health Sciences, School of Public Health at Walden University where he teaches biostatistics and mentors doctoral student. Patrick has a unique blend of knowledge and experience in healthcare, business development, software engineering, quality and research. Dr. Dunn is a clinical exercise physiologist and health educator with 35 years of experience in cardiac rehabilitation, preventive cardiology, and wellness with specific expertise in digital health literacy and digital coaching methods.

LuAnn Etcher is an Associate Professor at Sacred Heart University. She is also a nurse practitioner. Her research interests include examining the impact of trauma on health, distance monitoring and telehealth use.

Jessica Giraldo supports the instructional technology training needs of the Herbert Wertheim College of Medicine at Florida International University through the development and design of resources, workshops, as well as contributing to curriculum and training projects. Jessica is an FIU alumnus holding a B.A. in Communication, and has a variety of experience working with support services, information technology marketing, legal services, and instructional design.

Christina Gunther, EdD, is an assistant professor and chair of the Health Sciences Department at Sacred Heart University. Dr. Gunther's expertise lies within the fields of cultural literacy, diversity, equity, social determinants of health and social justice in the global arena. She presents and consults nationally on topics that include diversity, power and privilege, implicit bias, and stereotype representations.

Tiera J. Lanford holds a Master's degree in Higher Education Policy, Planning, and Leadership and recently graduated with a Master's in Public Health from The George Washington University Milken Institute School of Public Health. Her current research interests focus on community based participatory research, technology, mental health, and military family health.

Samantha Lemus-Martinez, PhD, is a faculty developer and assistant professor with a decade of experience in teaching at both the K-12 and post-secondary level. Having earned a PhD in Curriculum and Instruction with a specialization in research and curriculum evaluation, Dr. Lemus-Martinez utilizes her expertise to develop faculty and students, assist in the development and refinement of curriculum, provide guidance in program evaluation with a focus on integrating the practice of the scholarship of teaching and learning, in addition to designing and implementing innovative programs that elevate the quality of instruction and ensure the success of the 21st century learner.

Donna McHaney is an Associate Professor at Sacred Heart University. She is also a nurse practitioner and computer scientist. Her research interests include examining telehealth use in both practice and academia and innovative technology applications in graduate education.

Courtney Monroe is an Assistant Professor in the Arnold School of Public Health and a faculty member in the Technology Center to Promote Healthy Lifestyles at the University of South Carolina. She is a certified American College of Sports Medicine Exercise Physiologist and behavioral scientist. Her research focuses on technology-based physical activity promotion and behavioral weight control in adults, with an emphasis on how to best harness social support and social networks for those purposes.

Lisa Nichols is a Program Manager at the AIDS Program at Yale University. She received a Bachelor of Arts degree from Hobart and William Smith Colleges and a Master of Public Health from Southern CT State University. Ms. Nichols has been involved in HIV and Hepatitis C research aimed at re-engaging HIV clients into HIV care and curing hepatitis C among vulnerable populations. In her current role, her work focuses on Data to Care, capacity building, HIV, and hepatitis C treatment in vulnerable populations. Ms. Nichols has always had a passion for working with marginalized groups. Prior to her work at Yale University, she served as a Peace Corps volunteer in rural Madagascar. During her two years of service, she lived and worked alongside local community members on various projects ranging from sustainable environmental practices to maternal and child health and disease prevention. Through her work, Ms. Nichols aims to also improve access to care disparities within health systems for all patients, especially those at a disadvantage.

Erika Patterson earned a Doctorate of Education in Curriculum and Instruction from the University of South Carolina. She taught Middle School English for nine years and is currently teaching High School English. She has focused on the mental health of students as they navigate difficult school environments, finding ways to meet them where they are so they can be successful.

Danielle Provenzano is a first-year graduate student at Sacred Heart University, working on her Master of Science in Speech-Language Pathology. She is interested in working with children with ASD, dysphagia clients, and researching adult neurogenic disorders.

Melanie Reyes is a second-year Master of Public Health student at Sacred Heart University. Her interests are in health education, promoting physical activity and nutrition, and investigating health outcomes with acculturation and diet. Her goals are to help eliminate racial disparities in health care and serve marginalized communities as an aspiring public health clinician.

Katarzyna Sims is the Training Development Specialist at Yale School of Medicine. She trained at Quinnipiac University in Instructional Design. Her teaching and research interests focus on online learning, graphic design, instructional design pedagogy, and educational technology. She has experience leading educational efforts for various HRSA-funded projects, including multimedia and interactive curricula development.

Jill Stefaniak is Associate Professor in the Learning, Design, and Technology program in the Department of Career and Information Studies at the University of Georgia, USA. Her research interests focus on the professional development of instructional designers, designer decision-making processes, and contextual factors that influence design in situated environments. Dr. Stefaniak has experience leading instructional design and performance improvement projects in healthcare, medical education, higher education, and safety.

Merceditas Villanueva is the Director of the HIV/AIDS Program within the Infectious Disease Section at Yale University School of Medicine. Her career has focused on improving healthcare service delivery for vulnerable populations, primarily PWH. She previously established the Ryan White funded HIV clinic in Waterbury Hospital as a collaboration between community-based AIDS organizations and HIV clinicians. After recruitment back to Yale faculty in 2009, she established and continues to serve as the Principal Investigator for the New Haven Ryan White HIV Continuum, a collaboration between different clinics and community organizations which promotes service coordination to improve quality of care for PWH. She has been an ID/HIV physician for over 25 years and has been the HIV/AIDS Program director at Yale University since 2009.

Maximilian D. Wegener, MPH, is an epidemiologist with Yale University's School of Medicine, AIDS program. His previous work had focused on communicable disease case and outbreak investigation. Currently, his research is centered on hepatitis C and the impact HIV co-infection has on infected patients' treatment and cure. Mr. Wegener is a member of the International AIDS Society (IAS) and the American Public Health Association (APHA) and was a past member of the following: the International Society for Disease Surveillance (ISDS) and Nevada Public Health Association (NPHA).

Index

A

B

C

D

E

F

G

H

I

L

M

N

O

P

R

S

T

U

V

W

www.ingramcontent.com/pod-product-compliance
Lightning Source LLC
LaVergne TN
LVHW080536300926
849162LV00007B/1618